Praise for *Exploring Body-Mind Centering*

"Bonnie Bainbridge Cohen is one of the foremost explorers of the body's intricate subjective wisdom and its enormous potential for healing. This text has long been awaited by those who have had the good fortune to know Bainbridge Cohen and her work. It is an absolute must-read for anyone interested in a major contribution to the medicine of the future, and its availability now."

— Deane Juhan, author of *Job's Body: A Handbook for Bodywork*

"This book, so sensitively and deftly created, is a vast and rapid tour through the world of Body-Mind Centering. Inside, the reader will find treasures and wonders of vast and varied perspective and dimension."

— Susan Aposhyan, developer of Body-Mind Psychotherapy
and author of *Body-Mind Psychotherapy: Principles, Techniques,
and Practical Applications* and *Natural Intelligence: Body-Mind
Integration and Human Development*

"Bonnie Bainbridge Cohen and company guide and enthrall with a cornucopia of wisdom as they continue to unfold the magnificent spirals of life."

— Emilie Conrad, Continuum founder and author of *Life on Land:
The Story of Continuum, the Word-Renowned Self-Discovery and
Movement Method*

T0352887

Exploring
Body-Mind Centering

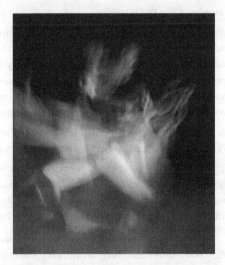

*An
Anthology
of Experience
and
Method*

**Edited by Gill Wright Miller,
Pat Ethridge, and Kate Tarlow Morgan**

North Atlantic Books
Berkeley, California

Published by
North Atlantic Books,
Berkeley, California

Cover photo by Mishele Mennett taken at the Doane Dance Performance Space, Denison University, Granville, Ohio
Cover and book design by Brad Greene
Printed in Canada

This is issue number 68 in the *IO* series.

Exploring Body-Mind Centering: An Anthology of Experience and Method is sponsored and published by the Society for the Study of Native Arts and Sciences (dba North Atlantic Books), an educational nonprofit based in Berkeley, California, that collaborates with partners to develop cross-cultural perspectives, nurture holistic views of art, science, the humanities, and healing, and seed personal and global transformation by publishing work on the relationship of body, spirit, and nature.

North Atlantic Books' publications are available through most bookstores. For further information, visit our website at www.northatlanticbooks.com or call 800-733-3000.

MEDICAL DISCLAIMER: The following information is intended for general information purposes only. Individuals should always see their health care provider before administering any suggestions made in this book. Any application of the material set forth in the following pages is at the reader's discretion and is his or her sole responsibility.

Library of Congress Cataloging-in-Publication Data
Exploring body-mind centering: an anthology of experience and method
/ edited by Gill Wright Miller, Pat Ethridge, and Kate Tarlow Morgan.
 p.; cm.
Includes bibliographical references.
ISBN 978-1-55643-968-1
1. Body-mind centering. I. Miller, Gill Wright, 1952–II. Ethridge, Pat, 1951–III. Morgan, Kate Tarlow, 1954–
[DNLM: 1. Mind-Body Therapies—methods—Collected Works. 2. Awareness—Collected Works. 3. Stress, Psychological—therapy—Collected Works. WB 880 E96 2010]
RC489.M53E97 2010
616.89'14—dc22   2010024447

3 4 5 6 7 8 9 MQ 25 24 23 22 21 20

This book is a testament to nearly forty years of research, exploration, and expression in a field that is grounded in what is real, what is present, and what is alive. To Bonnie Bainbridge Cohen, to The Body-Mind Centering Association, to the movers who stepped into the unknown, to the clients with whom we have worked, we dedicate this anthology to all of you.

❖

Acknowledgments

First, we would like to acknowledge the writers of these essays for committing to paper what is rarely described in words.

Equally, we appreciate the creative and responsive publishers and editors at North Atlantic Books: Richard Grossinger, Jon Goodspeed, Jessica Sevey, Kathy Glass, and Brad Greene among them. Without their wisdom, this book would not have been possible.

Finally, we are grateful for our families, friends, and employers, who allowed us the time and the space to make this book a reality.

Contents

Section Three: Applying Body-Mind Centering: A Presence Across Practices..... 235

Section Four: Embodying Body-Mind Centering: Being and Doing..... 367

Epilogue: Biographies, Historical Records, and Notes 399

Preface

In the second half of the twentieth century, a ferment of cross-pollinating research and discovery occurred across disciplines in the sciences, philosophy, the arts, and healing. The fruits of this ferment were visible in the United States in the landing of a man on the moon, advances in civil rights, a second-wave women's movement, emerging trends in the arts, and alternative healing forms. The influence of Asian thought and practices was also becoming more widely felt in America. The consequences of these developments grew out of earlier research and explorations happening as far back as the nineteenth century or earlier in the U.S. and Europe.

It was in this percolating atmosphere that Bonnie Bainbridge Cohen began her efforts to understand patterns of human movement. Her dance teaching and her therapeutic work with children unfolded in the larger context of the field of somatics,[1] the study and practice of approaches to mind-body integration. "Body-Mind Centering," the name she gave her work, has become a distinct somatic modality with almost unlimited applications.

Body-Mind Centering (BMC)[2] teaches us to be centered in ourselves, to be embodied. As an approach, it operates from two premises: one, that the mind is inseparable from and centered in relationship to the body; and two, that through the body, the mind can be explored and expressed. These premises provide a starting point for intensive, extensive investigation into the nature of our existence and its interrelationships and changes over time. Along with the resources of the traditional knowledge bases of medicine, arts, and philosophy, BMC utilizes, as a primary source, the individual's personal life experience with self, others, and the environment. The shared understanding derived from this form of empirical research is cumulative and transmissible.

We are incarnate beings in a physical body. The human form is a template evolved from prior life forms both similar to and different from others in Earth's history. From conception to death, we transform continuously in conformance with genetic patterns both predestined and unique. We also adapt to environments shifting and rebuilding in time. As our lives proceed, our sense of who we are, what our abilities and capacities are, and what we understand about life's changes is balanced by the awareness that some aspects of ourselves remain constant.

A characteristic BMC concept is the relationship between being and doing (a concept easily traced to Eastern thought), which can be modulated by one's relationship to desire, because *wanting to move* is fundamental to our nature, on every level. *To sense, to feel, and to act* become the means to self-knowing through this work of self-centering. For each individual, the journey is different. Bainbridge Cohen encourages mutual participation because this invitation or enticement itself becomes a protocol for discovery. Thus, her school became her laboratory. Through her collaborative teaching and learning processes, utilizing a body-based language, new material is always being generated.

Seekers of all sorts throughout the centuries have utilized various methods to address our self-unknowing. Many technologies have been developed, most of which emphasize one aspect of existence over the others. Many seekers come from a specific focus, like medicine, which imposes a particular lens or filter. Much later, the seemingly unimportant may be discovered to be essential, the missing piece which pulls the rest together. In contrast to this tradition, Body-Mind Centering is an approach that derives from several different sources and therefore has a wide lens. Both the field and its practitioners explore, as a process, movement reeducation and repatterning. They utilize information and perspectives from dance, occupational therapy, sports, art, Western anatomy, psychology, Asian philosophy and medicine, and Western esoteric philosophy, among other sources. The result is not a random amalgamation of information but a coherent understanding that can be systematically taught, verbally articulated, and personally experienced—even of otherwise mostly unconscious processes. And very often, because those who study BMC are searching for an access point for growth and development, this work is transformative. People become more fully themselves.

As an approach, Body-Mind Centering has developed outside the mainstream. Questions often dismissed or denigrated in the institutional context are welcome, and individual experience is accepted as personal testimony to the empirical nature of understanding, leading to meaning and resonance beyond lenses and filters. All these aspects are brought together in a community of seekers where dialogue and sharing of personal experience and insight are valued. Thus, a common body of knowledge has been developed that recognizes intelligence as an attribute not only of the brain, but also of the body, even at the level of the cellular membrane.

Bonnie Bainbridge Cohen has given a name, a focus, and a clarity of method to somatic explorations being conducted in different ways by many investigators of her time. She has a special gift for illuminating patterns of experience that give rise to insight, understanding, and integration. She facilitates the ability of individuals to recognize in themselves what is needed for healing and growth. Her focus, first, on the person who embodies a "reported problem" rather than on the problem itself, respects the humanity of the individual. It also acknowledges that individual's right to make choices regarding personal destiny and change. The choices we make change us. Bainbridge Cohen's astute and basic principle "support precedes movement" reflects this approach and requires a willingness to rest in unknowing and allow its nature to be revealed. For more than thirty years, she has explored her own questions and shared with others what she is careful to call "results" rather than "answers."

Those drawn to Body-Mind Centering find support, recognition, and clarity in community and through exchanging their experiences and understandings. Some of these individuals have worked with her for decades, some only for a brief time. In the beginning, the group was small and often met in Bainbridge Cohen's living room. In the last thirty years, the group has enlarged to embrace a professional community that has spread all over the world, communicating physically when possible and virtually when not. As the nucleus of the group grew, its practitioners developed more professional responsibility to the work, their clients, and each other. This resulted in the formation of a professional organization; the presentation of conferences and seminars to share discoveries in content, practice, and pedagogy; and a written newsletter and then a journal to record and refer back to some of this work. Both the larger community and the smaller professional membership continue to exchange applications of BMC principles in various arenas, thus extending the reach of the work.

Reading This Book

Although the earliest essay in this volume dates only from 1996, the writing as a whole reflects more than twenty-five years of investigation conducted by BMC practitioners, teachers, students, and advocates, recording the wider group's collaborative understanding for here, for now. Many individuals have written articles and books elsewhere, but this volume is intended as a sampling and not as a comprehensive review of all those writing about Body-Mind Centering.

The Prologue opens with Bonnie Bainbridge Cohen's original and ongoing answer to the question, "What is Body-Mind Centering?" Bainbridge Cohen explains the nature of this experiential work—that it is both ongoing and patterned, and that our movement reveals where we are along this journey. She confirms that there are many ways to work toward a centered alignment in the body and shows us ways to organize that exploration: through a cellular embodiment, a recognition of the many systems of the body, and a reinvestment with a spiraling, ontogenetic process that evolves over a lifetime. Bainbridge Cohen's introduction concludes by inviting the reader to engage with this approach and material through touch and repatterning.

The four sections that follow represent writing about Body-Mind Centering—as an experience, as a somatic practice, as a paradigm for other kinds of practices, and as an embodiment—which are intended to promote a conversation among practitioners, clients, students, and seekers new to the field.

In the first section, *Experiencing Body-Mind Centering: Systems and Development*, we have selected sample writings demonstrating a "way in" for those meeting BMC for the first time. The first essay, Catherine Burns' "The Active Role of the Baby in Birthing," proposes, contrary to received medical opinion, that it is vital to recognize the baby's activities in the birth journey as equally important as those of the mother and her birthing assistants. Each subsequent essay takes the reader through steps for an experience. It is not our intention to cover all of the "systems" nor all of the "developmental" material. Instead, this section introduces the reader to BMC practices through various topical applications: *e.g.*, Thomas Greil's evoking fluids, Annie Brook's finding support, Michael Ridge's vibration and pulsation, and Pat Ethridge's tuning in to our perception as it shifts between inner and outer. We anticipate that readers will make their way to the direct experience by ingesting this material slowly and methodically. As one of the essays instructs, "take time with this information. Allow it to move you to action. Do not rush."

In the second section, *Practicing Body-Mind Centering: Case Studies*, we offer writings that demonstrate different concerns and approaches within the BMC somatic discipline. The case studies show practitioners, scholars, and mothers working with "clients" of all descriptions. We witness both revolutionary moments of understanding and slow, steady progress over long periods of time. Through the writings of nine different authors from four different countries, this section is intended to introduce the notion that there are as many ways to access this material as there are people encountering it, and each has its place in the web of understanding. While each case study begins with desire—a hope or wish for the client—in all cases the "practitioner/teacher" is equally transformed.

The third section, *Applying Body-Mind Centering: A Presence Across*

Practices, illustrates the breadth of this work. Here, it has expanded beyond the boundaries of a personal journey of self-integration intended to address the Cartesian split between mind and body and enters the worlds of the arts, medicine, yoga, and academia. From the interview with an award-winning choreographer to tips for learning karate or piano, from working with a practitioner in yoga or using the Internet to create a distanced relationship with mentors, these essays invite the reader to imagine a world where all participants have access to their own ways-of-being and can live and grow to their fullest potential.

The fourth section, *Embodying Body-Mind Centering: Being and Doing,* concludes with the slightly more political yet still certainly personal. First, Maggie McGuire asks: What can we learn about our responsibility within the world? Then, Linda Hartley suggests that we ask: What can be learned about world politics by investigating these somatic practices? Finally, Martha Eddy asks: What are the benefits of a somatic arts-based community in the process of healing? These last three essays invite the reader to see a larger, more global picture and then to act on "the child" within our reach, literally and figuratively.

We conclude this text with an *Epilogue* filled with historical information not recorded anywhere else. There is a biography of Body-Mind Centering's founder, Bonnie Bainbridge Cohen, a history of her School that offers teachings in this modality, and a history of The Body-Mind Centering Association, an alliance of practitioners, teachers, and advocates that maintains the standards of this practice in the greater community.

The editors would like to thank all the members of the BMCA community who, through their creativity, support, and holding of the circle, have made this expression possible. And our deepest gratitude and appreciation to Bonnie and Len Cohen for their vision, their pioneering work, their commitment, and their friendship.

— Gill Wright Miller, Pat Ethridge, Kate Tarlow Morgan
January 2011

Prologue

Introduction to Body-Mind Centering (excerpt)[1]

~ **Bonnie Bainbridge Cohen** (2009)

Body-Mind Centering® (BMCˢᵐ) is an ongoing, experiential journey into the alive and changing territory of the body. The explorer is the mind—our thoughts, feelings, energy, soul, and spirit. Through this journey we are led to an understanding of how the mind is expressed through the body in movement.

There is something in nature that forms patterns. We, as part of nature, also form patterns. The mind is like the wind, and the body is like the sand; if you want to know how the wind is blowing, you can look at the sand.

Our body moves as our mind moves. The qualities of any movement are a manifestation of how mind is expressing through the body at that moment. Changes in movement qualities indicate that the mind has shifted focus in the body. Conversely, when we direct the mind or attention to different areas of the body and initiate movement from those areas, we change the quality of our movement. So we find that movement can be a way to observe the expressions of the mind through the body, and it can also be a way to effect changes in the body-mind relationship.

In BMC, "centering" is a process of balancing, not a place of arrival. This balancing is based on dialogue, and the dialogue is based on experience.

An important aspect of our journey in Body-Mind Centering is discovering the relationship between the smallest level of activity within the body and the largest movement of the body—aligning the inner cellular movement with the external expression of movement through space. This involves identifying, articulating, differentiating, and integrating the various tissues within the body, discovering the qualities they contribute to one's movement, how they have evolved in one's developmental process, and the role they play in the expression of mind.

The finer this alignment, the more efficiently we can function to accomplish our intentions. However, alignment itself is not a goal. It is a continual dialogue between awareness and action—becoming aware of the relationships that exist throughout our body/mind and acting from that awareness. This alignment creates a state of knowing. There are many ways of working toward this alignment such as through touch, through movement, visualization, somatization,[2] voice, art, music, meditation, through verbal dialogue, through open awareness, or by any other means.

The Body Systems

Our Cellular Foundation: Each cell in our body has living intelligence. It is capable of knowing itself, initiating action, and communicating with all other cells. The individual cell and the community of cells (tissue, organ, body) exist as separate entities and as one whole at the same moment. Cellular embodiment is a state in which all cells have equal opportunity for expression, receptivity, and cooperation.

Attuning ourselves to our cellular consciousness brings us to a state in which we can find the ground from which flows the intricate manifestations of our physical, psychological, and spiritual being.

When we embody or perceive from any cell as a unique individual, the feeling or mind-quality is the same for all cells. There is a one-mindedness. However, when we perceive from any cell within the context of its community of cells or specific tissue, the feeling or state of mind is unique to each tissue. Underlying this oneness or uniqueness are general feelings on continua between cellular anxiety and at-easement, rest and activity, inner and outer focus, and receptivity and expressiveness.

Skeletal System: This system provides us with our basic supporting structure. It is composed of the bones and the joints. The bones lever us through space and support our weight in relationship to gravity and the shape of our movements through space. The spaces within the joints give us the possibility of movement and provide the axes around which the movement occurs.

The skeletal system gives our body the basic form through which we can locomotor through space, sculpt and create the energy forms in space that we call movement, and act on the environment, in relationship with the other forms around us.

Through embodying the skeletal system, the mind becomes structurally organized, providing the supporting ground for our thoughts, the leverage for our ideas, and the fulcra or spaces between our ideas for the articulation and understanding of their relationships.

Ligamentous System: The ligaments set the boundaries of movement between the bones by holding the bones together; they guide muscular responses by directing the path of movement between the bones; and they suspend the organs within the thoracic and abdominal cavities.

This system provides specificity, clarity, and efficiency for the alignment and movement of the bones and organs. It is through the mind of the ligaments that we perceive and articulate clarity of focus and concentration to detail.

Muscular System: The muscles establish a tensile three-dimensional grid for the balanced support and movement of the skeletal structure by providing the elastic forces that move the bones through space. They provide the dynamic contents of the outer envelope of flesh encompassing the skeletal structure. Through this system we embody our vitality, express our power, and engage in the dialogue of resistance and resolution.

Organ System: The organs carry on the functions of our internal survival—breathing, nourishment, and elimination. They are the contents within the skeletal-flesh container.

Organs provide us with our sense of volume, full-bodied-ness, and organic authenticity. They are the primary habitats or natural environments of our emotions, aspirations, and the memories of our inner reactions to our personal histories.

Endocrine System: The endocrine glands are the major chemical governing system of the body and are closely aligned to the nervous system. Their secretions pass directly into the blood stream, and their balance or imbalance influences all the cells in the body.

This is the system of internal stillness, surges, or explosions of chaos/balance and the crystallization of energy into archetypal experiences. The endocrine glands underlie intuition and the perceiving and understanding of the Universal Mind.

Nervous System: The nervous system is the recording system of the body. It records our perceptions and experiences and stores them. It can then recall the pattern of an experience and modify it by integrating it with patterns of other previous experiences.

The nervous system is the last to know, but, once knowing, it becomes a major control center of psychophysical processes. It can initiate the learning of new experience through intuition, creativity, and play. The nervous system underlies alertness, thought, and precision of coordination and establishes the perceptual base from which we view and interact with our internal and external worlds.

Fluid System: The fluids are the transportation system of the body. The major fluids are cellular and interstitial fluids, blood, lymph, synovial fluid, and cerebrospinal fluid. Fluids are the system of liquidity of movement and mind. They underlie presence and transformation and mediate the dynamics of the flow between rest and activity.

Fascial System: Fascial connective tissue establishes a soft container for all the other structures of the body. It both divides and integrates all other tissues and provides them with semi-viscous lubricating surfaces, so that they have independence of movement within established boundaries of the body as a whole.

It is through the fascia that the movement of our organs provides internal support for the movement of our skeleton through space, and the movement of our skeleton expresses in the outer world the inner movement of our organs. Through the fascial system we connect our inner feeling with our outer expression.

Fat: Fat is potential energy stored in the body. It provides heat insulation for the body and electrical insulation for the nerves. Its synthesis, breakdown, storage, and mobilization are greatly controlled by the endocrine system.

Static fat is stored as repressed or unacknowledged potential power and creates a sense of heaviness and lethargy. Fat that is mobilized expresses strong primordial power and a sense of graceful fluidity. Fat that is embraced offers nurturing comfort.

Skin: Skin is our outermost layer, covering our body in its entirety and defining us as individuals by separating us from that which is not us.

Through our skin, we touch and are touched by the outer world. The outer boundary is our first line of defense and bonding. It sets our general tone of openness and closedness to being in the world—through our skin we are both invaded and protected, and we receive and make contact with others.

All Systems: While each system makes its own separate contribution to the movement of body-mind, they are all interdependent, together providing a complete framework of support and expression. Certain systems are perceived as having natural affinities with others. However, those affinities vary among individuals, among groups, and among cultures. We discover their voices by consciously and unconsciously exploring them in different combinations.

Developmental Movement

Underlying the forms of our expression through the body systems is the process of our movement development, both ontogenetic (human infant development) and phylogenetic (the evolutionary progression through the animal kingdom).

Development is not a linear process but occurs in overlapping waves, with each stage containing elements of all the others. Because each previous stage underlies and supports each successive stage, any skipping, interrupting, or failing to complete a stage of development can lead to alignment/movement problems, imbalances within the body systems, and problems in perception, sequencing, organization, memory, and creativity.

The developmental material includes primitive reflexes, righting reactions, equilibrium responses, and the Basic Neurological Patterns. These are the automatic movement responses that underlie our volitional movement.

The reflexes, righting reactions, and equilibrium responses are the fundamental elements, or the alphabet, of our movement. They combine to build the Basic Neurological Patterns, which are based upon prevertebrate and vertebrate movement patterns. The first of the four prevertebrate patterns is **cellular breathing** (the expanding/contracting process in breathing and movement in each and every cell of the body), which correlates to the movement of the one-celled animals. Cellular breathing underlies all other patterns of movement and postural tone.

Navel radiation (the relating and movement of all parts of the body via the navel), **mouthing** (movement of the body initiated by the mouth), and **prespinal movement** (soft sequential movements of the spine initiated via the interface between the spinal cord and the digestive tract) are the other three prevertebrate patterns.

The twelve vertebrate patterns are based upon: **spinal movement** (head-to-tail movement), which correlates to the movement of fish; **homologous movement** (symmetrical movement of two upper and/or two lower limbs simultaneously), which correlates to the movement of amphibians; **homolateral movement** (asymmetrical movement of one upper limb and the lower limb on the same side), which correlates to the movement of reptiles; and **contralateral movement** (diagonal movement of one upper limb with the opposite lower limb), which correlates to the movement of mammals.

Development of the Basic Neurological Patterns establishes our basic movement patterns and corresponding perceptual relationships—including spatial orientation and body image, and the basic elements of learning and communication. In **spinal** movements, for example, we develop rolling, establish the horizontal plane, differentiate the front of our body from the back, and gain the ability to attend.

In **homologous** movements we develop symmetrical movements such as push-ups and jumping with both feet, establish the sagittal plane, differentiate the upper part of our body from the lower part, and gain the ability to act.

In **homolateral** movements we develop asymmetrical movements such as crawling on our belly and hopping on one leg, establish the vertical plane, differentiate the right side of our body from the left, and gain the ability to intend.

In **contralateral** movements we develop diagonal movements such as creeping on our hands and forelegs, walking, running, and leaping; establish three-dimensional movement; differentiate the diagonal quadrants of our bodies; and gain the ability to integrate our attention, intention, and actions.

The developmental movement-perceptual progression establishes a process-oriented framework for the dialogue of the body systems.

Aligning inner cellular awareness and movement with outer awareness and movement through space within the context of the developmental process can facilitate the evolution of our consciousness and alleviate body-mind problems at their root level. As we are more able to experience our consciousness at the cellular and the tissue level, we are better able to understand ourselves. As we increase our knowledge of ourselves, we increase in understanding and compassion for others. As we experience the uniqueness of our cells within the context of tissue harmony, we learn about individuality within the context of community. As we gain awareness of our diverse tissues and the nature of their expression in the outer world, we expand our understanding of other cultures within the context of the Earth as a

whole and the awareness of our planet within the expanded consciousness of the Universe.

The Art of Touch and Repatterning

When we touch someone, they touch us equally. The subtle interplay
between body and mind can be experienced clearly through touching
others. The art of touch and repatterning is an exploration of communication through touch—the transmission and acceptance of the flow
of energy within oneself and between oneself and others.

In hands-on work, through touching in different rhythms, through
placement of attention within specific layers of the body, through following existing lines of force and suggesting new ones, and through
changes in the pressure and quality of our touch, we come into harmony with the different tissues and their associated qualities of mind.
We begin with cellular presence (cellular breathing) and focus on the
resonation and dialogue between client and practitioner. Each tissue
of the client is explored from the corresponding tissue of the practitioner,
i.e., bone from bone, organ from organ, fluid from fluid, *etc.* The initiation of intent, based upon what each person is perceiving, may be
shared consciously and/or unconsciously by both people.

Acceptance and curiosity guide the inquiry. Through mutual resonance between client and practitioner, attention is given to discovering
the primary tissues through which the clients express themselves and
those tissues which are usually in shadow, so that the supporting tissues
can be given voice and the articulating ones be allowed to recuperate.
This shifting of energy expression allows for more choices and
expanded consciousness of body-mind for both the client/student and
the practitioner/teacher.

Postscript

My description of Body-Mind Centering would be incomplete without acknowledging my continual gratitude to all the BMC teachers and students who have offered not only their experiences to the work but their thinking, articulation, and interpretations of those experiences. Beyond this, they have also given freely of their love and friendship through these many years.

And always by my side has been my husband Len. BMC could not have developed without his continual presence, penetrating questioning, steady guidance, and the profound caring for me and all the people who have come to share in this ongoing journey.

Articulating Our Experience

~ **Gill Wright Miller** and **Pat Ethridge** (2010)

In the twenty-first century, the work of Body-Mind Centering is no longer being steered solely by founder Bonnie Bainbridge Cohen. Teachers and scholars delve deeply into one aspect or another of the work; practitioners develop numerous applications and programs of their own; and students are now learning the work from BMC teachers other than Bonnie Bainbridge Cohen. As BMC has spread globally, its various constituencies are voicing a collective understanding of "the work."

In 2005 Ellen Barlow, a long-time teacher of Body-Mind Centering and a founder of the Body-Mind Centering Association (BMCA), created an initiative called "The Pool Project."[1] Prior to this initiative she had led two conference sessions, the first in 2003 considering our professional roles and how we represent our know-how to the public and to other professionals, as well as how we function in larger contexts requiring understanding and strategic participation. The second session, in 2004, explored examples of BMC applications. Barlow's recognition that professions self-define in order to set standards for best practices led to the Pool Project's first focus group. That group assessed common strengths and defining characteristics of the BMC approach by looking at four applications and one signature technique. This work was presented and elaborated upon by conference attendees in 2005, which led to the Methodology Focus Group. The focus group pooled their experiences and drafted summary statements about Body-Mind Centering methodologies, philosophies, theories, and principles. The scope of the work was intended to generate methodological criteria for assessing best practices and not intended to be a comprehensive or definitive analysis. Focus group members met five times via teleconference from August 2005 through April 2006 and fulfilled writing/reading assignments in between conference calls. The group worked initially on the BMC approach to somatizations, an orally guided technique commonly used in Body-Mind Centering with clients and students to give them a personal entry into embodiment. At the 2006 USA conference, the group conducted a discussion and writing session utilizing this material. From this, Barlow and the other group members developed the following preliminary descriptions.

Methodologies of the BMC Approach

At heart, the Body-Mind Centering Approach is an inquiry into the nature of our physical selves in relationship to our world—a belief in the inherent intelligence of the body in motion. When activated, this intelligence yields a transformative capacity for change and growth in the direction of health and balance, as well as respect and compassion for the highly personal and universal aspects of our research and discoveries. The methods of the BMC approach include somatizations; guided-movement exploration; structured improvisation; information relayed through talking and explaining; supporting materials (such as photographs or models); and assisted movement, movement demonstration, and movement repatterning.

This process utilizes a unique body-based language to describe movement and mind-body relationships through study and practice, through individual research, and through community. The two primary areas of focus are (1) the evolutionary and perceptual-motor basis of our human development and (2) the awareness of the structural, functional, and energetic nature of our human anatomy and physiology. Participants engage in the groundwork of somatic awareness, awakening pathways of developmental repatterning and the specificity of personal embodiment and integration.

Philosophy of the BMC Approach

The beginning premise maintains that the body has inherent reason. Each cell, each tissue, and each system has organic purpose, knows that purpose, and conducts itself to carry out that purpose. Communication with and from the soma—the mind-body—is directly available to us even when it comes to our awareness in the form of dreams or visions, meditations, or creativity. Communing with this soma (our own first, then that of others), in whatever form, supports a second premise: that inner/self is the ground for outer/group.

In our work to reconcile the physical world with human consciousness, or reality with awareness, the phenomenological experience of one's human body is tied simultaneously to a physical existence and the sensation of experiencing that existence.

Finally, as somatically awakened beings, we are existentially inclined toward taking responsibility for our choice to exist in the world in the way that we do, and that inclination invites authenticity, refusing to take things for granted, creating and shaping one's own reason-for-being, and continuing to try new approaches. Within this framework, individual discoveries are acknowledged and celebrated.

Theories of the BMC Approach

There is conscious experience in our soma, which we witness as consisting of live, present-tense bodily experience, revealed through movement expressions. The consciousness of soma teaches us to experience ourselves as alive, awake, and fully present. We choose to witness, be present, and let go of witnessing, taking in only as much or as little as we can at any given time, making our way toward reintegrating ourselves as wholly witnessed. Being seen teaches us to wholly see and increases our capacity for human awareness and relationship, and human empathy.

All living cells have consciousness or "mind," are breathing, and have the capacity to initiate movement, and this movement is perceivable.

"The mind moves as the body moves."[2] Therefore, the "mind" is perceivable. All cells have mind or consciousness and can be accessed and brought to the foreground of our experience.

We can and do directly experience and perceive ourselves somatically. We can locate ourselves in the consciousness of the body system/tissue/cell ("place") being focused on, as a direct experience. Via the exploration itself and the resulting information and discoveries, this process yields improved function, health, and vitality, both of the specific bodily place and of the whole organism. The organism thrives to survive and will gravitate toward better functioning if it is guided or inspired to do so.

Principles of the BMC Approach

The principles of the BMC approach have been articulated variously by teachers, practitioners, and students who have worked collaboratively over the years. Although there are many principles, some emerge as more "fundamental" than others. The following list was generated first through individual experiences of studying the work, gathered in a compilation by certified practitioner Alison Granucci in 1989, and then through condensing those ideas to form a short list agreed on by participants at the 2006 USA conference. The following nine principles attempt to articulate what underlies the approach.

1. All cells have consciousness (mind).
2. All levels of physiological organization (e.g., tissues, systems) have consciousness that can be experienced directly.
3. As we begin to make all systems more conscious, they become more accessible.
4. We can transmit to each other the embodiment of the group's shared learning.
5. The mind of the body system (e.g., bones, muscles, organs, nervous system) is reflected in the room when that system is touched.

6. It is possible to create, evoke, and titrate resonance.
7. Support precedes movement.
8. Embodiment can initiate movement; movement can initiate embodiment.
9. There is a difference between the map of the body and the territory of the living person's somatic experience.

Closing Note

In her report about the Pool Project, Ellen Barlow reminds us: "To our knowledge, a comprehensive analysis and presentation of the methodology of the BMC approach have never been attempted. The stuff of such an intellectual inquiry exists in many places: our collective consciousness and sub-consciousness; SBMC [The School for Body-Mind Centering] written materials; individuals' integration and expression of the BMC work over the years; more mature, related fields of study and practice from which we can learn; and interested academicians well-versed in aspects of methodology in their own subject areas."

While Bainbridge Cohen's essay above ("Introduction to Body-Mind Centering") grounds the practice of BMC as a discourse, this essay reflects on its methodologies, philosophies, theories, and principles from a practitioner point of view. We are outlining some of the thoughts currently circulating in this work because we trust it will support the reader's journey through this anthology. We know that support necessarily precedes movement. We invite you to continue the conversation.

Section One
Experiencing Body-Mind Centering: Systems and Development

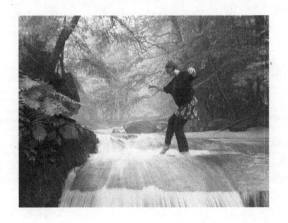

The Active Role of the Baby in Birthing

～ **Catherine Burns**, USA (1999)

What is the active role of the baby in birthing? I have carried this question with my babies nestled in my belly and wriggling in my arms. I have carried this question to other mothers, to midwives and childbirth assistants in my community, to my colleagues in Body-Mind Centering, and into my research of the medical literature. Join me in an exploratory investigation that will give us transformative images of the birth journey, where the baby is actively partnering with the mother.

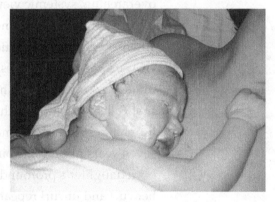

We can observe the mind of the baby in tonic labyrinthine response as the baby develops connection and trust in the earth and in mother as supports.

I am writing from the perspective of Body-Mind Centering, the groundbreaking work of Bonnie Bainbridge Cohen, which provides valuable insights for our understanding of babies and birth. Rooted in experiential explorations of human developmental patterns and anatomical systems, Body-Mind Centering informs us of the rich internal and expressive experience of the body-mind in the context of fetal and infant development. Bainbridge Cohen works with babies in the first year of life because "This is when the relationship of the perceptual process (the way one sees) and the motor process (the way one moves or acts in the world) is established. This is the baseline for how you will be processing activity, either in receiving or expressing, throughout your life. The importance of working with babies during the first year

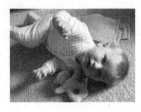

Reach of the eyes in an
adept roll.

is that . . . it helps set a broader baseline, offering more choices in not only how to see events or problems, but how to act on them; it gives [babies] the most multiplicity of direction . . . By working on these movement patterns with the baby as it's developing, you can help the infants on a continuum to have stronger, more balanced alignment, action and integration."[1]

By experientially investigating developmental patterns and anatomical systems, Body-Mind Centering identifies the mind states and movement qualities associated with the activities of specific patterns and systems. "I think that all mind patternings are expressed in movement, through the body. And that all physically moving patterns have a mind," states Bainbridge Cohen.[2] Through collaborative experiential research, BMC practitioners enter into the provocative inquiries and observations of body and mind relationships. With its overarching, systemic view of human development, BMC is evolving a cogent theoretical framework with high explanatory value in the emergent and disparate field of body-mind practices.

The appeal of BMC lies in its respect for the intelligence of both our minds and our bodies. This intelligence is a function of life, from the first cell's formation to the miracle of self-organization into a whole human being ready to meet the world. Having trained in BMC for seven years prior to the birth of my first child, I wondered at my newborn daughter's profoundly simple and essential activities. Watching her curl and uncurl repeatedly reminded me of her birth journey, and I was struck with the question: What is the baby doing in birth? What aspects of fetal development and the capacities of the newborn can be recognized as the baby's resources for the birth journey?

In vivid video-documentation of newborns, physician Lennart Righard and nurse-midwife Margaret Alade report research findings that overturn widespread perceptions of the baby as a passive object of birth. Their research demonstrates the newborn's ability, within the first hour after birth, to self-locomote to the breast, to independently locate the nipple, and to self-attach, when the baby is unmedicated and permitted to remain in uninterrupted, skin-to-skin contact on the mother's abdomen.[3] Lennart Nilsson's photo documentary "A Child Is Born" also shows a newborn pushing herself to the breast.[4] These strong demonstrations of neonatal capacity compel us to look at fetal development and activity to understand how they underlie newborn capacities. Only through gradual development of fetal capacity is the newborn able to undertake this first self-initiated action after birth.

From observing the newborn, I theorize the ability of the baby to actively partner in the birth. A picture of that partnering emerges from birth stories interpreted from the perspective of BMC. Physiologically, the baby's movements, developmental patterns, reflexes, body tone, hormonal organization, and alignment in the optimal birth position permit the baby to push actively against the uterine wall and to reach through the pelvic canal. From early hormonal signaling through the intensity of labor, the baby—if unmedicated and optimally positioned—works with the mother to bring himself out of the womb and into the world.

This article focuses on the physiological aspects of the baby's activities during birth. I also introduce here the principle of movement as an expression of mind, illustrating how fundamental psychological development of one's sense of self arises through movement.

Movement as Birth Preparation

Movement activities *in utero* may be regarded as functional precursors for next-stage development or *post-utero* survival. The baby *in utero* is physically active: swimming in his watery environment; kicking and punching reflexively; reaching through the mouth for his thumb; sucking; playing with his umbilical cord; pushing through all his limbs against the firm uterus; and flexing and extending his head, spine, and tail within the confines of the womb. The baby plays, interacting with and responding to her buoyant water world. These movement activities are important preparations for the baby's birth journey.

The influence of movement activities on the body-mind is indicated by the order of fetal nerve development. Bainbridge Cohen describes early sensorimotor development in this way: "The perceptual and the motor processes are not two separate things in the beginning. In the beginning, movement is perception. The first of the cranial nerves to myelinate (a sign of the importance of that pathway for survival) is the vestibular-cochlear nerve, which is the one registering move-

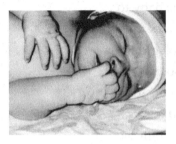

A newborn rests in cellular breathing.

ment and position in space (as well as vibration, velocity and tone—[both] muscle tone and sound). So the first perceptual nerve, and therefore sensory system, to myelinate is the one which perceives movement."[5] Through the movement of fluid in the semicircular canals of the inner ear, the baby senses gravity and direction in the three planes *in utero.*

By exploring movement and the uterine environment through moving her limbs, head, spine, and tail, the baby engages her internal sensory system, initially the vestibular nerve and later the proprioceptors of the muscles and joints. Through maternal and baby movements, and the compression and resistance of the uterine container, the baby learns the essentials of where she is in gravity and space, what her parts are and how they are connected, and where her body begins and ends. In the floating, mobile environment of the mother's womb, the baby also experiences gravity, as "up" and "down," felt through relative lightness and density of compression and the sense of weight through the internal organs.

In short, the baby begins to know himself through movement *in utero.* Kinesthetic knowledge, our first learning of ourselves and our environment, begins *in utero* through movement and touch. This kinesthetic knowledge is not of the conscious mind or high brain; it is instead the felt intelligence of the body knowing itself. For example, baby's legs rubbing against and then pushing off the uterine wall without preplanning are movements that underlie subsequent motor coordination. Just as we can touch our nose with our eyes closed, the baby's mouth and thumb can find each other without visual cues through his network of internal sensory connections.

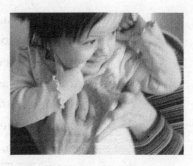

Exploratory play of fingers and mouth establishes kinesthetic self-knowledge.

The importance of this self-knowledge in birthing is that through these internal sensory connections, the baby is capable of aligning herself to the optimal birth position, given a relaxed pelvis and the absence of complications. The baby aligns herself head-down through her experience of gravity in the womb. At full-term compression, head-down permits the most movement and therefore is probably the most comfortable for the baby if the pelvic ligaments are soft, the bones are well aligned, and the uterine tone is well balanced.

Evidence from hypnotherapy studies and yoga, as well as successes in chiropractic and craniosacral alignment work and acupuncture, confirm the baby's ability to realign a difficult presentation.[6] Dr. Lewis Mehl-Madrona notes in his research findings that the baby's ability to actively move around *in utero* is itself critical to the baby finding the optimal head-down birthing position. His study concludes that hypnotherapy successfully results in spontaneous rotation of breech babies due to relaxation of the lower uterine segment.[7] In other beneficial modalities, such as combined chiropractic and craniosacral work, practitioners adjust bones, ligaments, muscles, and fascia to open and align the maternal tissues that then enables the baby to drop her head into the pelvic inlet.

Tone Arising through Movement

Just as the baby's capacity for movement is essential for aligning with the mother's pelvis, so too is movement integral to early developmental stages that prepare the baby for birth. Bainbridge Cohen posits that the emergence of tone, in the internal organs and subsequently in the muscles, is stimulated by the active baby.[8]

Tone is a description of the level of vitality in organs and muscles. "Baseline tone" is the readiness to function and relate.[9] Balanced tone is not a specific vibrational pitch but instead encompasses a broad range, just as our voices have vocal range. For the organs and muscles, this range arises through tissue movement. As the baby *in utero* explores all his movement possibilities, the organs glide like water balloons in suspension, each evolving the rhythm associated with its processing activities. These rhythms may be slow and irregular, as in early swallowing through the digestive tract, or they may be driving and steady, as in the heart. Fetal organs supported by their associated sensorimotor nerves evolve tone through gradual, ongoing stimulation and activity. Through this feedback loop, the tissues develop and refine the vibratory range of tone in the organs and muscles.

Organ tone underlies muscle tone, by either filling or collapsing the internal space, and so affects overall postural tone of the musculoskeletal system.[10] Bainbridge Cohen describes a baby with good organ tone as one who has vitality and resilience, like a balloon filled with water. A low-tone baby's skeleton is unsupported by the inner organs; they are like flabby balloons with insufficient air. Organ tone develops through movement. "Movement of the mother (and of the baby *in utero*) stimulates the baby's vestibular mechanism of the inner ear," says Bainbridge Cohen.[11] "This stimulation is the earliest sensorial experience of the infant, as the vestibular nerve is the first of the cranial nerves to complete its development [to myelinate] *in utero*. The function of the vestibular organ in the inner ear is to register and modify movement and postural tone in relation to gravity (which we reference later to develop sense of), space and time. Vestibular stimulation facilitates the development of tone in the organs, which in turn is reflected in the postural tone of the skeletal muscles," says Bainbridge Cohen.[12]

The vestibular nerve is closely allied with the vagus nerve, which serves the organs and cues autonomic nervous system function. Early movements and vestibular sensing provide vagal input for the lifelong balancing act of the autonomic nervous system. Autonomic decisions of where to dedicate systemic resources, either to rest and digest (toward the organs) or to active and alert states (toward the muscles for readiness to act) are moderated by our sense of support in the gravitational field. The nausea of what we call "motion sickness" is an example of vestibular-vagal-autonomic interaction. Here the dissonance among visual input, movement of the vehicle, and the body's senses of gravity and acceleration overwhelms the autonomic nervous system, throwing the gut off. Bainbridge Cohen's premise that support precedes movement reflects the importance of feeling grounded for both physical and emotional balance. Weak vestibular function and weak muscle are problematic for many children with developmental delay and behavioral problems, well researched by Sally Goddard Blythe.[13]

These conclusions are further corroborated by the studies of physician and psycholinguist Alfred Tomatis, a pioneer in auditory learning and communication. Tomatis observed that initial function is in the low-end range, in the sensory field of sound and vibration. Through his auditory-vocal research, we know that babies first perceive low-frequency sounds through the vestibular-cochlear nerve path.

In utero development of the vagus nerve and early swallowing movements elicit digestive tract tone, which provides the baby with support for her vertical soft body. In Righard and Alade's video documentary, newborns lift their heads and scan in search of the nipple, supported by the digestive tract and the reach of the mouth.[14] The unmedicated babies of this study who are allowed to stay in skin-to-skin contact with their mothers display very strong tone in their ability to crawl to the nipple and demonstrate baseline tone as a readiness to function and relate.

Low organ tone is expressed as poor and immature digestive function. Low-tone babies, such as those who are premature or who have Down's syndrome, are more likely to present breech than babies with balanced tone. Low-tone babies are often slow to birth because they do not adequately hold their own space within the womb in resistance to uterine contractions. At the other end of the tonal range, high-tone babies may also be more likely to experience difficulties positioning and birthing. Extremely high-tone babies may have impaired capacity to yield. Difficulty in yielding may be expressed in the baby who cannot tolerate settling down into the bony pelvic wedge, and so presents breech. In other babies, the inability to yield may potentially lead to a bruising struggle against the intense compression of contractions.

Because vestibular function underlies organ tone, extreme-tone babies may have impaired vestibular function, which affects fundamental bodily orientations in space, gravity, and time. In either extreme of low tone or high tone, the difficulties in presentation and birthing are due to the imbalanced relationship between the baby's tone and the mother's uterus. The mother's uterus may be low tone (due to multiple births or extreme obesity) or may be very high tone (due to trauma, stress, or other factors). Good positioning and good progress of labor are affected by balanced tone in the relationship between the baby and the mother's uterus.

Well-balanced postural tone arises naturally for the active, moving baby in her evolving development. This baseline postural tone is reflected in her fetal position through physiological flexion. Bainbridge Cohen states, "Physiological flexion is the pattern of total body flexion. It develops during the last trimester of uterine life, as the infant's size increases in relationship to the uterus and its boundaries are more defined. It is the process by which the flexor muscles on the front of the body increase their tone so that the infant's total body is curled into a posture of total flexion.... At birth the flexor tone is so strong that the baby's body will remain in a flexed C-curve, even when the baby is suspended in the air belly-down or belly-up. Physiological flexion reflects the newborn's basic postural tone."[15]

A baby with low postural tone and poor physiological flexion will be more likely to enter the birth canal with a face-down presentation instead of the optimal crown presentation. "In the mechanics of birth (the rotation of the baby's head as it travels through the birth canal), the baby needs to be in flexion with everything folded up," notes Susan Kroll, a certified nurse-midwife who teaches on difficult births at the

University of Minnesota. Babies who are not aligned in the optimal position have longer and more difficult births, with greater risk to themselves. A well-positioned baby enters the pelvic canal leading with his crown, the area where the top and the back of the head intersect. The crown presentation is the most compact shape for the baby to squeeze through the bony tunnel he must traverse. A well-aligned baby in crown presentation is able to engage in his full capacity to partner with his mother in undertaking the developmental task of birth.

The Song of the Mother and Baby

Organ tone, muscle tone, and vocal tone each arise from vibrations of tissues, as vocalist and dancer Marilyn Habermas-Scher elucidates.[16] High-frequency vibrations result in high tones, and low-frequency vibrations result in low tones, while ultra-low frequencies, which are below the range of hearing, characterize tissue tone.

Marilyn Habermas-Scher, Diane Elliot, and Gina Wray, each trained in dance, voice, breath, BMC, and Vipassana meditation, have explored Bainbridge Cohen's concept of tone relative to voice, movement, and body tissue. Their work and my dialogues with childbirth assistants Gail Tully and Kim Garret and childbirth educator/nurse practitioner Beverly Pierce inform my experience and understanding of tone.

Tone arises from the interplay of movement, sound, vibration, touch, and integration of these experiences within the nervous system. Tone develops incrementally *in utero* and can be affected by movement and voice. While *in utero* normal, individual differences in tone arise which may later appear as personality differences in high-energy or very calm newborns. The baby who has greater tonal range in its body has more possibilities of choice in response to the intense range of uterine birth activity, as seen in the baby's ability to both yield and hold her own space in relation to the mother's uterus during birth. Organ tone and muscle tone are resources *in their full range*. The key word here is "range." Good tonal range, observed in the vitality of the tissues, is a healthy continuum of vibration or aliveness in the body, allowing resilience and capacity for movement choices.

A pregnant mother can help her baby develop tonal range in several ways. By moving throughout her pregnancy, a mother helps her baby to establish a range of tone. Expectant mothers and fathers can support the vitality of their baby and the mother's uterus by singing to their baby and to the mother's uterus, or by simply toning vocally into the baby-belly. Toning vocally into a tissue increases its vitality because it vibrates the tissue, instructs Habermas-Scher. Toning or singing through a range of high and low pitches will develop high tone and low tone, which are both resources for the baby and uterus during pregnancy and birth. Toning is particularly valuable for babies at risk for premature delivery, such as twins.

Mothers experience a wide range of capacities and limitations in pregnancy, birth, and postpartum. Some women bear children easily while others are exhausted due to physical, hormonal, or energetic challenges. Women can also tone for themselves during pregnancy, in birth, and postpartum to sustain their energies or to be revitalized. Toning into the glands with an experienced teacher can access and balance hormonal resources.

The Baby Shares the Lead in the Hormonal Orchestra

The miracle of life unfolds from the joining of the egg and sperm to the emergence of an extraordinarily complex, complete, and unique human being. The baby's DNA blueprint and the hormonal mediators of both baby and mother initiate various stages in this process of creation and birth.

Medical science, in its quest to reduce the damaging effects of birth complications, has researched the endocrine system activities of baby and mother that affect birth onset. Recent research indicates that the baby's placenta develops a "timer" that determines the term of pregnancy.[17] The baby and mother meet at the cellular level in the placenta. At the placental interface, nutrients, oxygen, and hormones are exchanged across the semi-permeable membranes of the mother's and baby's intertwined capillary beds. Within the placenta itself hormones are manufactured, some of which appear to set the clock for the length of gestation.[18] Other studies look at the hormonal events associated with the onset of labor. Researchers conclude that "The initiation of a complex cascade of events resulting in the delivery of a healthy newborn appears to involve the integrated actions of the fetus, mother, and the placenta."[19]

An expectant mother's trust that her baby will begin his birth journey when he is ready is now mirrored in our scientific understanding of the birth process. In the wisdom of life unfolding, the cells becoming a baby also generate his first life-support system, the placenta. The placenta functions as a specialized, external organ of the *in utero* child. When the baby is ready for birth, he with his placenta and his mother, in concert, undertake the child's arrival into the world. Cascading hormones provide communications among the baby, the placenta, and the mother. These intermingling messengers stream together with rising momentum and, like a great tidal river, lead to the ocean-like waves of uterine contractions.

Fluid Rhythms Underlying Birth

In the first part of labor, while the baby is floating in the uterus, her active flexion is supported by her organ tone. Among the organs, the digestive tract is a soft vertical axis that supports curling inward. Bainbridge Cohen observes that "the skeletal-muscular activity of physiological flexion appears to be an outer manifestation of the digestive organ activity."[20] This soft, simple tube is sheathed by smooth muscle layers that alternately squeeze and release, creating the peristaltic rhythm that moves food down the tract. Global Somatics and BMC teacher Suzanne River notes that the digestive-tract rhythm underlies the baby's alternating physiological flexion and extension *in utero* and after birth.

This undulating peristaltic rhythm is a resting-state rhythm. We rest when our bodies shift into digestive mode: blood shifts from the limbs to the core, the entire involuntary nervous system orients inward, and we settle into internal processing with this rhythm. Both baby and mother come into this deep relaxation during early labor.

Then baby and mother arrive at a moment of readiness for the child to move out of his uterine home and through the final passage. A new wave of hormones floods the system, moving the mother's energy down and out, intensifying labor into transition. The baby also sends adrenaline to the mother's pituitary gland, augmenting her labor. The baby shifts into a new rhythm, the cerebrospinal rhythm, which underlies physiological extension.[21] This rhythm arises from the slow waves of the cerebrospinal fluid, which cushions and nourishes the brain and spinal cord. As the baby's head comes into the close bony passage of the birth canal, he is protected by amniotic fluid on the outside and by cerebrospinal fluid on the inside.

The baby's shift to the cerebrospinal rhythm brings a shift away from the internal orientation of processing and toward movement into space with the head-spine-tail. The baby's whole body readies for her compression through the bony passage, but this new orientation is not initiated from the bones of the head, spine, and tail, for they must yield for passage. It is instead initiated from the cerebrospinal fluid. By means of the integrated neuroendocrine system, the soft brain and its cord-tail swim with energetic, hormonally charged intent toward the pelvic opening.

Hormonal Alignment: Organizing around the Vertical Axis

When the great forces of nature are at work upon us, the skills we need most are piloting and navigation. When the ocean currents and wind

storms of contraction seize us, mothers must be capable both of sur-
rendering to forces beyond our control and of making those small
movements of rudder and sail—via the pelvis—that will enable the
baby to move out. The mother can do specific activities to help the
baby come into alignment as an active partner in birth.

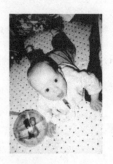

Alignment is the organization of a system or systems in relationships
that permit access to internal resources and a wide choice of actions.
Aligning and accessing the neuroendocrine system provides specific,
potent resources for baby and mother. Hormones provide the raw
energy necessary for mother and baby to birth, from the initiation of
labor through transition and emergence of the baby. Hormonal alignment through the vertical axis also supports structural, or skeletal,
alignment. During labor contractions the mother's body may go into
a protective "freeze" response. Sending vibration into areas of intensity
through toning can allow a woman to move through a contraction, as
toning gently awakens the tissues to their capacity to move at a vibrational or micro level. Our explorations indicate that focused toning
along the vertical axis can assist mother and baby in aligning for birth,
help a woman to move through the intensity of labor, support postural
alignment during pregnancy, and ease postpartum recovery.

A child finds con-
nection to gravity in
underlying yield
and individuation
in the homologous
push pattern.

Body-Mind Centering uses toning and breath to enter into specific
tissues and to access the endocrine system. Through BMC's embodied
explorations, the endocrine system has been described as loci of
intensely concentrated and specialized chemical messengers that can
shift the entire body-mind state. The endocrine system appears to parallel the yogic *chakras*, energy centers with specific qualities located in
approximately the same regions as the endocrine glands.[22] Each of
these systems describes a way of being vertically organized.

In BMC explorations, Bonnie Bainbridge Cohen and colleagues have
"found the joints, muscles, organs, and perceptions that are associated
with each gland, so that instead of tapping the glands directly in their
rawness, they are given a form, a structure. The neuroendocrine system
is the force through which the structure functions."[23] Bainbridge Cohen

notes further the importance of "integrating [the neuroendocrine system] with the skeletal-muscular system so that the [raw glandular] energy wasn't chaotic but had a vehicle through which it could be expressed."[24]

Mothers and birth attendants describe the presence and movement of birth energy, which from the perspective of BMC is interpreted, in part, as endocrine activity. Mothers, as well as home birth midwife Gail Tully, describe a laser beam of energy emitting from the baby's crown, guiding the baby as it heads down the birth canal. The well-aligned baby and mother are able to fully access this raw endocrine energy, allowing it to flow through them along the vertical axis.

As noted earlier, toning into areas of intensity can help a woman ride out contractions. Toning into the endocrine glands during pregnancy can support postural alignment, give a woman access to all her hormonal resources, and provide experience for reading internal cues and flows of energy. This internal tracking skill is invaluable for birth. We hypothesize that toning into the baby's endocrine glands *in utero* would also give the baby access to all of her hormonal resources for birth, supporting optimal alignment and energetic movement through the birth passage.

Toning into the glands should be undertaken with an experienced teacher because it can access and release potent hormones. As noted above, contacting the joints, muscles, organs, and perceptions related to a given endocrine gland is necessary to ground the raw energy of the endocrine system. Also, as Bainbridge Cohen notes, "We found that you have to open the channels between the glands as well as the glands themselves."[25] With such grounding and balance, toning can access the endocrine system for increased vitality for mother and child during pregnancy and for integrated and fine-tuned response during birth.

Fontanels: Windows of the Spirit

Once the baby has arrived at the optimal head-down position, typical of birth, his next activity is to refine his head alignment in relation to the pelvic structure. The easiest passage for baby and mother is when the baby leads with the crown, as most babies do.

The importance of this final refinement of positioning is described by midwife Valerie El Halta: "If there is no progress with good contractions, it is usually head position [that is the problem]."[26] The mother can help the baby move into an optimal position by walking around, by shifting her position, or by compressing her upper pelvis or sacrum, all of which help the lower pelvis to open. If these approaches are unsuccessful in enabling the baby to move into the best position, the midwife can "adjust the head at 3–4 centimeters, saving the woman a long and arduous labor," advises Nancy Wainer Cohen.[27] El Halta and Cohen, a midwife team, determine placement and make adjustments of the baby's head by locating suture lines and fontanels, which they declare "are God's directional signals for midwives!"[28]

Putting mothers on prolonged bed rest may impede a baby's ability to move and may result in malpresentation. Mother Colleen Ahlers Moore reports adhering to bed rest at the suggestion of her physician, in spite of ongoing misgivings. Her baby led with his brow instead of his crown, prolonging labor and resulting in chronic hyperextension by the baby while nursing and resting.[29]

In Native American traditions, the parietal fontanels are regarded as an opening connecting the Earth-bound baby with the Great Spirit. The Hopi view these fontanels as the window of the spirit, in the context of a system of vibratory centers. "The Hopi believe each person has five vibratory centers: the solar plexus, the heart, the throat, the forehead, and the crown. They also believe that the spot on the top of the head is soft, the spirit can go in and out," instructs Native American teacher A. C. Ross.[30]

While reference to mythology may seem like an extreme reach for understanding physiological function, once we enter into embodiment and observation, as in BMC, we find a great deal of coherence and wisdom in myth. Indeed, Joseph Campbell, the eminent student of world mythologies, concludes in his later works that all mythologies—

including religions, philosophies, arts, and customs—arise from the experience of embodiment. Campbell identifies the culmination of religious and artistic expression as an embodied spiritual journey through the energy centers along the vertical axis.[31] Multicultural manifestations of a pilgrim's progress up a metaphoric, body-referenced ladder range across the globe, in ancient Egypt, the cultures of pre-Christian Celts, pre-Columbian Aztec, Navajo, in yogic traditions and Buddhism of India, and medieval Dante. Campbell concludes that all expressions of mind and systems of thought arise from the universal human experience of being in the body.[32]

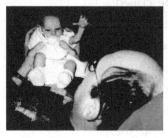

Physiological flexion provides infant Erin with core self-knowledge as she reaches into relationship.

In birthing each human undergoes his or her first rite of passage, with robust spirit and vibrant intentional body coming into the light and onto the Earth, eventually to take his or her standing as a creature of Heaven and Earth.

Coming into the Horizontal Relationship: The Earth Plane

Refining movements leading through the occipital-crown axis are also undertaken as the baby rotates her head while traveling down the final, close passage. These cardinal movements, as they are called by midwives, bring the baby into horizontal relationship with her immediate environment. Homebirth midwife Kim Garrett conceives of these movements as the baby coming into relationship with the earth—the horizontal plane—by orienting to the four directions. An alert, unmedicated baby is able to move and can use "the head to search and perceive the environment and make choices through the senses," says Bainbridge Cohen.[33]

Head-spine-tail integration underlies the refinement of head positions. This integration, along with the organization of the baby's endocrine system, enables the baby to move with the least expenditure of effort in the direction of the crown. During birth, the baby sends out a steady beam of hormonally-based energy originating from his vertically-aligned glands and streaming through his crown. This energy leads the baby through the birth tunnel. The final adjustment of crown presentation allows the baby to employ its resources of head-spine-tail integration and to energetically engage all the glands in alignment to navigate the narrow straits.

As the baby moves down into the birth canal, balanced organ tone allows the infant to have her fullness and so to "hold her space" in the intensity of uterine contractions. In labor the upper uterine muscle contracts while the lower uterine muscle segment, which has softened and thinned in late pregnancy, allows itself to be stretched. While the baby gets strongly squeezed during a contraction, the infant with balanced organ tone holds some of her internal space, so that the lower uterine segment and cervix slides over her head. Both movements happen at once: the baby is pushed by the upper uterus toward the lower opening while the lower uterus slides over the head as the baby holds her space.

Some births are long because there is not enough counter-resistance of tone in the interaction between baby and uterus to move things along well. (To imagine the action of counter-resistance, return to the balloon image discussed earlier in regard to organ tone. If you squeeze a firm water balloon, it wants to bulge toward one direction. If, instead, you squeeze an overstretched, flabby water balloon, it has no tendency of direction.) Low-tone babies, such as typical premature babies, Down's babies, and medicated babies, may be slow to come out, even if well positioned. On the other side of the relationship, maternal factors may include a low-tone uterus (as in a mother who has had many, many babies), or weak contractions due to interrupted oxytocin production (as in a mother who is stressed or constantly distracted by medical staff while in labor).

Pushing Off the Fundal Floor

A baby with well-balanced tone, who is holding his own space, propels himself through the birthing tunnel. Early reflexes enable a baby with an optimal crown presentation to push himself out by planting his feet on the firm floor of the fundus. Bainbridge Cohen states, "If the baby's head is down for birthing, it can use its feet to push or propel itself out, while guiding and directing with its head."[34] With these early, primary reflexes—survival mechanisms that almost all babies develop *in utero* between mid- and full term—stimulation of a specific area of the body (in this case, the fundus contacting the baby's feet) elicits an automatic response. I suggest that in contraction, the pressure of the fundus on the feet stimulates the primary reflexes of crossed extension (onset 28 weeks) or spontaneous stepping (onset 37 weeks), seen in the newborn when his feet touch a surface.

The newborn's capacity for movement is an extension of her *in utero* activities. The baby kicks and pushes with her limbs in the womb, both reflexively and voluntarily, as when she responds to sound and touch. In Righard and Alade's documentation of newborns self-locomoting to the breast and initiating suckling, the researchers conclude that the stepping/crawling reflex enables the newborn to crawl to the breast.[35] The mouth and the digestive tract provide organ support for this action, with the vertical soft-body providing the vital tissue tone to support the newborn's relatively weak leg muscles in the developmental pattern push-from-the-lower-limbs. The vertical soft-body also provides a head-to-tail connection, integrating the searching head with the pushing legs, feet, and tail.

Alert Babies, Engaged Bodies

Documentation by Righard and Alade as well as Nilsson demonstrates that infants are able to orient themselves through the head in relation to their environment—in this instance, in their search for the nipple. This capacity is based on the primary reflexes of neonatal neck righting, which develop *in utero*.

Neck righting can be observed when the newborn looks around for the breast.[36] The alert, unmedicated newborn is able to use his head, responding through its reflexes and engaging perceptually. The newborn who is able to seek, find, and self-attach to the nipple demonstrates capacities developed *in utero*.

We can study *in utero* development and newborn movement further for their contribution to our understanding of the baby's active role in birth. This understanding can lead us more fully into assisting newborns—for example, those who have had difficult or medicated births leading to problems with nursing, digesting, and other aspects of early infant development. Bainbridge Cohen comments, "If I see a baby (or an adult) where the head is dragging, then I would wish to awaken the senses in the movement of the head so they could dialogue more immediately with their environment rather than be isolated."[37]

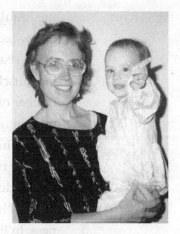

Reach and pull patterns: Erin reaches toward her father. The gesture arrives at completion when her father brings himself to Erin's hand. Erin then pulls him to herself.

Coming into the Light

The baby is first a creature of the ocean, a unicellular being evolving *in utero* into sea-like forms very similar to the pulsating jellyfish and then the radiant sea star. We carry the ancient memory of these forms in our cells. Having sensed herself in floating gravity *in utero*, the baby meets the intensity of being earthbound in the compression of late pregnancy and in birth. The baby swims down the canal, at one with the mother, as the great waves of the contractions carry the child from the inner sea. Like a fish gliding through the intricate maze of a coral reef, the baby undulates and maneuvers through the narrow passage of the birth canal out into a new realm of gravity, space, and air. After birth, the baby meets gravity fully through the yield response. Yielding, one of the reflexes and developmental patterns, is the baby's first move to relate directly to the Earth.

As we are creatures of the Earth, this relationship with Earth is essential to who we are. The baby moves from being carried within the mother to being carried by the mother. Then the baby extends the cellular trust of this experience into being supported by the earth below us.

The baby "magnetizes" toward the mother and the earth by increasing muscle tone on the surface of his body, which is in contact with the mother or earth. This tonic labyrinthine response brings the newborn into connection with gravity, which then supports the baby in pushing off and in individuating. Later developmental patterns take the child into the freedom of space through reach activities.

The developmental patterns express, in subtle and observable ways, the developing mind of each child coming into its fullness and uniqueness. In her activities, the baby shows the same unthinking grace as a tennis player returning a volley; she is not making conscious decisions. There is no thought, just the whole beautiful body going forward to meet the next moment. Bainbridge Cohen states, "Underneath ALL successful, effortless movements are integrated reflexes, righting reactions and equilibrium responses."[38] It is in these movements that we witness the mind of the baby; we see the outward expression of brain growth as neurological pathways are created and interconnected.

After birth, the infant replays his birth journey, integrating this major developmental step. We can see the newborn repeat rhythmic, whole-body flexion and extension. The deeply coiled strength of physiological flexion, along with intense compression by the uterus, provide a spring-loading for the newborn to energetically expand into the world upon birth.[39] Now the baby is free to move into space, with the spine, head, and legs uncurling, pushing into extension and returning to flexion.

In order to be born we must align ourselves, move with rhythmic and fluid energy, surrender to greater flows and forces that will carry us along, and find the opening to the selves we are to become through specific and close limitation. The baby is active and partners with the mother through this journey. While birthing, the baby takes her place between Heaven and Earth as inspired body and embodied spirit, ready to undertake her life journey and to share her gift of becoming and being with the world.

Evoking the Fluid Body

~ **Thomas Greil,** Germany (2002)

As human beings, we are an accrual of many life forms that have been shaped by our oceanic origins, still pulsating as the intrinsic world of our organs, our connective tissue, our nerve fiber. We are a process of millions of years of an open-ended experiment.

—Emilie Conrad in *Rolf Lines*, May 1998

For more than thirty years, Emilie Conrad has been exploring the vibrational field in sounding, breathing, and stillness. Continuum Movement, which she developed, works with a wide range of techniques to increase fluidity in the body, to dissolve patterns, and to evoke changes.[1] In this article I would like to present my ideas on how Body-Mind Centering (BMC) and Continuum can inform each other and bring more understanding to how vibration affects fluidity in the body. I will finish this article with a few explorations I have found helpful in discovering Continuum from a BMC background.

Body-Mind Centering and Continuum are both based on the concept of movement. Without movement there is no life, and with impaired movement health is also impaired. One characteristic of movement is that it is non-repetitive; direction and intensity change with each movement. The heartbeat, for example, is highly irregular. It is not predictable when the next beat will happen. The more regularly a patient's heart beats, the sicker the heart is. If it beats like a metronome, it is a sign that the person will die soon.

A sick heart reacts like the cruise control in a car. Set the speed and the car automatically accelerates, but this is the only parameter it is reacting to. It won't slow down if there is a truck in front of you. As a complex organism, the body needs to fine-tune its responses much more than this. This ability to adapt is crucial. Every cell, every tissue, and every body system needs to cope continuously with internal and external stimuli in order to accommodate changes—like the heart adjusts to the need for blood and oxygen, but also to emotional stimuli like stress or joy.

Life is dependent on maintaining an adequate balance between two states: a more fluid state and a more solid state. The body is constantly creating form and dissolving form, which can be experienced in rhythms, like the autonomic nervous system rhythm—the flow between the back side (extension, sympathetic) and the front side (flexion, parasympathetic) of the body; the "simultaneous condensing and expanding yield"; or in the breath—inhaling (creating form) and exhaling (dissolving form).

On the cellular level this flow is reflected by the exchanges happening on the cell membrane. Life started millions of years ago when specific molecules began to form membranes encompassing an environment where processes could occur in a controlled way. Without membranes no discrete spaces are defined, and without fluid no communication is occurring. Membranes can be found in the body on all levels, defining fluid spaces and separating tissues.

The tone of a membrane is its capacity to let exchanges happen. It is the ability to be informed by the environment inside and outside of the membrane. If the membrane tone is high, the level of communication is low. Fewer adjustments to stimuli happen. The body is in defensive mode; it is blocking out information. If, on the other hand, the membrane tone is low, a lot of exchanges are happening. The body can't control what it would like to take in. The sympathetic nervous system raises tone, and the parasympathetic nervous system lowers tone.

The fluid system is the main carrier for these informational processes in the body. Specific informational substances called *ligands*—hormones, neurotransmitters, neuropeptides, and so forth—bind to certain receptors on the surface of the cell.[2] Each cell has millions of those receptors, and there are two hundred to three hundred different informational substances in the body. The fewer the receptors a cell has, the less the information that is exchanged—for the heart, this means that it does not easily adjust to stimuli. These substances are not only produced in the brain or in the endocrine glands, but in every cell of the body, even immune cells. Also, the receptors are found all over the body. Each cell has the capacity to release and "sense" the ligands.

The "mind," therefore, is not only a function of the brain but also of every cell. With the focus on one part of the body—on a single cell or on a body system, for example—the mind of the whole body shifts, because the fluid system is distributing these substances, via the bloodstream, all over the body. One's entire perspective or awareness can come from that part. The body is a psychosomatic network, a field of information and energy that is constantly moving in and out of different mind (and fluid) states. Everything is happening at the same time.

This communication network is much older than the nervous system. Millions of years ago, single cells already interacted in this way— and they still do. Most communication in the human body is, in fact, chemical. Even in the brain, where we consider the "electrical nervous system" to be the most active, only two percent of the communication occurs at the synaptic gap. Ninety-eight percent of the time, substances act on cells farther away.

Because this "ancient" or "primitive" fluid-based communication system is by its nature vibrational, it reacts very well to sound and breath. The messenger molecules produced by cells to transmit information are changing shape all the time. Each shape has a different state, and the molecules are vibrating between those states. Each molecule is able to create different bonds with other molecules, depending on their vibrational states. The receptors, the "sense organs" of each cell, have the same ability. They are floating freely on the surface of the cell, picking up frequencies. This creates a dance between these molecules and the receptors.

Recent research from France has shown that simply applying the frequency of a ligand to a cell is enough to stimulate the receptors and create the same reaction as the ligand itself.[3] Sounding in particular, but also breathing, creates a resonance on the cellular level, increasing communication directly on the cell membrane. Sounding and breathing facilitate the exchange of information in the whole body. By "joining that dance," life is brought to body parts that have been deserted or that have become quiet or erratic in their functioning. The body can engage in the "creative flux" again, which makes life a celebration. When we join that fluid body, we can overcome our cultural limitations. We are not limited by boundaries anymore. We can "go under."

Touch

1. With a partner, put hands together to take a baseline reading.
2. Part from one another and begin sounding. Feel vibration expanding in your body.
3. Put your hands together again and feel the difference.

My experience is that with sounding, the awareness and vibrational quality in the hands increase. So every sound or breath you explore in Continuum can be transmitted through your hands. This can be helpful in cases where the client cannot do the sounding or the breath by himself, such as when working with babies.

Vibration

1. Lie comfortably on the ground, eyes closed.
2. Imagine swimming in the big ocean millions of years ago—molecules floating around, changing shapes, vibrating, communicating with each other.
3. Imagine the first cell forming, then chains of molecules forming a membrane and closing to create a discrete space—an inside and an outside.
4. Imagine the millions of receptors on the outside of the cell.

5. Imagine another cell and its relation to the first cell—two cells vibrating together in the fluids, exchanging information.
6. Let movements happen in the fluids and through the fluids.
7. Let the movement spread and inform your whole body.

With this exploration the amount of information exchanges in the body can be enhanced, bringing awareness of the "ancient nervous system" and movement to areas where there is none, such as with paralysis. You can add any sounds or breaths you like. For hands-on work, this exploration adds a lot of sensitivity and a feeling of connection.

"Theta" Breath

The "theta" breath is created by letting air out slowly through the mouth while the tongue is held behind the front teeth, like in the start of the word "theta." This exploration is structured with three participants—one person lying on the ground, one with the hands on the head at the sphenoid of the person lying, and one at one calf of the person lying (both hands have full contact with muscles and bones).

1. The person at the calf begins sounding and gently pulls, with a feeling of distributing the sound through the fascia.
2. The person at the head feels what happens to the sphenoid.
3. Now the person at the sphenoid begins sounding without moving.
4. Feel what happens at the calves.
5. Take your hands away and allow the person to feel their body without being touched.
6. Let movements arrive from the sensation.
7. Switch roles.

In my experience, the "theta" breath has a strong ability to disperse energy and to create space between the fascia. It also can be used to lengthen ligaments and tendons.

"Jacques"

The "Jacques" is composed of two sounds, JJJJ and ZZZZ, that alternate in a random, non-predictable way. You can experience the impact of its vibration by placing the fingertips on any of the bones while sounding—e.g., at the sternum, iliacs, cranium, knees, toes, etc. Its strong vibratory quality penetrates the bones, accessing sensation in the bone tissue.

1. Begin either lying on the ground or standing.
2. Put one or two fingertips on part of a bone that you can feel clearly.
3. Begin sounding.
4. Once in a while, stop sounding and feel the vibration in stillness inside your body.
5. Let movements happen from that place—slow, fast, smooth, jerky.

My experience is that "Jacques" brings fluidity to the bones; increases information; and invites small, unexpected, incremental movements. Try also with a partner.

Developmental Actions as Pathways of Support

~ **Annie Brook,** USA (1999)

In the field of body psychology, you often hear people speak of the sequencing of energy, meaning the flow down into the legs for grounding or into the heart for intimacy and contact. Psychotherapists often look at containment of energy and how to find support as important issues for clients to consider.

Body-Mind Centering (BMC) teachers and practitioners also look at these phenomena, viewing them from the lens of developmental movement and actions. We look at how physical development supports cognition and emotional integration. BMC correlates movement patterns with stages of brain development. Knowing these developmental stages and movement patterns allows us to support infant development and to assist repatterning work with adults. This repatterning supports our human nature of desire and need fulfillment, or attainment of pleasure.

To gain pleasure in our lives, we need to know how to feel our desire and to have the support to reach for what we want and to embrace it. Infants explore this when they learn to reach and crawl. It is an organic and often forgotten aspect of life. Remembering how to attain satisfaction and actually feel it in the body can transform the way we view our world.

A simple and effective tool of developmental integration is the developmental action sequence. This is a cycle of actions that an infant performs in task completion: actions of yield, push, reach, take hold, and pull. The cycle goes through each action and completes with a final yield, which starts the cycle anew. Having full range of the developmental action cycle allows someone to feel desire, to move into action, and to complete that action. By feeling desire and being able to sequence toward completion of desire, a person develops a sense of confidence and capability. He or she is able to participate in the world and to meet essential needs.

To understand how the developmental action cycle functions, watch this cycle in action. Take a small toy and play with a baby. As the baby becomes aware of the toy through stimulation of the senses, she yields and takes in the new information. As this information comes in, she will gather energy and push down into the support of the earth. A counter-push moves back up and through her body, sequencing out her head and tail and giving her the support to look with awareness at you and the toy. Watch as she reaches out and takes hold of the toy. Feel the strength of her grasp and the pulling force as she pulls this toy toward herself. Notice how she yields again as she explores the toy and then decides whether she likes it or not. She may take it further in, or push it away and explore elsewhere. This is the natural progression of yield, push, reach, take hold, and pull. It is repeated over and over as a young one explores her environment.

Let's look at the psychological implications of this sequence. Each action in the sequence needs the underlying support of the previous action. Push needs active yield underneath so that it is organic and healthy. If active yield is lacking—meaning that tissue tone is too taut or too collapsed—it will cause the push to be demanding or weak; the free-flowing energy is not available to push. Without proper push, the ability to reach is affected. A person will not go directly for what she wants, or can be incessant and never satisfied. Reach needs a free-flowing, supported push so that one can reach fully with support rather than overextending.

Imagine what happens when this sequence is interrupted, in both adults and children. Most often, the actions get interrupted through fairly normal circumstances. I worked with one person who had a brother two years older than himself. As an infant, this man had the experience of getting his hands on something, only to have it immediately pulled away by his brother. This happened over and over throughout childhood and resulted in the experience of a low-grade lethargy within my client about really going for what he wanted. This lethargy showed up physically as a push that was a bit resigned and a reach that was not fully extended. Another client's desire was self-thwarted; she moved away from what she actually wanted and toward something else as soon as she felt others were watching her. In her experience, it had been unsafe to go for what she genuinely desired. As a consequence, her reach became distracted and her taking hold had little energy.

Think about the impacts of these actions on behavior. Have you ever met people who don't know how to yield? They respond before processing all the information at hand. They may finish your sentences for you, or not listen fully; they may start things when only partially prepared. People who lead with a push without an underlying active yield are often unaware of the impact of their energy. They work very hard and push into life without getting much support. They may be obstinate or difficult to be around. They are often tired. They may try to dominate in conflicting or intense situations. Other people might have the opposite problem; they are not yielded but collapsed. They have no available energy to take in and process information. They approach life already defeated.

What about those who are always reaching yet never getting their needs met? Either they may not have enough underlying push, which gives the reach a place to anchor from, or they may not know how to take hold of what they reach toward. They may have the world at their fingertips yet cannot meet or enjoy it, because they cannot take hold. Perhaps they do not know how to pull in. Have you ever met people who have support all around them, yet don't know how to use it? They may not take hold of the support. What about those who gather a lot of material things, or are always very busy doing activities?

They may take hold of experience, yet not digest these experiences. They may compile numerous material things because they cannot yield into them. They can get frozen in a continuous cycle of reaching without satisfaction.

All these examples illustrate subtle symptoms that appear when the developmental actions are missing or not fully sequenced. By learning the simple progression of yield, push, reach, take hold, and pull, you can support people to make significant changes toward greater satisfaction and an improved ability to relate to others. Think metaphorically and notice when there are gaps in a person's sequence. Watch physically and see if posture supports the fullness of each action. Notice how the lack of flow through the sequence can produce an emotional effort.

To support change, you can help clients to repattern this sequence. I suggest supporting this through cognitive, emotional, and physical levels of awareness. As an example, I often lead people through the developmental progression and let them discover where they have gaps. I invite them to lie on the floor and go through the actions just as a baby would, or I model and talk them through the actions from a sitting posture. Sometimes I will hand them an object and notice if their ability to reach or take hold is fully developed. I look for the presence of motivation and desire in their lives.

We then explore the ramifications of developmental gaps on a personal and emotional level and practice repatterning the missing or limited action. This simple work produces significant emotional shifts. If a practitioner assists clients with the development of each action and then the overall sequencing, this will simply and instrumentally support a shift in their ability to feel satisfied and more responsive in daily living.

Explore this through the following exercise:

Find active yield. First, simply notice your connection with the floor beneath you as you lie on your back. Notice if you feel connected to the floor, collapsed into it, or pulled away from it. This will help you to become aware of your tissue tone, which directly influences your ability to yield. Now exaggerate the sensation in your tissue. First go for a high tone; tense your body from the inside and notice what happens to your breath. Notice if you can feel the floor supporting you, or if all the support is coming only from within. Lift your head off the floor and notice the level of effort it requires; notice how you feel as you look out through your eyes. Do you feel receptive or emotionally open with this inner tension?

Now lower your head, relax, and take a breath. Move into the opposite extreme by producing a collapsed state, which is a low tone. Imagine that you are like a broken water balloon. Exaggerate this feeling. Now, from this position, think about lifting your head. You may not be able to do it. If you can, notice how you must compensate to do so. Notice how you perceive the world emotionally from this state. A low tone means you will feel collapsed into the floor rather than supported by it.

Once you know these two extremes, find the middle ground, which is active yield. Go back and forth between low and high tone until you find a balance. Rest here a moment and allow this balanced tone of active yield to renew and support you. Once you have active yield, push down into the floor and let the push come back up through your body and out your head and tail. Use this energy to rise up onto your forearms so that your elbows are resting on the floor. Look out into the world; notice how push gives you the support to do this. Feel your desire. Look around. Notice what interests you. Now lower yourself back to the floor. Find yield, move into push, and again come up.

This time, as soon as you are up, feel your desire: locate something that interests or motivates you, and reach for it. Feel the force of your energy as you reach. Move your body until you can take hold of what you wanted. Observe yourself as you grasp it. Close your hand around it and feel the sense of taking hold thoroughly. Notice the satisfaction that might be growing inside you.

Pull the object in toward your body and embrace it. Feel the strength and delight of pulling. Bring it all the way in and feel the satisfaction of a full pull.

Now that you have the object, scan your tissue tone and sequence into active yield again. As you yield, take in the object and the sense of satisfaction that comes from noticing, desiring, and having what you wanted. Explore the object you grasped. Notice if you like it and want to keep it for a while, or if you want to let it go and reach for something else.

Repeat this cycle over and over until every phase of it feels easy in your body. Give yourself time to yield, push, reach, take hold, and pull. Allow enough time in each phase for you to feel it fully. Notice your emotional sensations once the entire sequence is easy and fluid.

Another interesting way to explore this is by sitting up and making contact with another person or object without touch. Here you reach and pull with your eyes. Explore this with a partner.

Sit up and find active yield. Feel the support of the floor as you push down through your sitz bones, letting that feeling rise back up through your spine and support you to sit in a comfortable manner. Reach with your eyes toward your partner; take hold of that person with your eyes. Appreciate the connection by pulling the energy in and feeling it. Yield as you take in this level of contact. Notice if you tend to defend, as in high tone, or collapse, as in low tone. See if you can return to active yield, letting your eyes be soft and aware. Notice how you feel as you connect in this manner.

You can use the practice of developmental actions throughout the day in various ways, such as opening a door or greeting and meeting someone with your eyes. Explore how many different ways you can use the sequence. Notice how it can support a sense of renewal and presence as you interact in the world.

Thinking in Place

〜 **Pat Ethridge,** USA (2000)

What is a balanced nervous system? Before we answer that question, let us briefly examine the structure of the nervous system. Our nervous system—which has a central component (brain, spinal cord, and retina) and a peripheral component (the structures outside the central nervous system which connect to the rest of the body)—provides command and control functions for our body and mind. The peripheral nervous system has both somatic and autonomic components. The somatic part is composed of sensory nerves and receptors that send incoming information to the brain and other nervous cells and of motor nerves and receptors that send outgoing information mostly to the body's muscles, bones, and skin, primarily to facilitate movement responses. The autonomic component of the nervous system governs our more "unconscious" functions, regulating organs, blood vessels, glands, and overall internal chemistry. The autonomic system has a sympathetic part, which prepares the body for outward responses, and a parasympathetic part, which focuses the body on its internal processes. The nervous system operates in conjunction with the other systems of the body. In Body-Mind Centering terms, it is "shadowed" or supported by the fluids, especially the blood.

When one functional aspect of the nervous system is predominantly active, we say a person is "in the mind" of that part, as when, for example, someone is "sympathetically" oriented. Being in "sympathetic mind" can be very helpful to someone trying to cross a busy highway, but if that same person were trying to take a nap, that state would interfere with the desired activity. If someone is "stuck" in one state of mind and cannot transition out of it, this is a state of imbalance. A person may have a preference for a certain state of mind as, for example, when one is extremely sensitive to external stimuli and thus perhaps overly situated in "sensory" mind at the expense of "motor" mind. One may be too much in the mind of the nervous system at the expense of the fluids, which can have either a slowing down or stasis effect on the "fluidity" of nervous system flow, or a speeding-up effect of jitteriness. Or perhaps trauma has created conflicts or "reversals" in function.

So what does it mean to be balanced? Sometimes we know what this feels like within ourselves. We can monitor the status of our nervous-system functioning by bringing our attention to our internal state, by focusing our sensory nervous system in a motoric way. We can do this by observing neutrally our thoughts, our feelings, and our physical sensations and by comparing this experience with previous observations. Over time, we can learn to distinguish when we are in balance and when we are out of balance. When we are in balance our experience is less stressful because we are not using more energy than necessary or using energy in conflicted ways. Consequently, we feel more restful in our functioning. One of the goals of meditation is to create a balanced internal state; meditation, or internal observation, is itself the means to that goal. A balanced internal state can then support external functioning.

We can also monitor our experience of nervous-system functioning by bringing our attention to what we are doing externally—specifically to the ease or difficulty with which we are operating. A moving meditation can permit the fluids to integrate nervous-system information and thus "clear the decks" for new experiences. We can know when we are "in the zone," that place of being in which everything we do is effortless and perfectly performed. At such moments there is a sense of buoyant flow caused by the fluids' support of the nervous system. We feel free to invest our psychic energy in what we are doing. There is a seamless interaction between sensory input and motor output and the integration of our experience. We are using no more energy than is necessary and yet as much as we wish to accomplish our tasks. We can take in as much information as we need, being neither overwhelmed by too much nor stressed by too little. Our challenges seem neither so great that we are made anxious nor so small that we become bored. We can utilize our learned skills to meet new difficulties successfully, and we can expand and develop our selves to a higher level of complexity.

What does a balanced nervous system look like? One image that has been offered by artists through the centuries is the image of the Buddha in meditation. It can be very instructive to view a collection of these images. These Buddha figures, or images of related beings, are almost always presented in the vertical (or *door* or *coronal*) plane, facing front. This plane is associated with thinking and decision making, weighing two sides of a problem. This notion implies the person as the central force supporting two invisible scales of consideration (or duality), one on either side, which seek stability. Variations from this format are sufficiently rare to emphasize the importance of this primary image.

While the iconography of the various artistic traditions is usually quite proscribed, creating an apparently monotonous similarity between one image and another, it is often possible to discern varying states of mind and body presented by individual artists. With some images there is no sense of the figure's internal state; the exterior physical presence is dominant and the inner mind workings are impervious to view. With others, the internal mind state is the strongest presence. Occasionally the figure seems lost in a dream, and the physical body seems like an un-lived-in appendage. Or the figure focuses his gaze on the viewer with a powerful outer-directed force. Frequently the hand gestures express a lymphatic precision. Sometimes the figure hardly seems human at all, but more like a supernatural being. This type of figure does not seem to have organs or fluids or even bones, but only a giant force of brain/nervous-system/gland mind. And yet a few convey the central state—exactly between inner-outer, mind-body, or other dichotomies—where there is nothing that is too much or too little, and all is held in exquisite balance.

An interesting example of the latter is offered in the statue *Guanyin of the Southern Sea* at the Nelson-Atkins Museum of Art in Kansas City. This figure, created in China about a thousand years ago, seems quite human in appearance, with both body and mind present—not that different from a person in a similar state of balance whom we might meet. The figure sits calmly meditating. The overall muscular tone is balanced equally between tension and relaxation, creating an easy postural support. The spine is erect without stiffness, allowing for free breathing. The joints are relaxed, and weight falls to the underside of the limbs without creating limpness. The glandular energy is awake but not overactive, adding that quality of support to the overall tone.

The figure is alert but not hypervigilant, relaxed but not collapsed or sleepy. There is an equilibrium between the sympathetic and parasympathetic branches of the autonomic aspect of the nervous system. Although typically inwardly focused, the figure is not lost in a dream. The outside world is not lost to awareness; a fly buzzing by would be heard, without distracting the figure from meditation inner and outer are equally balanced. The figure could respond with movement should it be required but is not anticipating that need. The senses are monitoring the internal and external environments but are not overactive. The motor and sensory components are in equal relationship to each other.

The particular position that the figure assumes is very interesting. The gall bladder meridian (a concept from Asian medicine) is activated by the posture shown, with the limbs open to the side. This meridian, which runs along the sides of the body from head to foot, provides a valuable image for people in our society. We tend to be overactive and/or constricted in the gall bladder and related liver meridians. Together these meridians comprise the Wood element. This element relates to the free flow of energy throughout the body and in one's life, governing planning and organization, decisions and competitiveness; when functioning in excess or when blocked, it can give rise to tension and anger. The right hand seems to extend this flow of energy into space.

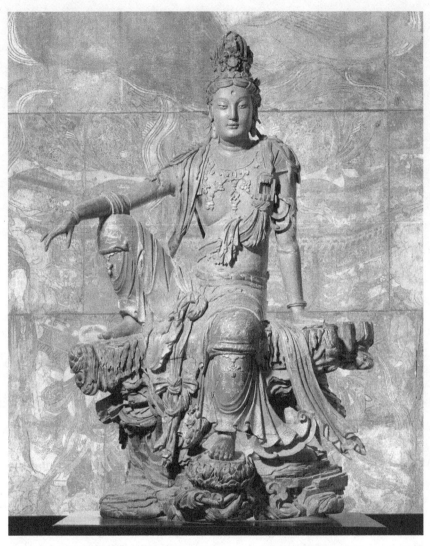

Guanyin of the Southern Sea, Liao (907–1125) or Jin (1115–1234) Dynasty.
Nelson-Atkins Museum of Art, Kansas City, Missouri.

Similar figures may hold in the right hand a small scroll, which often looks more like a stick. This adds a slightly defensive or lymphatic cast to the "woodiness" of the image; with it the figure looks a little less like a thinking scholar and a little more like a warrior with physical power held in abeyance. But for this image, the hand is open, emphasizing the traditional "at ease" posture. It is apparent that, despite the lifted knee—which in many people would cause a corresponding lifted hip—this figure has both sitz bones resting on the ground; there is no deviation in the energy flow from head to tail. Likewise, although the left arm partially supports the weight of the body, there is no loss of the figure's central connection with the earth. There is a slight spiral created by this position but, together with the position of the right arm, it serves primarily to manifest the three-dimensionality of the being in space. This also demonstrates organ support, while simultaneously giving a sense of personal energy field. The freedom and ease in the energy shown by this figure create a restful image of balance for the viewer.

When you view this image, can you feel in yourself the state of mind and body that this figure presents? Is it easy or hard for you to do this? Does this give you clues to your own state of being? What do you usually do to balance your nervous system? Are you usually in balance or out of balance? Are you aware of what is happening when you are out of balance? Can you remember what it feels like to be in balance?

Many images in art and elsewhere can be helpful in creating states of balance in various systems. Analyzing exactly why an image has this effect depends on our understanding of the underlying principles of Body-Mind Centering and how they may apply to our own functioning and that of other people. BMC also helps us to understand the appearance of cultural imagery, in which these principles may or may not be operating.

Are there favorite images for you that you can analyze in this way? Is it easier to analyze images that are not so familiar? Do you feel drawn to certain images over others? Does analyzing them help to explain why? What do these preferences tell you about yourself?

Vibration and Pulsation

~ **Michael Ridge,** Australia (1996)

On July 12, 1996, The Body-Mind Centering Association held a Teaching Seminar at Stillpoint Center in Hadley, Massachusetts, during which certified practitioner Michael Ridge gave an experiential presentation on the early patterns of vibration and pulsation. What follows is an excerpt from Michael's presentation.

I have been working on these patterns for a long time, but in the process of deciding what to do today, I realized I came up with an approach that is completely the opposite of what I do in my own exploration, but I'd like to present that anyway, just for the fun of it. It will be great to do it with a group of people who are also exploring. I'm very excited about that. I don't want to say too much. I just want you to have your own experience, so during the next part I'm not going to speak at all.

I'll play twenty-three minutes of music to which there are three elements: the first piece is very brief—it's a prelude or an introduction—then there are two main sections. Between all three pieces there is a return to silence. I left a short time at the end for feedback and discussion. The only other thing I want to say is that my own experience is usually done alone. It's very personal. Also, I'm not into words, because how I perceive vibration and pulsation is not about words. I feel that words emerge much later. Phylogenetically, words and language are way down the line of evolution. One of the ways that I more commonly explore is through voice, and that was interesting for me to notice about myself. So through just listening I got some new insights, and that is what I wanted to present today.

This exploration is about being receptive to vibration and pulsation through sound. So the only guideline I would give for this exploration is that you really focus on *"active listening"*—what is your experience of listening? Listening to silence and listening to sound, notice when you leave your listening—where do you go? Why did you leave? How do you come back to active listening?

When I played this music in the studio, I realized that my organic resonance or response to the first section was to be still, and in the second section, to move. But you should feel free to learn however you explore and to have the experience you choose to have.

Find a comfortable spot on the floor and we'll begin. Let's start by relaxing.

[Exploration begins]

Silence

Opening Piece (Impulse)

(Prelude from "Das Rheingold" by Richard Wagner)

· Silence

Section One (Vibration)

(Selections from "Himalayan Bowls II" by Karma Moffett)

Silence

Section Two (Pulsation)

"Bolero" by Maurice Ravel

Silence

[As people slowly come out of the exploration and up to sitting or standing, Michael says:]

Just notice how you come out of silence and listen. What pathway do you use to emerge? Notice all the different qualities of stillness: stillness when we're resting, stillness when we're moving. As everybody is slowly taking his/her time, I'm just going to say what it was for me. So you have all the time you need.

Over the last year, when I played with these patterns so much, I really did it more from the perspective of the fluids and layering, i.e., separating out vibration, adding pulsation to the underlying vibration, then finding the radiation coming out of the relationship between vibration and pulsation, and so on, all the way through to locomotion and free movement through space. So my initial idea of how to share this exploration was to take the same approach, using different pieces of music that I felt transmitted the sense of vibration only, then vibration and pulsation combined, and then vibration, pulsation, and radiation or emanation, etc., sequentially adding the next pattern and progressively building up all of the layers. I also thought about how we might include voice, sounding, movement, and touch. But as I was listening to different pieces of music, I started to feel how they contrasted in different ways. And as I listened more closely, I began to separate out the pieces that most clearly loaded my attention toward awareness of either *physical resonance* or *psychic resonance*. So for this exploration, instead of doing all the different blends and combinations, I wanted to contrast these two principal qualities of vibration and pulsation.

In the first section, with the Tibetan bowls, the pieces that I chose had a strong psychic resonance for me. They felt out of body, or they took me out of my body or away from my physical perception. That was where I felt I resonated for the whole first section. I also noticed that the higher the pitch, the stronger the effect it had on me. It was a hard place for me to hang out sometimes. I didn't really enjoy it. I could listen to it and it was OK, but I didn't really like it. Either it was too much of that kind of stimulation, or maybe I have a lot of that already and I didn't want any more.

The second section, "Bolero," is pretty self-evident—is there any better musical example of pulsation in the universe? It has such a strong physical resonance for me. What I really see here is that there are psychic and physical elements to both pulsation and vibration. They are mirror reflections that counteract each other, and all the other patterns arise from the dynamic relationship between these two. That is what I tried to show through these three examples of music.

When I heard the first short piece of music that I played as the opening ("Das Rheingold" prelude), I realized that at a very deep level, vibration and pulsation are not separate. You can hear that they are different but they are not yet differentiated, and that together they underlie what eventually becomes radiation and polarization. Then, the Himalayan bowls piece is clearly about vibration. We have this ground of silence out of which the sounds come as a sudden initial impulse, reverberate, and then slowly diminish or dissipate back into silence and stillness. And then in "Bolero," there is this rhythmic ground, out of which pulsation gradually emerges, this strong slow rhythm, building and building to a final impulse, which suddenly disperses into silence and stillness. So in comparing vibration and pulsation, we find one supported by silence and stillness (space) and the other supported by rhythm and activity (time). One suddenly appearing at full intensity and then slowly disappearing, and the other, slowly appearing, building to full intensity and then disappearing suddenly—two complementary ways in which an impulse (energy) comes into and out of manifestation (material existence). For me, that's the interconnecting loop, so we're back to the image of the lemniscate [infinity symbol], which I drew on the board.

The other thing I wanted to mention is that being present at a birth five years ago opened up something for me that was the beginning of this exploration. What I experienced at the birth was the intense physicality of it, how primal it was: the archetypal bodily expression of pulsation. Beautiful, profound, and frightening, all at the same time. Then recently I was at a death, which was also very moving. I was deeply affected by what I experienced energetically. I always imagined birth and death as the two polar opposites of one continuum, but during these two experiences I began to feel the same difficulty that came up in trying to differentiate vibration and pulsation—that both of these experiences were connected in a way, but that I didn't have all of the pieces yet. Now, over time, these four pieces have emerged—*orgasm, conception, birth, and death*. I'll never physically experience conception or giving birth, but having witnessed both, I feel that orgasm and birth are intimately connected to physical resonance, and conception and death are intimately connected to psychic resonance. It's interesting to me, with regard to fertilization, that orgasm and conception happen quite separately in terms of time, and that one is more pulsatory and the other more vibratory. And I feel that a lot is revealed by looking at these experiences in this way, especially how they are expressed as patterns of experience in our minds and bodies as men and women. And I leave that exploration to each of you.

One of the reasons why I put conception in the psychic resonance category is that the perception of vibration, which I experienced over many years, both within myself and within others, came to me, I feel, through conception. And that is all I know to say about it. I perceive it as my *life force*. It came to me, or arrived in some way in manifestation into matter, through conception. I am aware of it, I can trace it back, and ultimately, I feel that it will leave. This is also what I felt at the death of that person. That is what I felt left. I would say the physical rhythms ceased, but there was something else that was still leaving, that didn't die with the last breath or the last beat of the heart. It was *that* which was connected with conception, like a quota of vibration. It was so strong in the room, probably because it had become isolated out from all of the physical rhythms. The person had ceased pulsating but was still vibrating, maybe even more so. And so then, beyond birth and death, I leave that to everyone's personal exploration. This is just a piece, and it's where I am in my own exploration.

So, this is what has come to me over the last few years. I have been around Bonnie so long and absorbed not the road map but her joy of investigation. In fact, whatever Bonnie comes up with I usually don't understand, so I have to pull it apart until it makes sense to me. Breaking it down into pieces allows me to get the gestalt of what it represents. Then I can put it back together in a way that has meaning for me. It's that process of doing (or undoing) something with the material that ultimately gives it meaning for me. Over the last few years, whenever

I was exploring the patterns and the cellular material, I would always end up getting confused. At the level of the cell, I was always aware of two things happening at once, both pulsation and vibration. I couldn't make sense of it in a certain way, and so that became a curiosity to me. Finally I realized that we have all these names like "cellular breathing" and "navel radiation"—always these combinations of a noun and a verb at the same time, and that's where I kept getting lost. Bonnie has a way of being able to blend everything she organizes into a soup, and yet she is still able to identify all those pieces within the soup as a whole. It's actually a way that she organizes her experience; it's one of her strengths. I needed to separate out what was substance and what was vibration.

The motion of energy is what brings matter into manifestation. At the atomic level, matter is energy moving in a circular pathway—underlying all forms is really just energy vibrating. Over the last two years, I started separating out the elements of these two categories and mapping them separately. Evolution is the pathway that consciousness is taking as it is coming into manifestation in matter as form, so I might call these two categories mind (or energy of consciousness) manifesting as patterns of motion, and mind (or energy of consciousness) manifesting as patterns in form. The elements of each are still constantly changing, but they make my own exploration clearer for me. This was also my response to the new way in which Bonnie began presenting the developmental material two years ago, more through layering the integration of the patterns. I love that. It came from her fluids epiphany, when she was finally able to link up all the patterns with the fluids and their target tissues. At that point the old map of Basic Neurological Patterns no longer worked for me. I wanted a map of the patterns that correlated *all* of the forms of biological life that we see around us and their diverse expressions of movement, one that met the level of integration of the map of fluid affinities and the body systems—evolutionarily, that met the level of the map of the fluid affinities and the body systems.

Many years ago, when I first looked at the traditional studies of evolution, biology, and the natural sciences, I recognized that there were all these developmental gaps that we don't acknowledge in the Basic Neurological Patterns, primarily with the prevertebrates. I felt that key elements were missing, and it was the jellyfish that opened everything up for me. Seeing the jellyfish moving through the water showed me the importance of pulsation as the complementary shadow of vibration. We can see in the pulsating movement of the jellyfish the first effort of early life to separate out these elements of reach and pull and yield and push, but they are still so closely interconnected you can hardly distinguish between them. In the sphere of the cell, they are still unified or undifferentiated. They are unmanifested, but they are all present and expressing equally as potential. Then with the hemispherical form of the jellyfish, they're starting to differentiate out and, with this movement, differentiate their intention, which is what gives the jellyfish its ability to move through space. In humans, we can see how clearly these elements of reach and pull and yield and push have become differentiated, and how profoundly they articulate with both locomotion and perception in relationship to our environment. So we can begin to distinguish these various stages in the unfolding of the patterns themselves, from unity (through co-emergence) to duality (through individuation) to multiplicity, in the development of both the different animal forms and the different qualities of their movement.

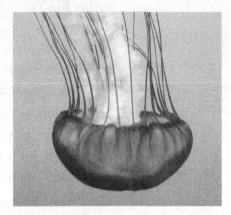

Sea nettle (jellyfish).

Clarifying this process of how the patterns themselves emerge helped me to resolve the earlier cellular confusion I was experiencing. It gave me a bridge from the cellular sense of stillness, or not doing, and containment, to radiation and the beginning of activity, initiation of movement, and intention. This is one of the main contributions of the jellyfish. They were the first to actively explore movement through space, and pulsation was the key. But my insight was not exclusively about the jellyfish. It was also becoming more consciously aware of our relationship with all life and wanting to embody that—not that we have to, but that we can and, in fact, we have. We are all one family—all evolutionary life is reflected in us as aspects of our nature. Being part of life itself, we carry their inheritance. As I looked at these earlier life forms, I became more and more grateful for their extraordinary gift to us.

In closing, I would like to say that this is what the study of Body-Mind Centering is for me—the unceasing exploration of relationships and embodiment. When I am exploring alone, I am the material. When I am exploring with others, we are the material; it's a shared exploration. Over the years, I have heard Bonnie say many times in hands-on sessions, if the person is not changing under your hands moment to moment, then do something else. And that is my vision for the study and teaching of BMC—like life itself, a vital structure in which we are the material, every aspect of ourselves—physical, psychological, emotional, and spiritual. Through the teaching, we are able to experience change and transformation moment to moment, class to class, while at the same time the material of each class changes along with us. So at the end of a session, a class, a workshop, or a summer intensive, not only have we embodied new experiences and evolved new empathy and understanding of both ourselves and others, but the material and the curriculum have also been changed. How can we create a forum of both teaching and learning in harmony with the deepest principles of life itself? How would that function?

Lumbrical Movement of the Feet and Hands: Sensory Integration from Core to Periphery

~ **Annie Brook,** USA (2007)

For Yoga Instructors, Physical Therapists, and Movement Educators

Listening to exquisite Middle Eastern music while doing slow-motion forward bends, comprises an evening of Sufi meditation with Master Teacher Adnan Sarhan. To ease muscle strain, I brought my attention to the lumbricals. Many years ago, Bonnie Bainbridge Cohen, the founder of Body-Mind Centering, demonstrated initiating forward bends starting with the lumbricals. These tiny muscles are the innermost layer of the feet, and moving them relaxes the sacrum. As I initiated with my lumbricals, the outer muscles of my legs softened and lengthened. I moved into the deepest and most relaxed forward bend I had ever experienced.

I realized that this would be good news for students of yoga and Pilates. Forward bends are often called for in these disciplines and often limited by tight hamstring muscles. Lumbrical initiation, however, can change those limitations.

Lumbricals are basic connectors, being both flexors and extensors. They underlie basic actions such as push and reach, curling, early in-utero movement, and primitive reflexes. Lumbrical movement supports the breath, grounding with the earth, and one's ability to be present in the world. For anyone interested in body wisdom and movement, they are worth exploring.

To find the lumbricals, one must find the innermost muscle layer in the feet and hands. Lumbricals are the only muscles in the body that connect muscle to muscle, instead of to muscle via tendon to bone. These tiny muscles might be seen as what would be the webbing if we had "duck feet" and "duck hands." Because they are located on the innermost layer of the feet and because we stand with our feet upon the earth, the movement of the lumbricals is essential to allow us to feel the pulse of the earth, to push and pull against gravity when walking, and to have full inhalations and exhalations in upright breathing.

Early Origins of Flexion and Extension

When a baby is *in utero*, the last six weeks are spent folding and curling in. As the baby grows, it is forced into a curl. It must tuck the head, fold in the arms and legs, and curl the spine from head to tail. This curling is called flexion and occurs on the trunk of the body through the digestive tube and along the front of the spine, all the way from head to tail. Even the brain is included in this flexion. Flexion is the powerhouse of movement. We use it to gather energy at the core. The baby *in utero* is gathering potency and tone in the muscles during this condensing, curling flexion.

Birth is the first activation of flexion into extension in relationship to gravity. When we push into extension we move through space. The next important flexion and extension action, post-birth, is nursing. In the sucking/swallowing reflex, the upper palate must extend and reach to grasp the nipple and then flex and pull on the nipple to release breast milk. This action occurs in the mouth and the trunk of the body, and if you watch closely, you may see the response in a baby's feet.

Once we start moving, we need the force of propulsion, and for this we need our limbs. We move forward and back in the sagittal plane, and we run, curl, reach, and leap. We flee for safety and chase or gather food for survival. Our basic flexion and extension through the arms and legs support these actions.

I have always been interested to notice that the flexor muscles of the legs are located on the back of the limbs, while the flexor muscles of the arms are located on the front. This is due to the rotation of the limb buds *in utero* and allows for pushing down against the earth for running, or reaching and pulling through swinging locomotion. Like our monkey relatives, we can flee by using our arms, by pulling tree vines down from the heavens to swing forward. We gather by pulling fruit from the tree or plants from the earth. In this case, flexion is related to a pulling action.

During uterine development, the limbs begin as buds. They stick straight out from the torso. Picture that the front half of the muscle tissue of the embryo is programmed for flexor tone and the back half for extensor tone. This is how early muscle tissue is oriented.[1]

Picture flat muscle tissue curled around a horizontal axis. This is the baby flexed along the front, curled in the sagittal plane. Its front is flexed and its back is extended. That is the basic beginning. Through cell growth and maturation, the muscle tissue of the limb buds lengthens and spirals into arms and legs. The limb buds of the arms rotate laterally as they grow, changing their original orientation. The flexor tissue of the front moves a bit laterally and the extensor a bit more medially through this rotation, still allowing the arms to flex in the sagittal plane. In contrast, the limb buds of the legs rotate medially. The extensor tissue moves to the front and the flexor tissue to the back of the legs, allowing the legs to fold for springing and pushing away from the earth. Now we have limbs that are functional, able to flex and extend in the sagittal plane and propel us away from danger and toward safety and food. Flexion and extension meet in the hands and feet through the lumbricals.

Lumbricals as Diaphragms

Another focus of lumbrical movement is its support for breathing. Diaphragms could be thought of as horizontal muscle dividers of an upright body. I like to think of them as being like heads of a drum. When they are functional they can move, stretch, vibrate, and respond. Diaphragms are directly involved with breathing, and we have five major diaphragms in the body. I think the lumbricals' action makes them a sixth "diaphragm."

In simple terms, we extend the front surface of the body to inhale. This gives us a full breath and maximum oxygen to feed the muscles needed for movement. In a full breath, we extend the muscles all the way from the pelvis through the trunk and out the limbs to the lumbricals, those final intrinsic muscle endpoints of the hands and feet. When all the horizontal muscles move, they support us to fully oxygenate our body.

Tough fascial tissue inside the skull, called the tentorium, is one diaphragm. It supports the brain like a sling. Another diaphragm is the vocal one in the throat area. It supports the flow of breath into speech. We have the familiar thoracic diaphragm, which helps to open the breath. We have a urogenital diaphragm of muscle tissue in between the trunk and the genitals. We have the pelvic floor diaphragm, which holds our bowels and uterus. And, in my opinion, we have a final diaphragm at the endpoints of our limbs. The hands and feet contain the lumbricals, and their movement allows us to feel and respond more fully to our environment.

In drumming, when you push down on the drumhead it will spring back up and release sound. If one drumhead is played, all other drums in the room will have a slight response. This is also true in the body. If you move one diaphragm, all the other diaphragms will respond. If muscle tone is optimal and emotional energy allowed to sequence, the diaphragms are responsive. We then have a fully sequenced movement that initiates with the breath and moves out into our brain, genitals, pelvis, voice, and our hands and feet.

Diaphragms (except the tentorium) are made of muscle tissue. Muscle tissue is a microcosm of fibers bundled into macrocosms of movement groups. All muscles are interconnected through fascia. This fascial web holds its own memory. Once formed, it could "stand on its own" if the muscle tissue were removed.[2] For effective muscle movement, we must attend not only to muscle tension but to the state of fascia, ligaments, fluid, and organ tissues as well. Attending to all tissue brings in full movement support and integration. The disciplines of BodyMind Psychotherapy and Body-Mind Centering promote this tissue awareness as the basis for all life.[3]

In the microcosm of muscles, the intrafusal fibers are the "sensory organs" of muscles. They communicate to the extrafusal fibers, which are the "action organs" of muscles. If we expand out from this microcosm to view muscle groups, we have intrinsic muscles and extrinsic muscles. Intrinsic muscles are closer in toward the spine and smaller. They are capable of the fine motor skills and can finely tune and adjust movement. Extrinsic muscles are closer to the surface of the body and are larger and more powerful. They are responsible for moving the body through space. To move our muscles most efficiently, we initiate with intrinsic muscles, power and move with extrinsic muscles, and fine-tune again to completion of movement using intrinsic muscles.

Muscle and Lumbrical Action in Relation to Movement and Breath

Now let's return to our discussion about flexion, extension, gravity, breath, and presence. The lumbricals are the intrinsic muscles of the hands and the feet. When muscles extend, they move in an eccentric or lengthening contraction. When muscles flex, they shorten and move in a concentric contraction. These are, in essence, the antagonist and agonist muscle groupings that support joints. Contrary to standard anatomy, however, Body-Mind Centering suggests that both muscles are in motion.[4]

Pilates places attention on the lengthening support of muscles.[5] Most weight training and body-building does the opposite, with a focus on the concentric shortening contractions for strength. Yoga can be practiced either way, depending on the awareness levels of the practitioner and teacher. Movement is best taught when instructors know that balanced joints occur through balanced muscle action and teach students to engage both the lengthening and condensing of muscle groups.

Muscles need oxygen. In efficient movement we want the breath to sequence all the way to the limbs and to reach the lumbricals. We want the lumbricals to flex and extend and to support us to push upright and, finally, away from gravity as we step and leap. As the lumbricals gain more flexibility, the other diaphragms move and breathe more easily, and the body becomes more present to support our awareness of life.

Please explore the following exercise to awaken lumbrical movement.

Lumbrical Exhale-Inhale Standing Exercise

Stand with feet hip-width apart. Compress the air out of the body by curling or flexing all the way through the body. Starting with the palms of your hands, curl the lumbricals. Draw in the little finger and the subsequent fingers sequentially as you flex your hands in and across your body at the level of the heart. Continue curling down the front of your spine until your legs are bent. Engage the inner lumbricals of the feet by curling the bottoms of your feet as well.

Next lengthen the lumbricals of the feet and hands. Follow this extension out the toes and fingers and all the way through the back of the legs and up the arms, all the way into the trunk. Follow this extension up the front of the body all the way out the top of the head. As the heart lifts, feel the air flow into the lungs as you push against the earth and reach toward the heavens. Repeat a number of times until this becomes effortless.

Lumbrical Forward Bend Exercise

Sit upright with legs in front, feet flexed and hands at your sides. Extend your lumbricals while your feet are still flexed, lengthening through the backs of the legs and reaching the arms up to the sky on an inhalation.

Exhale, curling in with the lumbricals and folding forward. Notice that you can curl the lumbricals of the hands and feet while still maintaining straight arms and legs. This will help to straighten the legs into the earth and to reach the arms toward the heavens. Start by keeping the spine straight and feeling the sequential curling of the intrinsic muscles of the spine as you bend forward. Go only as far as you are comfortable. Come up by extending your lumbricals and following this motion through the body.

If you practice forward bends regularly, explore the difference when you initiate with your lumbricals and when you don't. You might notice how this lumbrical initiation takes pressure off the hamstring muscles and allows muscle movement to sequence through the lower legs into the hips and core of the body. During inhalation, flexion (concentric shortening of muscles) occurs on the back of the body and sequences into concentric movement of the front of the legs. (Remember that the muscles on the front of the legs are extensors.) This helps to stabilize the trunk while bending and supports the feet to remain flexed in a forward bend. During exhalation, the concentric support (shortening of muscle tissue) moves to the front of the body for stability, and the back of our body lengthens (eccentric contraction) for ease of movement. It is the concentric shortening of the muscles on the back of the legs that brings our legs into the earth, and the curling of the lumbricals (related to the front of the spine) that keeps our feet flexed.

Once you have awakened your lumbrical movement, explore walking using the reach and pull of the lumbricals against the earth. Walking becomes both efficient and effortless using this support.

Conclusion

Lumbrical movement through the hands and feet is movement of the endpoints of the body. These "diaphragms" support all the other diaphragms to move when we breathe. The movement of the soles of the feet gives us greater response to the pulse of the earth. Actions that involve running or swinging benefit from lumbrical movement. When we oscillate attention in and back out (an essential skill for staying present and in contact with others and the environment), lumbrical movement supports the most complete sequence of curling into the core and extending back out.

To apply lumbrical awareness to movement, use the above exercises. To apply lumbrical awareness to body psychotherapy, use the information and movement exercises to educate clients to feel and release tension of muscles. Have clients practice exercises to reach and pull through the palms and soles of the feet. You can help them to translate this moving, pushing, and pulling into the ability to stay grounded and engaged with the world.

Storming/Calming:
Living the Autonomic

~ **Pat Ethridge,** USA (2003)

We all know people who like to "burn the candle at both ends." Perhaps you are like this—always seeking out intense, exciting experiences in the outside world of new people, new places, and new sensations, the more the better. Or perhaps you do not focus so much on intensity but still prefer to be out and about, choosing to interact socially with others rather than to work quietly on your own. If so, you have company: there are about three times more extroverted people than there are introverted people.

However, "extroverted" does not just mean outgoing, as many think, nor does "introverted" define a person as necessarily shy or antisocial, although the introverted person might be the one who prefers to stay home and read a book rather than attend a crowded, noisy party. "Extroverted" and "introverted" are descriptions of different types of temperament and are the most reliable reflection, in language, of a person's personality and way of being in the world.

What these two types are really about is different ways of handling energy. Extroverts expend energy and look outside themselves for stimulation and refueling, while introverts conserve energy, refueling by going inside themselves and limiting outside stimulation.

These differences are inherited and are based on the dominance of one pathway over another in the autonomic nervous system in the brain. Extroverts have a dominant sympathetic pathway, while introverts have a dominant parasympathetic pathway, which results in significant differences in how people experience themselves and the world.

The focus of the extrovert is more outside—on activities, people, and places—while the focus of the introvert is more inside—on ideas, emotions, and impressions. Although extroverts are energized and refueled by external stimuli, they can expend themselves with too much activity and burn out; they need to balance their doing with just being. Introverts prefer to refuel and energize by processing their stimuli inwardly; they can easily become over-stimulated and drained by the external environment and, at the opposite extreme, limit themselves too much by avoiding such overstimulation. The need is to balance being and doing according to the individual's temperament.

It is important to distinguish over-arousal of the nervous system in general (by too much external stimulation) from anxiety and fear triggered by specific stimuli. Arousal is a response to stimuli of many kinds (oftentimes called "stress"), but arousal can also be caused by many emotions, including fear, joy, curiosity, or anger, as well as by low but constant levels of excitement with no obvious emotion. Being aroused and feeling aroused are not necessarily the same. Too often a "sensitive" person will recognize that he or she is experiencing arousal—sweating, blushing, trembling, pounding heart, shaking hands, confused thinking, upset stomach, muscle tension—and label that inner experience as fear, when in fact it might not be. But the perception of fear causes further over-arousal in an escalating progression.

Short-term arousal responses (from the sympathetic nervous system) will be amplified by the production of cortisol if the perceived stress becomes chronic—that is, if it becomes frequent or constant. This is why it is important for a stressed person to reduce the overall level of stimuli—it is important to lower the cortisol hormone level, which when high seems to set a lower threshold for an arousal response in general.

"Extroverts like to experience a lot, and introverts like to know a lot about what they experience."[1] Extroverts like breadth—they collect experiences, they have many friends, they enjoy many activities and travels and tend to be jacks-of-all-trades, or what some call generalists.

Introverts like depth—they have a few, very good friends and prefer to focus on one or two things. They are specialists.

Extroverts are quick to respond to danger while introverts are better at thinking before acting. This may be a reason why there are more extroverts; in terms of natural selection, the ones who were faster at dealing with predators would be more likely to survive. On the other hand, those extroverts who risked themselves more often in new or dangerous situations would have died off more rapidly.

The two types complement each other well: extroverts tend to be the leaders, the warriors, the "do-er" types, while introverts are the advisors, the counselors, the ones who slow down the extroverts and offer the thought, planning, and reflection that a particular situation calls for. American culture certainly favors extroverts, in school and in business, because they are action-oriented and get results. But introverts understand more from reflecting on their experiences and so have more wisdom.

Extroverts have a longer D4DR gene (sometimes called the "thrill-seeking" gene) which affects sensitivity to dopamine. Extroverts are less sensitive to dopamine and need more of it to feel stimulated—at the far end of the spectrum we see the "extreme" sports enthusiasts and risk-takers. Introverts have a short D4DR gene and are very sensitive to dopamine; hence they are easily overwhelmed by too much stimulation.

While basic parasympathetic and sympathetic reactions are the same in both extroverts and introverts, brain activity differs. Extroverts have more blood flow in the brain areas where sensory processing occurs, and the pathways are short and simple. They operate more from short-term memory. Introverts have more blood flow to the brain generally and therefore have more internal stimulation, along with more complicated pathways relating to internal thoughts and feelings. They operate more from long-term memory.

Sensory information arrives in the brain mostly via the spinal cord. The reticular activating system ensures that in extroverts more stimuli, and in introverts fewer stimuli, are transmitted to the brain. But at the hypothalamus there is a divergence: for the extrovert, information is sent via the sympathetic pathway to the posterior and lateral parts of the hypothalamus, whereas for the introvert information is sent to the anterior and medial parts of the hypothalamus via the parasympathetic pathway.

In extroverts the information then proceeds to the posterior thalamus, which sends stimuli to the amygdala, an emotional brain center that tends to merge feelings and actions. The information is then sent to the temporal and motor areas (which are also involved with short-term memory), and to centers for learning and processing sensory and emotional stimuli. Extroverts learn quickly but they also forget quickly. They often speak without thinking, or think and speak at the same time—they think out loud and tend not to hear others' comments, and they prefer face-to-face communication over written communication.

In introverts information moves from the hypothalamus to the anterior thalamus, which then forwards that information to the frontal lobe while dampening down the stimuli level to some extent. It then goes to Broca's area, which activates the internal monologue, and moves through the frontal lobe, where thinking, planning, learning, and reasoning occur. From there it moves to the hippocampus, which connects with long-term memory, and finally arrives in the amygdala, where emotions become attached to thoughts.

Overall, the brain pathways are longer in the introvert than in the extrovert. Introverts take longer to learn something, but they almost never forget it. They need time to think before speaking and become frazzled or "blank out" if called upon to speak quickly, without thinking. This is also partly because when under stress, the reticular activating system causes the emotional (limbic) areas of the brain to assert more dominance than the cortical, memory-linked areas; hence the inability to retrieve memories or to think clearly. Introverts are often better at writing, which is a more interior-directed activity, than speaking. (If they are left-brain-dominant, however, they may be very good at speaking.)

Each individual has a place of rest between the sympathetic and the parasympathetic. The challenge is to regulate inner and outer awareness so that this balance between the two can be maintained and supported. When the balance is achieved, the sympathetic provides a clear, calm state of awareness, and the parasympathetic provides a whole sense of self in the present.

The tone of this balance is regulated by the hypothalamus, which modulates the interface between the parts of the brain related to conscious and unconscious processes. For extroverts, this means pacing themselves by reducing their schedule of activities, spending more time with fewer people, and consciously setting time to rest and reflect. If they are doing work that requires concentration and single focus, they should take periodic breaks to chat briefly or to walk around. For introverts, this means paying attention to how much stimulation they are taking in from their external environment and preparing themselves when they know they will be going into a highly stimulating situation. It also means consciously choosing to seek out new experiences and people, within limits, in order to broaden their perspective and to challenge and strengthen their zone of comfort (habituate themselves), as well as seeking support from the usually few individuals with whom they are in intimate relationship.

As people grow and develop over their lifespan they tend to learn social skills and emotional coping mechanisms, so many of those beginning life at an extreme end of this temperamental spectrum can achieve a midrange balance in adulthood between being "in" and "out" that enables optimal functioning in the varying situations of their lives. For both types of individuals, leading a regular life is important in maintaining nervous system balance: drinking enough water, eating nourishing foods, getting regular restful sleep, engaging in appropriate exercise, and balancing work with the rest of life. Identifying the causes, triggers, and effects of stress and doing something to mitigate stress are also very important.

What happens when we are faced with an acutely stressful situation?

Our sensory apparatus conveys to our central nervous system information that is interpreted as "danger." Our sympathetic nervous system becomes more active, preparing for an active response by increasing energy flow to the somatic nervous system via norepinephrine from postganglionic fibers and epinephrine and norepinephrine from the adrenal medulla, which prolong and amplify the effects of the postganglionic neurotransmitter. (Norepinephrine also helps in memory formation, which is one reason why traumatic experiences, which engage the sympathetic nervous system and elicit the production of this transmitter, are remembered so vividly.) A single preganglionic axon in the sympathetic pathway can synapse with twenty or more postganglionic fibers (the parasympathetic axon synapses with only four or five fibers), which explains why so much of the body can be affected at once.

The classic description of sympathetic activators is "exercise, emergency, excitement, and embarrassment"[2]—there is preparation for physical activity, ATP production is increased, and the body ceases storing energy. In the "fight, flight, or freeze" sympathetic response, which is basically a reaction to a predator, the pupils dilate; the blood pressure, heart rate, and force of heart contractions increase; the airways dilate; the body temperature increases; and the blood vessels to the skeletal muscles and the organs related to energy production expand. For energy production, the liver releases glucose and commences glycogenolysis, the adipose cells commence lipolysis, and all nonessential internal activity, such as digestion, decreases.

If a fear reaction is experienced, the result is rapid respiration, sweating, trembling, palpitations, muscular tension or weakness, breathlessness, nausea, and dry mouth. In "paradoxical fear," an extreme state associated with the perception of imminent death, the sympathetic and parasympathetic systems are activated simultaneously, which can result in involuntary defecation and urination due to the release of sphincters. The third branch of the autonomic nervous system, the enteric (or "gut-brain") nervous system in the intestine, may be the primary "alarm" register of a dangerous situation to the rest of the nervous system and has an amplifying effect on the action of the other two branches.

Our earliest arboreal primate ancestors co-evolved with and faced three types of predators: snakes, cats, and raptors. The automatic "fight, flight, or freeze" reactions developed in response to the threats these predators posed, and elicited different responses according to whether the threat was on the ground (the snake), in the tree (the cat), or in the air above (the raptor). These responses can still be seen in monkeys today. As humans evolved and learned to operate in defensive groups and then developed more advanced cultural and technologically complex societies, these predators became less of a daily threat. Nevertheless, the responses to these predators are "hardwired" into the brain on a deep level.

The brain tends to merge related ideas into single units of information through chunking according to psychological significance for more efficient processing. (Seven items at a time is the maximum that people can handle.) At the same time our ancestors were adapting to life on the ground, the patterns of predator recognition became lumped into a general predator category, known culturally as "the dragon." This category, created after the initial stimuli were no longer an immediate threat to survival, retained the salient characteristics of each predator for more efficient storage and retrieval by the brain. The "dragon complex"—fear of snakes, cats, and birds—is the strongest in children between two and six years of age, but animal phobias are the easiest to cure, indicating the decay of these stimuli in evolution. The dragon complex resides in the limbic structures, the primitive mammalian brain, and can be seen in every culture in the world through the ages, including those that do not have one or more of the three types of predators in their environment.

The height of the dragon expression in Western Europe occurred between the eighth and the thirteenth centuries, when political group structures were shifting from bands and tribes to more unified kingdoms or states. This was a major and rapid shift in human-as-primate

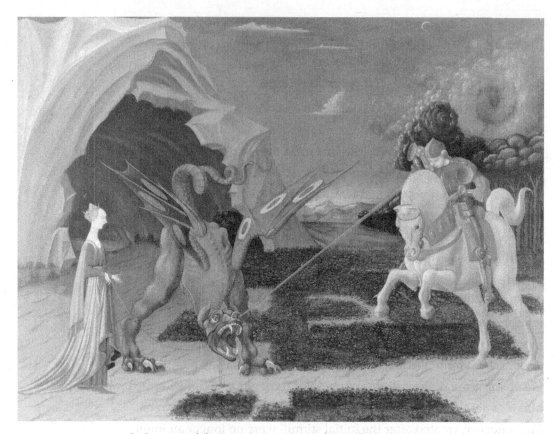

St. George and the Dragon, (c. 1470), Paolo Uccello (1397–1475).
Oil on canvas, 55.6 x 74.2 cm. National Gallery, London, Great Britain.

group relations that clearly caused much social stress, with accompanying warfare and social dislocation, the rise of monolithic religions, and much individual psychopathology.

The dragon represented a common enemy that was defeated by the culture hero, the dragon slayer, who was a stand-in for the new single head of the unifying state or religion. Once defeated, the dragon was adopted as an emblem of the state. But during this period the dragon response was called forth because "learned (cultural) responses no longer solve biopsychological problems, the human organism is upset at its deepest physical levels ... and these emotions are brought forward from a brain-space where the dragon lives."[3] (The Asian dragon is benevolent, since it expresses a later stage of cultural history. The threat is no longer perceived as imminent.)

In the classic image of *Saint George and the Dragon* by Paolo Uccello, the reptilian, snakelike quality of the dragon is quite apparent. Reptiles are older in evolutionary terms than raptors and cats, so their qualities predominate. In most dragon images worldwide the dragon looks basically like a very large snake. The circle spots on the dragon's wings are similar to those of spotted cats, but they also mimic the "staring eyes" of the predator.

The dragon has wings and taloned feet like a raptor. The open, fanged mouth and glaring eyes reflect the facial image in a close-range attack by a large cat. In most depictions of dragons and slayers, the dragon is shown five times the size of the slayer, which recapitulates the size ratios of predators and early primates. It is shown in front of a cave, a typical lurking place for a predator (and often is shown near a well or pool, similar to the watering hole that early primates would have to visit at risk of attack). The young female of childbearing age represents the future of the group, which is threatened by the dangerous dragon. Most animal phobias in adults appear in women in this age group. The culture hero in this painting, Saint George, who conquers the dragon and the danger it represents, is armed with a spear but usually appears with a sword, a similar weapon.

And what of the other side of the continuum? The parasympathetic response has been called "rest and digest." The focus is inward, on conserving and storing body energy. The activities expressed in the sympathetic state, such as heart rate and blood pressure, are decreased; the pupils and airways constrict. Food is digested and absorbed as the smooth muscles contract and glands secrete; salivation, urination, and defecation increase. There is more awareness of the general state of being, of a deep, overall unity of consciousness and a feeling of peacefulness and calm, or actual sleep. Being, rather than doing, is dominant.

The parasympathetic is the restorative, supporting background of the entire nervous system.

While acetylcholine is the primary neurotransmitter associated with activity of the parasympathetic system, there is another hormone involved with the activity of this state: oxytocin, sometimes called the "lust and trust" chemical.[4] Oxytocin is associated with uterine contractions and lactation in female mammals, but it also modulates both male and female social behaviors, such as infant and pair bonding. It is produced during pleasant sensual experiences, such as sexual activity, eating, bathing, and gentle vibration. In reptiles it assists mating by reducing stress, aggression, and fear of strangers. In mammals a social role has evolved, with oxytocin facilitating attachments and altruistic behavior, not only between parents and children but also between other kin and even between strangers. Generosity and positive reciprocity—and the good feelings and trust that result—promote cooperation, which leads to family- and community-building and stability.

Oxytocin functions as a hormone in the brain cells and the blood and as a parasympathetic neurotransmitter. The receptors for it are located in the hypothalamus, which regulates both the autonomic nervous system and the emotional centers of the limbic system. Although the development of trust can be aided by oxytocin, it is based not only on unconscious and emotional responses, of course, but also on cognitive, conscious processes that require, among other things, the capacity to evaluate differences of viewpoint and intention between oneself and another. But oxytocin may elevate the more unconscious aspects of trust (which would facilitate community living) over more conscious, purely self-seeking behaviors. Hostility, threats, and the resultant distrust suppress the release of oxytocin. When people feel themselves in a "trustworthy" environment, the parasympathetic aspect of the nervous system is more likely to be dominant than the sympathetic aspect.

What is a cultural image historically associated with the parasympathetic state? There are many possibilities, but one of the more common is that of the angel. Angel images and descriptions appear in the earliest

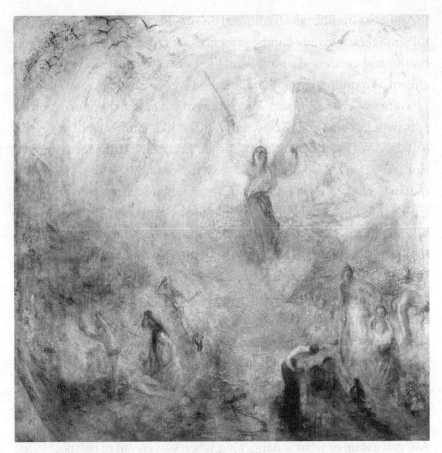

The Angel Standing in the Sun, Joseph Mallord William Turner (1775–1851).
Exhibited in 1846, oil on canvas, 78.7 x 78.7 cm. Tate Gallery, London, Great Britain.

forms of art and writing. Some believe this image is a regressive projection of a rescuing and comforting parental figure, since the angel
often appears at times of acute distress or danger. Typically, angels are
messengers; they bring a message that causes a shift in consciousness,
usually from a state of distress to one of calm and serenity. Their first
greeting is usually "Fear not" or, more colloquially, "Don't be afraid."
This initiates the shift from sympathetic to parasympathetic, as does
the warmth and gentle light they characteristically radiate. Sometimes

they appear in culturally traditional lineaments and other times as helpful strangers, invisible hands, presences, or thoughts, but always their beauty and gentleness disarm, and their visit is experienced by the percipient as a unique event that initiates a significant change of state.

Here is a characteristic description of such an experience: "There was instant Peace inside my mind, it felt like lamb's wool, it was so soft inside of me. It was a warm rush of Peace." Note the focus on interior sensations. Also, "They embody the peaceful, loving state; they radiate serenity . . . You find an inner connection, a deep knowing. Your worries are dissipated. A peace comes over your heart."[5] In this description the angel seems to be modeling a state of being. Also, "it is not that skeptics do not experience the mysteries and divine, but rather that the mysteries are presented to them in such a flat and factual, everyday, reasonable way so as not to disturb; for this is the rule: no one receives more information than he can bear." Here the emphasis is on the limits of the nervous system to incoming stimuli, while still introducing a new possibility for one's state of being.

What images operate this way for you? Do they help you become aware of the extent to which you are inside or outside the limits of your nervous system balance? Are you an extrovert or an introvert? Are you aware of what is happening when you go out of balance? What do you do to return to balance? How do you feel while you are doing this, and how do you feel when you have accomplished this? Does paying attention to this make it easier to return to and stay in balance?

Seeing and Perceiving

~ **Pat Ethridge,** USA (2001)

One evening I visited the Metropolitan Museum of Art in New York City with Body-Mind Centering teacher Ildiko Viczian. The museum offers sophisticated and educational examples of visual art from around the world. We walked through the galleries and viewed paintings and sculptures, mostly from Europe, dating from prehistoric times to the present. We observed how the range of human experience is depicted through visual history, as reflected in the expression of culture from a particular age. We saw that what is present and what is absent in an image can give us clues as to what was considered important in understanding both personal and cultural experience.

In writing down my impressions from that evening, I chose to discuss two paintings by artists from the Netherlands; the works represent the sacred and the secular sides of life in the artists' time. The first, *The Nativity* by Gerard David, dates from about 1515; the second, *The Harvesters* by Pieter Bruegel the Elder, dates from about 1565.

Looking at *The Nativity*, Ildiko expressed her thoughts: "I am attracted to the gentle beauty, peace, and faith emanating from medieval religious paintings. I only briefly evaluate the composition, the spectrum of colors, and the brush strokes, which are the technical aspects. I linger and allow the artist's reverent vision of the Divine Birth to elevate my feelings. Then I lift my gaze up to the hovering angels and feel transported by their lovely, pure facial expressions to the heavenly worlds conceived by the artist. I transcend the physical faculty of sight and, on the wings of imagination, join the company of angels, the symbols of goodness, benevolence, and love. They are weightless because they don't carry

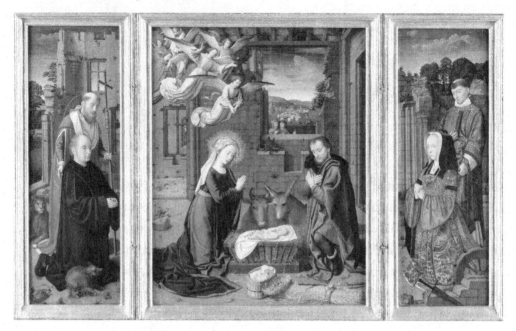

The Nativity with Donors and Saints Jerome and Leonard (painted c. 1510–1523), Gerard David (c. 1450–1523), oil on canvas, transferred from wood; central panel 35 1/2 x 28 in. (90.2 x 71.1 cm); each wing 35 1/2 x 12 3/8 in. (90.2 x 31.4 cm). The Jules Bache Collection, 1949 (49.7.20a-c). The Metropolitan Museum of Art, New York.

earthly concerns, and because they are selfless they can wholly adore the Divine Child. I feel the angels are our spiritual aspect, which is capable of flight. In BMC terms, the artist's imaginative reach into the realm of the supernatural can be expressed as a 'glandular reach' initiated by the pituitary. The pituitary itself is housed by the wing-shaped sphenoid bone which, as Bonnie Bainbridge Cohen once remarked, 'will one day enable us to fly.' The sphenoid might be the chariot, and the pituitary—the third eye—the driver, enabling us bodily to rise."[1]

The Nativity was created from the perspective of the Age of Faith and the lingering paradigm of the medieval world. Life is seen through the prism of an idealistic rendering of a religious event considered to be historical but shown as being outside time, like a crystallized—one might say glandular—image of the mind's eye. The angels are bright, flashing creatures who seemingly cannot be exactly located in space, but who hover suspended in an eternal realm. This quality of timeless suspension is characteristic of the cerebrospinal fluid. Very little is "bloodful" about this image. No one is actively doing much in this picture except the angels, which indicates that the state of being of the central figures is more important than any task they might be performing. Everyone regards the central child, who is celebrated for simply being. In the spiritual dimension of life, faith is more important than practical knowledge, and the individual is subsumed in the relationship to God. The scene takes place inside a building, a metaphor for the internally focused life of faith, in which the heavenly world to come takes precedence over everyday human life and physical reality. The crumbling walls indicate that the birth of a new spiritual order is taking place on and within the ruins of the old one.

In *The Harvesters*, painted only fifty years after *The Nativity*, the worldview is completely different. The Renaissance was already underway, and "the 'upward' movement [toward God] (which reached its climax in the late Middle Ages) went into reverse; man turned back to the earth … art became more realistic and sensuous … and embraced the whole visible world."[2] The scene depicts a specific place in a certain season and even a specific time of day and weather. We see the land curving across the painting and the ocean in the distance, with the hazy sky above. The Earth itself is the dominant form, with people as small creatures in relationship to it. In contrast to the exalted angels of the previous painting, who all look very similar, each figure in *The Harvesters* is a distinct individual. These people clearly have muscles and organs and fat. Also in contrast to *The Nativity*, the central figures are actively performing specific tasks—what they do is who they are. Each individual is a working part of a human community. The practical, physical side of life is shown, as opposed to the spiritual, idealized image in *The Nativity*. Although this is one particular day in which certain things happen in certain ways, the image represents one variation of the constantly repeating rhythm of natural life unfolding in time on the Earth.

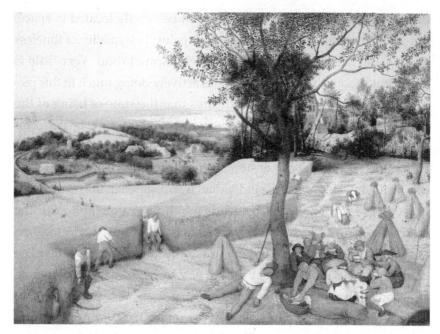

The Harvesters (1565), Pieter Brueghel the Elder (c. 1525–1569). Oil on wood; overall, including added strips at top, bottom, and right, 46 7/8 x 63 3/4 in. (119 x 162 cm); original painted surface 45 7/8 x 62 7/8 in. (116.5 x 159.5 cm). Rogers Fund, 1919 (19.164). The Metropolitan Museum of Art, New York.

What can we learn from these paintings? We can compare these images of almost five hundred years ago with the images of our own time and realize the extent to which our experience today differs from or resembles theirs. Many people today still carry in their minds idealized images of medieval Christianity like those shown in *The Nativity* and feel the support such images give to their beliefs. While a majority of the people in the U.S. no longer work in the fields, we can still relate to the feeling of physical work and of being physically connected to nature and its cycles, as shown in *The Harvesters*. We can sense how we are the current expression of the rhythm of life on Earth.

The sheaf of grain by the child's manger in *The Nativity* is a reference to scripture: "I am the bread which came down from Heaven" (John

6:41). Thus the infant, who will grow up to be the man who says, "Take, eat, this is my body," becomes a symbol of the food for the soul that religion represents. In *The Harvesters*, the grain being reaped will be made into bread and thus is the food of the earth, which feeds the body. The fields are being harvested at the peak of the earth's abundance, the height of midsummer, represented by the rich gold color that dominates in the painting. But the grain that is the food of the spirit manifests in the dead of winter for this painter, when the earth is dormant and covered with snow. So in these two paintings we see how the image of grain, which becomes bread—the food of life—feeds human life on both physical and spiritual levels, which in the culture of the time were held to be separate spheres.

What happens when we look at a painting? A technical explanation helps us to distinguish vision from perception and to understand the process of seeing.

Vision refers to the physical act of seeing or sensing by the visual sense organs, the optical structures that enable light to register in the brain; *perception* refers to the process by which the brain interprets what we see, and it ultimately permits understanding. Both operate in a sensory-motor feedback loop that includes our preconceived expectations and the feedback we receive during our experience. It also includes, of course, the fact that our visual experience is not isolated; we are also hearing and touching and feeling from our viscera and many other things, with varying levels of awareness. Visual sensory input is received; there is interpretation, which includes a sorting and comparison of the input previously received; then pre-motor planning or organization of the sensory information occurs; pre-motor planning is followed by the motor response, which generates sensory feedback regarding the motor response; and finally there is interpretation again, this time of the whole experience. This process recycles itself continually and is two-sided: in classic BMC terminology, one can motorically focus to sense and sensorially focus to motor.

Art is often described as having the power to inspire. I think that inspiration is an advanced part of the sensory-motor feedback loop, which begins with vision. Since one is generally inspired to *do* something, inspiration can be considered part of pre-motor interpretation. It involves the linking or cross-connection of other aspects of the body-mind self to the visual information, which enlarges one's field of awareness in the experience. Inspiration is often considered to be an emotional or spiritual state, which suggests cross-linkage with organs or glands. Things "come together" and one is inspired or motivated to act, and this moment can occur early in the loop or after many, many recyclings. People feel a "rush" of inspiration and act on it; this can also describe the moment when the fluid system shifts from being the support of the senses to being the mover, or the integrator. Artists have carefully rendered their paintings to capture the viewer's attention and initiate this process.

I offer this description of my museum experience as an example of an approach to awareness. Gazing at paintings is the sensory component and responding to them in verbal dialogue with others is the motor component. Our perception and understanding develop through such engagement and the subsequent recycling through the loop.

I'm sure those reading this will have their own comments about my preconceived notions and interpretations of my experience. But the point is that these differ according to the individual. "Art is not a descriptive statement about the way the world is, it is a recommendation that the world ought to be looked at in a given way."[3] Even photography, which is sometimes considered an exact reflection of reality, can be presented in that spirit.

To which images do we attune ourselves today? Many people live their lives in a hastening blur, uncritically watching flickering pictures that flash by on screens, and rarely taking the time to absorb the deeper meaning of what they are seeing or to consider whether it is congruent with their inner beliefs and feelings. Very often the cultural image of reality that we are presented with is designed to limit our perception, not to enlarge it. The sense of something missing that this engenders leads people to believe that true reality is somewhere "out there" and is something they are rushing to catch up to, instead of reality being inherent in themselves, in their own experiences. Slowing down and taking the time to see and understand how we perceive our own world brings people back to themselves and to their own essential wholeness.

I still remember how shocked I was when I reencountered television after not having it in my life for several years. It seemed to me that all sorts of highly political statements and unexamined assumptions were being thrown in my face one after another, with no space left for me to respond. I was initially stunned, then I wanted to jump to my feet and argue with everyone about what was being presented on that screen. Not only was no one interested, they didn't even see the point. And now that I have been watching TV again for several years, I have mostly lost that capacity to perceive and react—I am caught in the cultural trance again. I would have to "detoxify" my perception to regain my former perspective.

Most people, I observe, have no glimmering at all of the extent to which they are being held in that trance—like a fish not being aware of water because the water is everywhere. Most people will vociferously deny this. And yet so far as I am now in thrall, I can sense the way cultural attention flows like water—it flows here, then there, with its own rhythmic current and energy that affects me even though I have no control or influence over it. The sense of containment and the direction of focus are controlled by someone else.

From following that flow of attention I do have a sense, through my viewing, of becoming a member of an invisible herd, a vast group moving vaguely in quick time if not in space. But there is no development of meaning because that dimension is lacking, and there is no room for response, for reflection. The perceptual operation is interrupted; people are held at the point of intake and are not allowed to process. Since it all flows away with no interaction, no dialogue, all the politics and assumptions embedded in the images are allowed to flow by in unquestioned monologue, and that leads to unconscious acceptance. The extreme restriction on what is presented also leads to the normalization of certain images and the narrowing of what is considered acceptable. Different ways of viewing and imaginative presentations are pathologized if their underlying assumptions do not conform to the prevailing, controlled norm.

One could say that in earlier eras art did the same thing—the viewpoint of the Church or of a wealthy patron determined the imagery. But there was always more to great art than mere propaganda—it was about perceiving beyond the received image, understanding that we are more than just cultural objects or consumer units. The presentation of the prevailing image was a means to reflection and understanding of human nature, of oneself and the world on a deeper level, and on concentric levels of relationship. In the interaction of perception with image an internal dialogue was encouraged, a dialogue that developed inner awareness beyond the limitation of the cultural norm to the larger experience of life as a whole, even in its great subtlety.

Matthew Fox has observed that "imagination is very connected to memory, to the past, and to the future. That's its power but also its weakness. People can live only in imagination in a culture like ours, even in other people's imaginations, such as advertisers.' Imagination can be a distraction from living in the now—but it does not have to be ... The gift of healthy art is that it takes the power of the imagination and brings us back to the now, to the depth and truth of what really is."[4]

Paintings and other art forms offer insight into the spirit of a society, past or present, as well as into individual human nature. This insight can then grant us a more complex understanding of our own experience, awakening us from our trance to the possibilities of the new in every present moment. I highly recommend visiting the great art museums for a direct interaction, to experience the immediacy and intensity of seeing and perceiving of which we are all capable. Creating your own art is even better!

Section Two
Practicing Body-Mind Centering:
Case Studies

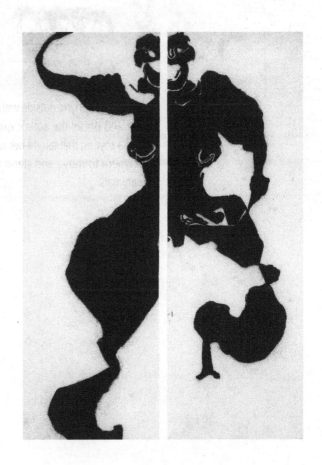

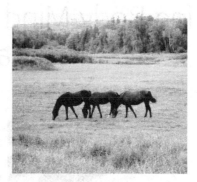

Growing up working outside with her father and uncle, the author experienced a rhythm that taught her when and where to move and stand with the animals.

Simon, Jennifer, and Me:
A Foot in a Sock in a Shoe

~ **Lee Saunders,** Canada (2002)

Who We Are and How We Met

There is something that happens when you grow up working outside.
The movement and rhythm of the day are determined by the animals,
crops, and weather. With the sounds of the birds and wind constant
in my ears, I became aware of placement, timing, and center of gravity
while mirroring my father and uncle as we did the daily chores. Anticipating the flow of movement between the tractor, bales of hay, and
our family of workers, I developed a bird's-eye view. Among the horses
and cows I learned where and when to speak, stand, or move in order
to guide them along their way. And with a simple touch at a strategic
point, they would lift a leg, drop their head, and align their spine, walk,
stop, turn, stand, or lie down. Empathy and the resonance of life flowed
richly between us and the other animals, as we assisted them to heal,
give birth, be born, walk, grow, and die.

I grew up and moved away, became a professional dancer, and studied anatomy, movement, touch, and voice with many, including Body-
Mind Centering founder Bonnie Bainbridge Cohen and her team of
teachers. The BMC understanding of the evolution of movement from
in utero to walking, and the facilitation of neuromuscular and perceptual
repatterning through movement, touch, and voice resonated perfectly
with my experience growing up on our farm. I took to BMC like a fish
to water and became a certified teacher of the work.

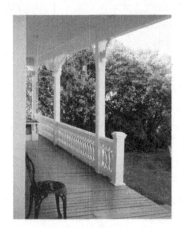

Returning to the family farm as an adult, the author found the comfort of the porch to be the place to receive Jennifer and Simon upon their first visit.

Several years later, like the cows returning home in response to our call, I moved back to the place where the seeds for my studies were planted—the family farm. It was January 1995, and it was a long and difficult winter. Several members of my family were unexpectedly and seriously ill. Seeking emotional and spiritual support through this turbulent time, I found a skillful guide and friend in my parents' minister. During the course of our numerous conversations Albert mentioned that his daughter Jennifer, who lived in Europe, was a single parent with two children. Her oldest child, Simon, had autism. I told Albert of the work I did as a Body-Mind Centering practitioner and somatic movement therapist and educator, and offered my services if they should ever come this way.

Now, several months later, it is high summer and I am sitting on the porch swing waiting for Jennifer and Simon. It is to be our first meeting. Jennifer and Simon are here visiting family for three weeks. We have agreed to meet for two hours, to see what happens and then take things from there. I will charge no fee. Jennifer's father helped me for free and I will do the same.

Meeting the Unknown Together

When they arrive at our home, Jennifer unfastens Simon's seat belt and helps him out of the car. He is seven years old, slight, with short light-brown hair. They hold hands as they walk toward me, the direction of their path veering slightly to the right, following the lean of Simon's body. He is bent to the side, as if his head, shoulder, spine, hips, and legs are braced against an invisible impact, and he looks out from the corner of his eyes.

Jennifer looks to be in her early to mid-thirties, about ten years younger than me. Still jet-lagged from their transatlantic flight two days before, she is impressively competent, patient, and calm in her communication with Simon. His voice is a humming sound that comes from the back of his mouth, and as we walk to the house he drops into a squatting fetal position that stops all movement.

I am used to this response from young children at our first meeting, especially from those who have gone through a lot of medical or therapeutic care. Simon's lack of interest in my presence is oddly reassuring; it is a normal response to the situation. If I follow his leads to help him find a greater sense of comfort, and to help Jennifer expand her skills for assisting Simon in his daily life, he may have a therapeutic experience with me that is different from what he has had before. My value in their world will come through the fruits of our efforts, nothing more and nothing less. We must work together like a foot in a sock in a shoe.

It is a cool grey day with a threat of rain, so Jennifer and I decide to work inside. Jennifer explains to Simon where we are going.

I ask, "Simon, would you like to come inside?" With my fingers I lightly brush the back of his hand, offering him my hand, and he takes it.

With Simon in the middle, we walk up the stairs. As we approach the landing where the staircase divides, leading to the two sides of the house, he collapses into his squatting fetal position, refusing to move, like a three-year-old in the middle of a mall. I know this is a recurring pattern for Simon that impedes his family activities. This was clear from the moment they arrived at our farm.

"Do you have a solution for this?" I ask Jennifer.

She replies, "No, not really, just a lot of gentle coercion or a battle of wills."

"Would you like to try my suggestion?" I ask.

"Yes," she replies.

I explain, "Simon is taking the lead here. So rather than seeing this squatting position as a problem, it is an opening to facilitate his movement. He is giving us the chance to meet him where he is rather than where we think he should be. We don't have to go upstairs to begin. We can begin right now."

With the three of us balanced halfway up the staircase, we continue to hold Simon's hands so that he does not fall. I ask Jennifer to place her free hand on the base of Simon's sacrum while I place mine on his knees and explain that, by focusing our touch on his bones, we can reinforce Simon's sense of structure and stability and ground him in the moment.

"How do you focus your touch on his bones?" she asks.

"It's like this," I say. Then, placing my hand on Jennifer's arm, I lightly press the bones in my fingers along the edges of the bones in her arm.

"Can you feel how the bones in my fingers are moving on the bones in your arm?" I ask.

"Yes."

Then, moving my hand to her sacrum, I repeat this bone-to-bone touch.

"Like this?" Jennifer asks as she places her hand on my arm, mirroring my touch.

"Yes, that's it."

Following my lead she places her hand on Simon's sacrum and slowly, lightly, presses it in an upward direction toward his head and a forward direction toward his knees. At the same time I slowly and lightly press his knees in a downward direction toward his feet and a backward direction toward his sacrum. As we simultaneously push our hands toward Simon's center—his navel—I speak with him in a friendly, adventurous way, pausing between phrases to allow time for his thought process, and for the subtle sounds or movements that are his response. Occasionally I mirror his sound, humming in quiet affirmation. "Simon, do you feel my hand on your legs? These are your legs. That's right, m-hmmm. These are your legs. Feel how strong they are." Simon's eyes begin to focus.

I place my hand on his feet and lightly push. "Feel your feet, Simon, these are your feet." Simon's head begins to lift. "That's right, these are your feet. Can you feel how they push into the stairs? That's right." As Simon's feet and legs push into the stairs his body begins to rise.

"Feel how the bones in your legs are helping you stand. M-hmm. That's right, Simon. Feel how you move." As Jennifer's hand and my hand draw closer, his sacrum and knees line up over his feet, and under his shoulders and head. Then voila! Simon is standing, surprised to be up, and more alert than when he was squatting on the stairs.

Next, I stand behind him and place one hand on his navel, the side of my thigh supporting Simon at his sacrum. I lightly slide my hand from his sitz bone down the back of his thigh toward his knee. Simon lifts his leg and begins to walk up the stairs toward the landing, holding Jennifer's hand. Curious and involved in the prospect of being in a strange house, Simon takes off by himself to explore.

Keeping him in our peripheral vision, Jennifer takes Simon's role and I work on her, explaining what we just did. Then we switch roles and she repeats the process on me, receiving my guidance and verbal cues.

Jennifer tells me, "In all my years of getting help for Simon, this is the first time a therapist has ever included me in the sessions. You've shown me how to handle him more humanely and efficiently. This is empowering, not just for Simon but for me too. The other therapy sessions may have been an emotional therapeutic outlet for Simon, but they left me outside, unable to help him on a day-to-day basis.

"As a professional musician I studied the Alexander technique to help me with my body alignment," she continues, "so I understand the principles about posture that we're working with here. It feels great to use what I learned then to help Simon now. What is new for me is understanding how to facilitate his alignment and movement using touch."

"So, Jennifer, you have an excellent foundation for understanding what we can do together. If you and Simon decide to continue working with me, this review process is a routine that we can repeat at every session, and as your skills and understanding increase we will work more and more as a team. This will give you more skills to access when you're at home."

"I would like that a lot," says Jennifer. "And I can tell by what we have just done that as an added benefit this is going to help me get back into shape. I must say I tend to neglect myself with all the demands of being a single parent."

Jennifer calls Simon, takes his hand, and we make our way to what she calls "Lee's special white therapy room." It is a simple space on the second floor, big enough for movement, yet cozy and small. The only piece of furniture is a dresser. Jennifer and I sit on the wood floor with a folded blanket beneath us to cushion our bones. There is a thin futon the size of a single bed for Simon. Standing facing the wall with his body about two feet from the surface, about two feet away Simon rocks from side to side as he slowly travels around the perimeter of the room checking out the picture, walls, window, and dresser. He doesn't touch anything. Occasionally he taps his head, smiles, and makes sounds as if questioning or commenting on what he sees. When he becomes agitated, the rhythm and intensity of his movement increase, and his voice takes on a more anxious tone.

As Simon explores the boundaries of the room, moving in a nonlinear path from one point to another, Jennifer tells me their story. I listen and watch them both, and as their history unfolds the rhythm and tone of Simon's movement and voice travel between calm and irritation.

"My pregnancy with Simon was my first and it was not easy. I was touring as a classical musician, and my marriage was in difficulty. I developed gestational diabetes, and by my ninth month I had edema that was so severe I could hardly walk.

"During Simon's birth I had what they called 'failure to dilate,' so they gave me epidurals and pethadine. After twenty-five hours of labor they discovered that Simon had a posterior presentation. They lost his heartbeat for about one minute and then it came back again. After thirty-two hours of labor they did a Cesarean section.

"At birth Simon had bruising on the left front lobe of his brain, the center for communication, and they had to suck fluids from his lungs to get him to breathe."

"Was he able to nurse?" I ask.

"I had a huge blood loss from the delivery and then developed an infection in my uterus. I could not nurse because of the antibiotics in my blood, so he was bottle-fed."

"And how did he do?"

"He had no problem feeding. When they tested his reflexes at birth his Apgar was 10, which is pretty normal. After his first inoculation, at three months, Simon developed a high fever and was almost unconscious. After that I noticed that he began to look from the sides of his eyes. When I spoke to the doctor about this he brushed it off. At nine months, after his second set of inoculations, Simon started having night terrors and eerie rhythmic screaming, as if something neurological was firing off in his vocal cords. Then he started fixating on his hands and twisting them in repetitive movements. Again, when I spoke to the doctor he took little interest. My husband and I were too inexperienced to question his response. So Simon had his third inoculation at twelve months. He had a large, localized reaction to the jab, and after that he had his first in a series of seizures, which grew worse over the year.

"Between his first and second year he was diagnosed with infantile spasms epilepsy. When I spoke to the doctor about the connection to the inoculations and Simon's difficulties, the doctor refused to admit a connection. Up until the third jab, Simon's developmental milestones were there at the right time, but they never seemed to be sustained."

"The impulse was there but the integration wasn't," I suggest.

"Yes," Jennifer says, and then adds, "In hindsight he should never have had those shots, but we didn't know that then. I was young, he was my first child, and we trusted the doctor's opinion." She pauses. "Now it is what it is and we have to move on.

"Simon's dad could not deal with Simon's injuries, and our marriage continued to falter. When Simon was two years old, his father left. At age five Simon was diagnosed as having pervasive developmental disorder and autistic tendencies. His dad continues to see Simon, but his presence in his life is sporadic and vague."

As their story unfolds Simon's level of agitation increases. He paces sideways around the room, slapping the right side of his head with the flat surface of his hand, making moaning sounds that match the rhythm of the slaps. I ask Simon if there is something bothering him, then ask Jennifer for her opinion.

"Yes, he woke up this morning with a headache—I can tell by the way he slaps his head."

I ask, "Do you think he might be upset by what you are telling me?"

"Yes, that's possible," she says. "He has had a very hard life and then on top of that, divorce is difficult for all children ... so it makes sense that he would be upset."

Watching Simon, I consider my next step. I feel deep empathy and understanding for his pain and life struggle. Why? Because as a result of a birth injury and several accidents, pain management and physical rehabilitation are a constant part of my life. I have improved my condition and contradicted my doctors' prognoses that I would be debilitated by pain forever. Now, in this moment, I wonder how to bridge the gap between Simon and me, how to gain his trust to let me work on his head, share the knowledge of my experience, and help him find a way out of his pain.

I let go of my reservations.

Moving to squat beside him, I mirror Simon's movement. We are about three inches apart. Over his sounds of discomfort I begin to speak, pausing for him to absorb the meaning of my words. "You know, Simon, I have had a lot of pain in my life with headaches. . . . I can't say that I have the same headache as you, but I know what it is like to live with a headache all the time ... When my head hurts I have someone put their hands on my head and hold it ... this has helped me a lot ... Would you like me to do that for you?"

He is quiet and still, no movement, no voice. I ask Jennifer, "Do you think he would like that?"

She asks, "Simon, would you like Lee to hold your head and see if she can help your headache go away?" He makes small, gentle hand movements on his head and equally small sounds. Then Jennifer says to me, "Yes, go ahead."

I gently cradle Simon's head between my hands and feel the force of his living, his vitality, the texture of his hair, the heat of his body, the meeting of my skin with the skin that covers his skull. Simon puts his head in my lap. It is far too heavy and hot for someone so young and so small. Silently I grieve for the weight of his injury.

Through my hands I feel the bones of his head. They are landmarks indicating the trauma of his birth and a container for his present pain. They are the recipients of his hits and the specific message that each hit carries. Focusing my attention inside his skull, I feel the craniosacral fluid as it circulates around his brain. There is a restriction of its movement on the right, in the region that Simon hits. This restriction reflects a torque in his structure that begins with compression in the bones of his skull and travels down through his body to his feet. No wonder he veers to the right when he walks.... In response to my feather-light touch, I feel the area of restriction in Simon's brain begin to unfold. His cranial bones release and the fluid begins to circulate more freely. Simon crawls into my lap and curls into a fetal position. His body relaxes, his breathing is slow and even, and he is still. It is less than ten minutes since I first put my hands on his head.

Jennifer looks at me and says, "I have never seen him do that with anyone other than me before. Never."

We sit in stillness and absorb the impact of our meeting. Quietly holding Simon in my lap, with my hands on his head, I explain to Jennifer what we have just done. "With a traumatic birth like Simon's, his journey from *in utero*, being one with you, to being born and separate from you, was not completed on all body-mind levels. And then there is his reaction to the inoculations. Simon's movement patterns and vocal sounds indicate that developmentally he is still trapped in the birthing process somewhere between the comfort of your uterus and life outside your womb. Consequently he is separate from both worlds. The meeting place for us is where he last knew a sense of wholeness and wellness: *in utero*, at one with you. When Simon is overwhelmed he squats, like he did on the stairs, and that squat is a fetal position. Combined with gentle interaction through touch and the mirroring of his sounds and movement, I could meet him, hold his head, and reduce his discomfort. Ideally, by continuing to meet Simon at his developmental place, you and I can help him create a neurological bridge that will enable him to literally move on in his life."

Jennifer responds, "Before today, no one ever mentioned that Simon's reactions to stress were fetal. In fact, many practitioners have looked at his obsessive and self-hurting habits as an 'issue' that had to be dealt with. I think it's a literal assault on the sensibilities of neurologically injured children like Simon to expect behavior from them that is inconvenient, and I feel unbelievable relief to hear you describe Simon's movements as his way to communicate normal reactions to life, and to communicate the frustration he must feel from living with his injury and its limitations."

While we wait for Simon to surface from his nest, we agree to meet twice a week during the time they are here.

The Swing

It is our second session, and we are having fun playing with Simon on the swing. It is the small children's swing, the one that hangs on the lowest branch of the spruce tree in front of our house. A single plank with a hole at each end for the rope to pass through, it is a very tippy seat. Simon is sitting on it, holding the ropes in the same way that he squats and stands, spine bent to the side with his head forward and tipped to the right. His pelvis is twisted on the seat. His elbows are bent and his shoulders lift toward his ears, with his left shoulder and hand higher than his right. His knees are bent, with his lower legs and feet gripping the bottom of the seat. He is staying on by sheer force of will. If he slips off, he will land on the lawn that is compacted from generations of play around the roots of the tree.

The swing does not move unless Jennifer and I make it go, and as we do, it twists to the right as Simon swings forward and to the left as he comes back. Simon is a little frustrated because the swing is not moving well. He needs more balance in his body, vision, and hearing, from left to right and front to back.

Jennifer is in front of the swing facing Simon, close enough to ensure he does not fall off, yet far enough away to entice him to reach with his feet, which is one of our goals. Right now he is not reaching at all, which is fine. Following my instructions, she places one hand on each of Simon's knees and lightly pushes to propel him back toward me. Following my directions, her touch is focused on the direct line of his bones, from kneecap through thighbone to pelvis.

I stand behind Simon. He has a beautiful view of his mom as he swings. Behind her I see the vegetable garden, which is coming along nicely. Everything is up and thriving: corn, beans, peas, beets, and broccoli. Beyond the vegetable garden, a field of alfalfa stretches toward a hedgerow of trees at the top of a small hill, about three hundred yards away. The summer drought has not hit yet, so we are surrounded by a deep, vibrant green as far as the eye can see.

My hands are above Simon's on the ropes as I gently propel the swing toward Jennifer. She lightly pushes his knees in response. We do not want him to fall off. With the swing still in motion, I move my right hand and grasp the rope under his right hand so that they are touching. He moves his right hand up. Then I drop my left hand down the rope so it touches his left hand and he moves his left hand down. We repeat this dance until his hands are level on the ropes and his shoulders are more balanced. The swing is twisting less.

Simon is making sounds of pleasure with his voice. As he swings back, I join in with popping, clucking, or humming sounds that attract his attention. His head starts to lift, searching for the sound, and his legs begin to unfold. He swings back and forth and I keep singing to his right ear or left, depending on the direction I want his head to go.

Simon's head flops back so he can see me, and he looks from the sides of his eyes. I move to be more visible, stroke the back of his neck in an upward direction and stroke the front of his throat in a downward direction. He brings his head up to balance evenly on his spine. He swings toward his mom. She smiles, calls his name, looks him in the eyes and pushes on his knees. As he comes toward me I lightly stroke him on the right side of his spine in an upward direction, from his pelvis to his shoulder blade, and his spine begins to straighten in response. He swings toward his mom. Each time he comes toward me I repeat the stroking action, moving it from the left side of his spine to the right, choosing his lower back or base of neck as the place to stroke, depending on the direction his spine needs to go for balance.

With each stroke Simon's body moves closer and closer to plumb and his legs continue to unfurl. Jennifer can push him from below the knees now and, with each push moving up through the bones to his pelvis, his legs begin to push into her hands in response. As they do, they begin to reach toward her.

Jennifer mirrors Simon's alignment and joins in with our sounds. He focuses his attention on her, with the presence of me behind. Mom front, Lee back, Mom close, Mom far, left ear sound, close, far, right ear sound, close, far, Mom front, Lee back, Mom close, Mom far. . . .

Our popping, clucking, humming sounds surround him and pull on his ears, like a moving train blowing its whistle—at first far away and faint, then closer and louder, passing by loudest, then leaving, fading and gone. Combined with the natural smells all around us, we are working with space, movement, time, hearing, vision, touch, balance, and intention as one.

Simon's body posture and tone are balanced. With each push, Jennifer's hands inch down Simon's legs until his legs are fully unfurled. She pushes on his feet, the compression travels to his pelvis; the swing rides up and back. Yielding into gravity, Simon's spine and head balance forward and his arms bend. I push on his sitz bones; the swing drops forward to Jennifer. Yielding into gravity, Simon's spine and head balance back, his arms extend. He pulls on the ropes and reaches to meet his Mom's hands with his feet.

Jennifer pushes him back to me and Simon begins to actively pump the swing through the reach, push, yield, and pull of his head, hands, feet, and tail. I lightly push on his back or shoulders. Simon and the swing arc through space on a straight and vibrant course. His feet reach

Mom. She lightly pushes on them and Simon arcs back on course to me. We are laughing, talking, and singing together. As the swing slowly comes to a halt I ask, "Simon, do you know about yoga?" His head is cocked at a listening angle. "Jennifer, does Simon know about yoga?"

"Yes, he sees me do it."

"So Simon, if you know about yoga, do you know what a yogi is?"

Jennifer shakes her head no.

"Well, a yogi is a great teacher of yoga, and people come from all over the world to study with them." He is still listening. "I think you are a great yogi, Simon. I think you are a very gifted and very smart boy. You have a big injury and it is amazing that you do all the things you can do." Simon laughs and smiles.

Jennifer laughs. "No one has ever said that to him before. Do you hear that, Simon? Lee says you are a great yogi and a very smart boy!" He laughs and smiles more.

"It's true, Simon, that's what I think. It's easy to learn how to swing if you don't have an injury, but you, Simon, you have a big injury and you just learned how to swing. I am very impressed. You should be proud. You are a very brave, gifted, and intelligent boy. I have great respect for you, Simon. You are a great teacher."

Simon is rocking from side to side, laughing and looking at his mom and me. I start to push the swing and we resume our game once more.

When we're done, Simon goes off to play around the garden. Jennifer and I review the session, and as we work with each other on the swing I ask, "Have the doctors talked about Simon in front of him?"

"Yes," she said. "One in particular said he would always function at a very low level."

"And how did you feel when he said that?"

"I was angry, very angry. I felt he was totally missing Simon as a person, that it was awful to say those things in front of him, and that he was missing the things Simon could do."

"And Simon, did he have a response to the doctor's comments?"

"His general response to almost everything at that time in his life was freaking out. His world was not a secure place, at home or with the doctors. Now it's clear that Simon knows what we are saying to him, so I'm sure he understood what that doctor said, and I am sure it upset him. His world was a pretty horrible place, and he had his one way to respond, which was freaking out."

"Well," I said, "it's very clear that Simon is a long way away from functioning at a very low level for the rest of his life. He knows what's going on. He understands everything we say. I said what I did about a yogi because I thought he would enjoy it. And the other reason I said it was because I wanted to give him a context, to help him see his accomplishments in relation to others. He is very smart. The fact that he responded so quickly tells me that he has a lot of potential. With the right interaction, his nervous system is available and responsive. I have no idea how far he can go, but it is very clear that he has not reached his limit."

Halfway through our next session Jennifer says, "Oh, I forgot to tell you—the day after we did the session on the swing, Simon called me 'Mom'."

"Has he called you Mom before?" I ask.

"It's been several years since the last time he called me Mom. In fact, it's been several years since he has spoken with words."

"How did it feel to have him call you Mom?"

"It felt wonderful."

Head-Hitting

Today Simon is frustrated and angry. He is squatting and hitting his head. Hard, very hard. *Bang bang bang* with his closed fist on the right side of his head.

How can we help him without restraining his arm? I look for an opening and see the triangular space that is formed by his arm, shoulder, and neck when his hand hits his head. I extend my arm into the triangle and, starting at his shoulder, I glide it perpendicularly along his arm, directing his hand down to the earth. He returns to hitting his head and I redirect his hand to the earth again, saying, "You know, Simon, it's not your fault. Go ahead and be angry, but don't hit yourself—it's not your fault. Hit the earth, Simon, not yourself. Hit the earth—feel the earth and push."

As Simon's hand makes contact with the earth, I lightly push it on the ground to help him understand what it is I am telling him to do. The focus of my touch is through the bones. We repeat the process several times and then Simon begins to push on his own. The resulting action travels up his arms, through his shoulders, and down his spine into his center. He is being physically moved to his center, his navel and core, by the push from his hands and arms on the earth.

Now, rather than a helpless, self-defeating, imploding hitting, there is an external direction and action for his frustration. His attention begins to shift to the outside world, and his frustration turns into curiosity and participation. His fingers start touching the grass and rocks under his hands. The focus in his eyes changes and he is more present, thinking and looking at what is around him. He hears the sound of the tractor far off in the field. He gets up and walks away to play in the backyard.

At our next session Jennifer says, "Last night Simon got angry and I saw him walking around the house searching for a way to hit the floor. He was trying to do what you had helped him do, but he could not do it on his own. I tried to show him but I was not sure how to do it either." So in our reviews, Jennifer and I practice this move, over and over again.

Rebirthing

We are on the lawn in front of the house today, and Simon is angry. He is lying on his back, eyes closed, kicking, screaming, and banging his head on the ground, with his arms bent and flailing by his sides.

"Jennifer, we need to bring Simon back into his body and we must work quickly. I'd like you to squat about one foot away from the top of Simon's head, facing him. Then I would like you to place your hand on his head, like this." I place my hand on the birthing crown of her head and apply a slight pressure that travels down through her spine to her navel. I feel the subtle response of her spine pushing back. "Can you feel how your spine responded to the compression and pushed back?" I ask.

"Yes," she says.

"That's great. Would you like to try?"

Jennifer positions herself and places her hand on Simon's head. He is still screaming and flailing. With my hand over hers we take a few seconds to adjust her touch, then feel the response of Simon's spine pushing back. She says she is ready.

"Great. Now I'd like you to speak to Simon, reassure him and call his name. You are his mother, you are at his birthing crown, and we are going to try and help him find a way out of his frustration and bring him back to us."

Facing Jennifer, I stand above Simon so that he is lying between my legs. He is still on his back, his body arched like a bridge with his navel the keystone of the arch. Jennifer applies a slight pressure at Simon's head; I place one hand on his heart and the other on his navel. He feels like sprung steel.

In response to our touch Simon's body begins to flex toward his navel, like the petals of a flower closing for the night, or a fetus curving toward its umbilical cord.

At the moment his head, spine, and legs touch the ground I take my hand off his navel, place it on the side of his right hip, and roll him over to the left. Now he is lying on his belly, elbows bent, hands flat on the ground and silent. He seems surprised and a bit confused.

The silence ends. Simon's voice is less angry but the frustration is still there. He tries to arch his back like before, but can't because he is on his belly. So he looks for a way out. My hand is on the base of his skull and my other hand is on his tail. By lightly pressing and directing my hands away from each other, I offer him a lengthening of his spine and he takes it.

As Simon reaches from his head, he meets Jennifer's compression and begins to push. He wants to travel and wriggles on his belly, searching for mobility. We remind him of his hands, arms, legs, and feet by lightly pressing them into the ground. He follows our lead, makes a connection with the earth, and begins to crawl. He's not aggravated anymore. He is traveling and his voice is subdued.

We are moving as a unit. Jennifer's hands are on Simon's head, gently reassuring him through her touch and the encouragement of her words. My hands are at the base of his skull and tail. Like a turtle, Simon extends his head to see the world and rises through his spine. His arms and legs come under his body to provide support, and he is creeping, looking at where he is going—the swing! We move as a unit. Jennifer maintains constant light pressure at Simon's birthing crown that he pushes against, while I move my hands to touch him at his heart, navel, base of head, and tail. As his spine lengthens, he reaches further with his head and rises higher. His hands come off the ground, his feet come under his hips, and he rises to a walk, and then peacefully goes to the swing, leaving our hands behind.

"That was amazing!" Jennifer says. "He went from a defenseless baby on his back to a baby still agitated but on his front, wriggling like a snake, then he crawled and crept. Simon has never crawled or crept before."

Several times over the summer Simon went through this developmental movement sequence, and every time he did, he evolved to walking with an inner calm, an alert level of participation, and an ability to separate from us with a secure and inquisitive mind. We never used forceful touch or confrontation. We merely redirected his movement by offering another choice. He took the choice every time.

Taking a Walk

It is a clear, warm day and we are looking for a change. We spot the horses in the field and decide to go see them. Hand in hand, with Simon in the middle, he pulls us toward the arched footbridge that connects the yard to the fields.

As we reach the high point of the arch on the bridge, we are surrounded by space—above, under, and around. The view is clear and descends before us. Simon begins to collapse to his fetal squat. I place one hand on his navel and the other on his sacrum to help him feel the secure structure of his bones. Jennifer speaks to him and reassures him that everything is okay. His descent stops and he straightens his spine.

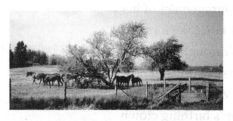

While walking, Simon finds himself attracted to the horses, and pulls Lee and his mother Jennifer toward the footbridge to go see them.

"Can you see the horses, Simon?" I ask. His eyes focus in the direction of the horses. We can see them from here, six of them grazing between a pair of gnarled, hundred-year-old apple trees on the side of a small hill. "Would you like to go see the horses?" Simon takes the lead and we move on.

Stepping off the bridge, we enter the pasture and walk toward them. We are in the horses' space. The air is dense and still. They lift their heads, turn, and come toward us. We stop. Symphony, the youngest, is six months old and still mouthing. She comes closer to us than the others, looking for something to nibble. Jennifer and I pat her and Simon lets go of our hands to mirror our movement.

Symphony's back is level with Simon's head. She is curious and relaxed, sniffing us, then nibbling the grass. Simon is making small, quiet sounds of contentment as he rubs Symphony's side. Then with a burst of enthusiasm he wraps one arm under her belly, the other over her back, and gives her a full frontal hug, humming with delight! Symphony's head arches high, and with an alert, startled look in her eye she snorts. The older horses move in with concern, their heads high and nostrils flared. Their bodies encircle us. I know we are safe. Simon moves like the horses, raises his head and releases his arms. His eyes are wide, assessing the situation, and he is making quiet sounds of concern from the upper back of his throat. He is standing free, with Jennifer and I as his protectors.

"Easy now," I say, "Easy." Then I wave my hands to shoo the horses away, and they scatter like a swarm of giant flies. The tension breaks and we three stand alone, watching them as they run into the distance, shrinking before our eyes.

"Simon, you were great—you handled that situation very well. You gave Symphony a great big hug. She was surprised; she has never had a big hug like that before. Especially from something the same size as her. You were strong and tall." Simon's head is tilted to listen, his body relaxed. "She was surprised, you were surprised, we were all surprised! Even the other horses were surprised. Are you okay? You look okay."

Jennifer nods her head in affirmation.

I ask, "Shall we go back to the house?"

Simon takes our hands and pulls us to return. As we cross the bridge, he does not collapse. It is a lovely day for a walk.

The Last Day

It is the day before Jennifer and Simon leave for England, and it is our last session. When they arrive the car doors fly open, and Simon comes roaring out of the car. Jennifer follows, saying, "What a time—he has been screaming and fighting all night long!"

Simon lies on the ground. He is hitting his head, moaning, crying and writhing in isolation. His eyes are closed, his hearing is shut off, and his body is rigid and tense. We work with him, repeating the developmental facilitations we have done before, and he comes out of his turmoil more calm, externally focused, and present. But the tension in his body and voice are still there.

"You're leaving tomorrow, aren't you?" I say. His head rises to focus his ears and he listens. "I know you know you are leaving, so I want to tell you that I have a colleague in England who has studied at the same place as me, and if you want, you and your mom can continue work like this with her. She is a very nice person." His restless movement and sounds of irritation stop.

Jennifer and I look at each other with surprise, relief, and satisfaction. "Well, that's clear," she says. Then Simon gets up and goes for a walk.

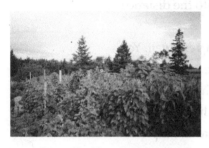

Venturing out by himself, Simon heads toward the hedgerow on the other side of the garden, and then connects across the distance by calling to Lee and his mother Jennifer.

"I'm afraid I won't be able to reproduce what we have done here when we return home," Jennifer says. "So, like Simon, I find it reassuring to know there is someone there we can work with."

"Yes," I say. "I can see it's reassuring for both of you. At the same time, I think it's important for you to trust what you know and to work from your place of strength. You understand the alignment of the body very well and you understand how a touch in a strategic place on Simon's body can offer him a movement choice that he might not be able to access on his own. Every time we offered Simon a choice to move beyond his pattern, he took it. This is a very important and wonderful thing. Obviously he wants to be helped, is very willing to be helped, and recognizes when someone can help him. He is still, relatively speaking, young. And this is good, because the younger the tree, the easier it is to redirect the growth of the branches. You and Simon have a lot of personal resources."

Simon is on the other side of the garden, headed toward the hedgerow. This is the farthest away he has ever been from us. We can see by his gait that he is engaged in what he is doing. And then he looks at us and makes a loud and beautiful call. Matching his call, I answer him back and wave, letting him know that we are here with him, listening and watching, even though we are far away.

He turns and continues to explore. Jennifer says, "Like so many parents, I have searched for and exposed Simon to many forms of therapy and have always scrutinized for the tiniest measures of visible improvement. Working together in this way with you, I feel we finally found our oasis. Now I understand how Simon's every movement is a valuable source of information. I want to move back to Canada with Simon and his sister Sarah so that we can live in the country, be with my family, and work with you. It would be much better for us than living in Europe, in a large city, but before I can move I must have the permission of their fathers."

Jennifer and I discuss this further and agree that it will be a long process, but well worth it. She calls Simon in and he returns of his own free will.

Jennifer's mom arrives to take them home and is amazed at the change in Simon's emotions. Simon gets in the back seat by himself and quietly waits for Jennifer and his grandmother. He is peaceful and still.

We say goodbye, they drive away, and I wonder when I will see them again. I feel sad to lose my direct input into their lives and find comfort in knowing they will contact my colleague in England. Knowing that client/practitioner relationships are highly particular, I hope it works well for them.

Later that summer I see Simon's grandfather and he tells me, "You know, this summer when Jennifer and the children were here, we went down to the kitchen one morning and Simon was quietly sitting on top of the kitchen table watching the birds outside. He had never done that before. After that, Simon would often go downstairs in the morning by himself and get his breakfast. This level of independence was completely new."

"Ah yes," I thought, "the fruits of our efforts are good."

Summer '97

It is August 1997, and Jennifer, Simon, and Sarah have come from London to visit their family. I am leaving town on business, so we only have two days to meet. It has been two years since we last saw each other, and we are excited to be working together again.

The car drives into the yard and Simon gets out as quick as a wink. He is very different from the first time we met—taller, older, and obviously more independent. There is no question that he remembers the place, and me. He taps his head, looks at me with his sideways glance, and makes a small sound in my direction as he goes to the swing. We follow.

He has grown so much, the swing doesn't fit! Making aggravated sounds, he expresses his frustration. I show him the grown-up's swing. Simon sits on the seat, Jennifer and I take our places, and we resume where we left off two years before. Only this time there is a big difference. Jennifer and I don't have to push because Simon pumps the swing on his own!

"Wow, Simon, look at you! You're so strong and straight in your seat! And look how high you can swing! This is such an improvement! You could swing well before, but look at you now. You are doing it all on your own! You and your mom have done such a great job! I am very proud of you both." We all smile broadly, taking pleasure in our accomplishments. The three of us work together like a foot in a sock in a shoe.

"How did it go with my colleague in London?" I ask.

"We liked her and the sessions went well, but Simon was disappointed. He was expecting the same experience he had here. You know, the trees and horses and swing. I never thought to prepare him about the difference of location. And then there was the empathy between you and Simon. He didn't have the same connection with her. I have never seen him crawl into someone's lap like he did that first day with you. I thought it was a good thing that Simon could recognize the difference and express his disappointment and preference. I know I certainly have preferences when it comes to working with a therapist. And there was the reality of the long trip across London to get there. It wasn't the short drive from Mom and Dad's house to yours, and I was ill. So Simon and I decided to put our efforts into working on our own and doing what we did with you rather than adjusting to someone new and a different style of work. In the end I think it was good thing to do. It gave me more confidence to integrate into our daily lives the informed touch and informed perceptual interaction that you had shown us."

"Yes, I agree it is normal to prefer one way of working to another. I don't hear criticism in your decision; I hear observation, communication between you and Simon, and choice. And I hear your need to assimilate and integrate the work we did into your family and your life-style before you took on anything new. Judging by how well Simon can swing, I would say you both did very well in realizing your goal."

Simon makes pleasing sounds. It is clear that he understands. Just like before, he takes part in our conversation. As he rides the swing, we continue the same alignment games and vocal games we have played before. Occasionally Jennifer tries to fill me in on where she is now in her life, but we are cut short. Each time Simon feels my attention wander, he shows aggravation through the disruption of his balance, aggravated sounds, and turning to look at me. Simon is proud of his accomplishments; he wants my acknowledgement, and he wants his time with me. Anything less is unacceptable. Happy to oblige him, Jennifer and I agree to talk later.

At our meeting the next day she tells me, "After yesterday's session Simon called me 'Mom' again. He hasn't said 'Mom Mom Mom' in a long time. In fact, he stopped calling me Mom a few months after we stopped the sessions with you. So there's got to be a connection.

"Once you started to work with Simon in the summer of '95, we never looked back. To this day, he still searches for the stimulation and perception stretching that you did with him on the swing, and he actively and willingly engages me in the process. This is still a measurable, significant milestone for Simon and me."

Simon's Place

It is May 2001, and I am sitting with Jennifer in her kitchen. It is a three-hour drive from my home to hers. She and the children have just moved to Canada and are living in the village where her parents grew up and now live. With the help of her extended family, they are all adjusting well to the quiet rural life. After the stresses and pollution of city life, the move is a very good thing.

Even though we have kept contact by phone, last night was the first time Jennifer and I had seen each other since 1997. We have just made a presentation on the work we did with Simon at the Provincial Learning Disabilities Association's annual conference. It was an interesting group of occupational therapists, physiotherapists, parents, foster parents, caretakers, and special-ed teachers. Our presentation went very well and we are debriefing.

Leaning against the wall is a beautiful poster that Jennifer has made for the presentation. She calls it "Simon's Place." It is a collage made from photos of Simon. In them he is laughing as he swings on a swing. The underside of his sneaker is visible and reads "natural world."

Simon passes the kitchen door and Jennifer calls him in. "Simon, do you remember Lee? Come say hello." He is twelve years old now, a young man. Standing at 5'4", he has the air of a teenager with things on his mind. His hair is rumpled from an afternoon nap. I smile and wave my hand. "Hi Simon! It's good to see you."

He enters the kitchen, looks at me, lightly taps his head, waves his hand, makes his sound of greeting, and then leaves, moving on to his original destination. His entire greeting is one continuous flow of movement.

"He remembers," Jennifer says.

"Yes, he does."

Meeting a Child: Somatic Approaches to Developmental Delays

~ **Darcy McGehee,** Canada (2003)

Under-stand-ing the Underpinning of Movement

Most of us have a sense of self and of the world. We perceive our place in our environment and we act, and the synchronicity of those sensing and motoring events allows us to relate to the world and to survive. We reach a place in our development where we stand on our own two feet. We under-stand. Standing on our own two feet allows us to add the -*ing* of active movement choices to our repertoire of actions; we move toward, we move away, we change direction, we change pace, all in relationship. Through reading the movements of others we are able to understand, to some degree, their lives and their perceptions. We have under-stand-ing, which dynamically weaves both self and other. This is what I hoped for my son.

Science and somatics agree that the way we move in relation to our internal and external environments impacts the development of the nervous system, and the development of the nervous system greatly influences behavior. A conscious sense of self, or being present in the world, depends on the representation of physical states of being, processed, often unconsciously, in subcortical brain areas.[1] In typical development, maturation of the cerebral cortex follows subcortical maturation. Where this developmental choreography is interrupted, cortical function is unsupported. A dynamic systems perspective explains the neural consensus that defines consciousness as a social phenomenon depending on both reflexive (subcortical) and voluntary (cortical) action. New stimuli change all previously existing patterns of neural consensus and contribute to neural plasticity.[2]

Autism has traditionally been described as a condition wherein a child is in his own world. Jack's comfort and learning were interrupted because he did not have a reliable, balanced sense of his own internal world. The processing and communication of Jack's internal state of comfort through early (lower) neurological centers was compromised and did not support his higher cortical abilities. His neural growth did not have a strong foundation. It was as if his cerebral cortex was forced to make up for this lack of foundational support by maturing out of sequence, processing more information than it could handle and making executive decisions without pertinent information. This compromised Jack's ability to relate in the world.

Assessments and therapies commonly used with autistic children aim at age-appropriate task completion and controlled behavior, without addressing the foundational developmental sequences that support these tasks and behaviors. They do not effectively address what a child is experiencing or how a child completes a task; instead, they attempt to correct the problem from the top down. Jean Ayres pioneered research in developmental movement repatterning in the field of sensory integration. She states, "As long as subcortical structures remain poorly integrated, resolution of the impairment through a cognitive approach will be limited."[3] Developmentally based somatic techniques that use relational touch and movement address early, subcortical development from a dynamic systems perspective, honoring a child's moment-to-moment experience. Embodied movement offers a child a template for expressive and receptive communication. When a child understands how to move in a way that is connected to his needs and desires, skills are then transferable and can be adapted to many learning situations.

There is no simple formulaic, therapeutic approach to neurodevelopmental delays, but there is a universal sequence to the emergence of basic neurological movement patterns in typical development. I support a theoretical model that connects the emergence of these Basic Neurological Patterns with the development of specific areas of the brain; future interdisciplinary research is needed to clarify this connection. Movement repatterning offers movement and behavior choices to stimulate neurological development. Basic neurological patterns, inherent in the nervous system, that emerge in a well-orchestrated sequence in typical development may be elicited where development is atypical.

Neural plasticity—the flexibility and potential of the nervous system to develop and change throughout life—allows us to call forth the expression of early patterns that support emergence into the world.

Jack's Story

I have an eight-year-old son. When Jack was eighteen months old I could no longer ignore his lack of ability to pick up verbal or kinesthetic cues. Jack glanced at people out of the corner of his eye, unable to share another's gaze. He slept in short spurts and had the climbing skills of a mountain goat. He was in constant motion. Try as I might to schedule him, Jack's impulse was the only clock he could follow.

By age two, Jack could memorize the entire texts of documentary videos and identify by topography all the moons of Jupiter, but he had no conversational language. His strengths were eerie. His deficits were heartbreaking and exhausting. I felt my child was being sucked away from me.

When Jack was almost three and his world seemed more chaotic than ever, I sought help. I was told that, while early intervention was crucial, we might be on a waiting list for a year and a half before Jack would receive treatment. I then began a long process to have my son admitted to the specialists who might help him. I gave long telephone interviews; I filled out forms. When I was told the evaluation process alone would take a year, I got busy. I found the necessary people to grant the necessary diagnosis to admit Jack to a preschool for high-functioning autistic children. We began speech and occupational therapies. I read and learned and researched.

My previous background has been useful. For many years, I have danced and worked with dancers, elite athletes who pursue movement for creative expression. I was interested in both theatre and dance, and my MFA studies focused on the connection between voice and movement. I have studied traditional anatomy and kinesiology as well as somatic therapies, which investigate the connection of mind and body.

Autism is now classified as a neurodevelopmental disorder; these are basic deficiencies or perceived lack of connection between areas of the brain that present with increasing insistence as the infant is developing. When my son was diagnosed with PDD—Pervasive Developmental Disorder or High-Functioning Autism—I began looking where I was most familiar: I began exploring how movement affects neurological development, and how neurological development could be facilitated through movement.

Jack has a developmental disorder that involves a lack of synchrony and maturation in his sensory and motor development. It made sense to approach this disorder from a developmental movement perspective. This approach respects the incremental sequence of early learning that supports relational behaviors. It also sees these sequences through the lens of multiple interacting body systems.

Somatic Pioneers—Touch, Movement, and Meeting a Child Where He Is

Jack lived in a body very restricted in its movement choices and its abilities to make transitions or engage in relationships. A developmental, somatic-movement model addresses the many incremental, early movement patterns commonly observed in PDD and autistic children: toe-walking, side-to-side gait, restricted gaze shift, an inability to cross the midline of the body, a propensity for holding the arms up, and late or absent language development.

In exploring the best ways to support Jack's development, I have had the unique opportunity to be mentored by and to observe the work of three of the top researchers in somatic and developmental therapy in North America: Bette Lamont, Martha Eddy, and Bonnie Bainbridge Cohen. These therapists and somatic pioneers look at my son for who he is, not for who he isn't. This is rare in the world of disabilities. Jack has a disorder that affected his early ability to be in a relationship. These therapists placed themselves in relationship with Jack, moving with him and touching him. With their guidance I too learned to work with Jack. Soon I held him and he held me.

I remember clearly the first time Jack placed his hands around my neck and held on to me. I cried with joy when he finally looked deep into my eyes. My husband looked to me with tears rolling down his cheeks when Jack was asked to call his brothers to dinner and, for the first time, he did.

Bonnie Bainbridge Cohen, occupational and neurodevelopmental therapist, is the founder of Body-Mind Centering, an established and evolving somatic practice taught at The School for Body-Mind Centering. Martha Eddy, EdD, is an educator, researcher, and somatic practitioner certified in Body-Mind Centering. In responding to neurodevelopmental disorders, Eddy delves into the somatic work and compares it to more traditional scientific inquiry. Bette Lamont is the therapy director at the Developmental Movement and Education Center in Seattle. All three of these practitioners are certified in Laban Movement Analysis, a qualitative, comprehensive system of movement observation. Each of these women stresses the individuality of any child's presentations in developmental delays.

Jack's difficulties with navigating environmental and social relationships and responding with appropriate actions reflected his inability to come to a place of comfortable focus and to make and sequence decisions. Bonnie Bainbridge Cohen's book *Sensing, Feeling, and Action* explains how the Basic Neurological Patterns of movement give us the basis for attention, intention, and action. If we have the comfort to attend, we can follow our curiosity and desire with intention and action. Underlying the Basic Neurological Patterns is what Bainbridge Cohen refers to as the "alphabet of movement": the primitive reflexes, righting reactions, and equilibrium responses. Reflexes provide a developing infant with a subcortical template for movement. Bainbridge Cohen was the first researcher to point out that all the traditional reflexes have a modulating reflex. Even in the earliest phases of life we see a precursor to choice in movement, which evolves into an ability to make conscious, modulated transitions based on new information.

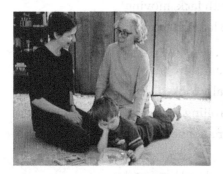

Bonnie Bainbridge Cohen with Jack and Darcy.

Many of Jack's early reflexes had failed to emerge or had been poorly integrated, limiting his movement choices. Incoming or sensory information from both his body and the environment could not be efficiently processed and screened. He could not come to a comfortable, grounded place of midline orientation, a milestone typically achieved around three months, and at the same point an infant develops a social smile. Without reliable sensory information and proprioceptive information (about position, movement, equilibrium, and resistance), Jack is unable to discern the temporal and spatial coordinates that underlie the ability to have intention in time and space. His actions are not supported by an integrated sensory-motor loop—where moving, sensing and perceiving, and moving again are in constant relationship.

The Ability to Be Inside—Yielding, Gravity, Cells, and Support

The reflexes that underlie movement are expressions of a primary relationship with gravity. In a sense, a highly skilled mover takes movement to a more reflexive place, relaxing conscious control and trusting the body's innate wisdom and subcortical proprioception. My work with

Bainbridge Cohen and Eddy has made this clear to me. This is part of my journey as a dancer and dance educator: learning to be present and responsive in the moment to support qualitative movement range and creative decisions. Without the proprioception of gravity acting on the body in space, we lack the support to venture into space and cannot transition between experiences.

In the fall of 1998, while I negotiated the bureaucracy of diagnosis, I searched online for Martha Eddy. Martha taught a Body-Mind Centering workshop I attended in 1996. When Jack and I first meet Martha, he is running through life at the age of three and a half. At this point, Jack does not read simple emotional or social cues through gesture or facial expression. He does not understand danger and is terribly confused by social motivators. Jack cannot shift his gaze and can barely turn his head. He does not bond to people, places, and things through his senses. He is hypersensitive and vigilant and yet sometimes appears to be unaware. He does not use the pronoun *I*, cannot express need, and cannot attend to others.

The first thing Martha asks me is what I want for Jack from the sessions. I timidly reply that I would like him to be able to express his experiences and his needs. (I had not been encouraged by the literature or specialists to expect these gains.) I want to know Jack. Martha nods.

Many autistic kids are great climbers; where they get into trouble is their inability to descend. Synchronizing weight shifts and behavior shifts challenge Jack. His abilities to change level and direction are ungrounded. His extended little frame just cannot curl into flexion. He cannot sense midline or descend through the midline. He cannot rotate his spine. Moving on the transverse (rotational) plane requires the support of weight-sensing and the ability to flex toward center. Research indicates that autistic babies present in an unusual rolling pattern of hyperextension, or they fail to roll over.[4]

Martha, Jack, and I go to the park a lot—many different parks with an assortment of apparatus to evoke losing one's balance in supported ways while ascending, descending, running, and jumping. Martha teaches Jack and me about the time and space of relationship—the phrasing of the pause at the bottom end of each delightful descent, whether it be in the microcosm of breath or the release into someone's perceptions and finally their arms. In our first session Martha makes

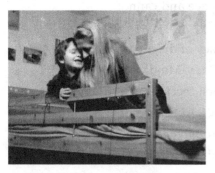

interesting sounds through a simple game of hide and seek. The enjoyment of discovering the source of these sounds allows Jack to direct his gaze, share his gaze, and experience being seen and heard in a pleasurable way. Jack begins a journey from defending to bonding.

Martha Eddy and Jack exchange bunk hugs.

Marin County, January 29, 1999

Jack and I meet Martha in the park. Jack and Martha form an immediate connection, which is unusual for Jack. Martha works with modulating tempo and rhythm in speech and movement. They engage in a game that requires Jack to track Martha's location in space, under the climbing equipment. Martha observes Jack's tiptoe walk, the lack of rotation in his spine, and his cerebellar problems with side-to-side balance. She offers cellular touch to bring out tone in Jack's arms and hands and invites softening in Jack's thoracic region, allowing the heart to pour to the back. Martha comments on the need for vestibular stimulation, prior to stimulation of the other senses, for adequate bonding.

Opening and Closing

Respiration occurs in every living cell of an organism. In the Body-Mind Centering model, cellular breathing is a fundamental developmental movement pattern, and it supports a discriminate pattern of the autonomic nervous system. Bainbridge Cohen speaks of the rhythm of the autonomic nervous system that is reflected in a simultaneous condensing and expanding yield, expressed in a starfish-like pattern from the center through the head, tail, arms, and legs that describes a cycle of going out and coming in. This autonomic rhythm supports the initial reflexes of bonding and defending.

The very basic choice of opening and closing defines primitive relationship in the choice of moving toward or away from stimulus. We establish the vital link of the extremities to the center by moving away from center and recovering stability, both physiologically through homeostasis and in our movement.

The simple action-recuperation cycle of expanding and condensing is interrupted in Jack. His sympathetic nervous system is very high-toned. He moves up and out in an extensor pattern without a sense of himself or the ability to transition back to a restful, parasympathetic state.

We have all experienced a "fight/flight" reaction in response to adrenaline, where the sympathetic nervous system (the actioning part of the nervous system) takes us into motion; it takes a while to recover into the "rest and digest" phase of a more parasympathetic state. Yielding and sensing his body weight are difficult for Jack. He has had digestive problems since birth, and his sucking reflex was less connected than I remember with my first two sons. The enteric nervous system (the nerves to and from the visceral organs) is the third division of the autonomic nervous system; it is intricately linked to transitions between sympathetic and parasympathetic states.

Martha engages Jack's curiosity to help him find stillness. She helps us both find the blood-full presence of the organs and a sense of weight, through cellular touch that acknowledges both container and contents, and through touch that acknowledges both support and movement in cellular breathing. Martha very quickly notices the absence in Jack of primitive reflexes, such as physiological flexion/extension (a whole-body movement toward and away from the navel center) and flexor withdrawal and extensor thrust (folding and extending the limbs), that are the reflexive support for moving toward and away from stimulus. The enteric nervous system piece of this is profound in initial sessions as I witness Jack begin to connect to the core of his central nervous system. Martha picks up on Jack's need to come into flexion and his system's inability to yield into that more parasympathetic place of nurture and comfort. She is able to provide the stimulus to cue flexion reflexively as well as the container to support yielding into that flexion.

In one of our sessions Jack is able to come to midline, clear his gaze, and express the discomfort of his past experiences. He then can yield into my arms and my body. This is my first experience of Jack's tonic lab reflex, a reflex signaling a cellular, vestibular, and proprioceptive relationship with gravity. Experiencing this remarkable change of tone makes me conscious of the cellular level of meeting someone where they are. I learn that I can help Jack to integrate his vestibular and proprioceptive reflexes by improving my own tone, relationship with gravity, and my cellular awareness, so that Jack no longer needs to respond to transition and change with hysteria. Jack starts to come in for a landing. So do I.

When yielding is present, a sense of self begins to emerge with the early push patterns.

Berkeley, January 30, 1999

Jack is upset about the transition of leaving the park. He is struggling in the stroller and crying out, "I can't stop." Martha works through touch and voice to meet him where he is and to help him modulate to stillness. He has definite breakthrough; he shudders and releases into her support, after which he is calmer than I have ever seen him while awake. The change is profound. I feel that the part of Jack that was being sucked away is attempting to emerge.

Oakland, January 31, 1999

We meet Martha at the studio. Martha encourages Jack to roll in both directions. When the "I can't stop" theme reemerges, Martha reinforces Jack's ability and gives him permission to stop. Jack plays piano and Martha drums out the rhythm of what he is playing on his body. When he begins to climb, she encourages him to push with his legs before reaching with his arms by giving resistance to his pelvis.

Oakland, October 17, 1999

Martha works on referencing body parts and on developing an awareness of the body in space. Jack enjoys marching about saying, "My feet are on the ground." She works on a softening through the shoulders and on Jack's forebrain-to-hindbrain connection. Later in the day, Jack says he wants to go to Jack's house, to Mom's house. This is the first time Jack has expressed anything like homesickness or acknowledged a sense of home. Jack wants to cuddle and tell me things. His torso has softened since Martha first worked with him in January. His increased ability to yield and flex the spine has made hugging a lovely part of his repertoire. His gaze is quite clear.

Yield and Push before You Can Reach and Pull

"In spinal movements . . . we develop rolling, establish the horizontal plane, differentiate the front of our bodies from the back of our bodies, and gain the ability to attend."[5] Through embodiment and observation, Bainbridge Cohen has associated movement patterns with specific regions of brain development. Nerve tracts in the spinal cord and brain stem control the spinal push patterns. The Basic Neurological Patterns of push of the head and push of the tail freely move and integrate the head, neck, jaw, spine, and pelvis. The push patterns utilize gravity to make weight shifts and develop the nervous system to record and communicate these changes of weight. Yielding and pushing into gravity provide a strong spring from which a child will unfurl, encouraging the spinal curves to develop in a balanced way. Pushing develops tone to support reaching. Specific, spatially directed vertebral patterns of the spine and limbs emerge from and echo the round, more whole-body experience of earlier, prevertebral patterns. Infant movement development follows an evolutionary progression.

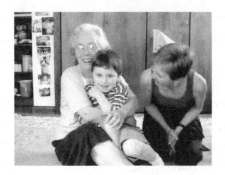

Bonnie Bainbridge Cohen with Jack while Darcy looks on.

Jack had a very prolonged delivery; he finally emerged with the cord wrapped three times around his neck. His head, neck, jaw, spine, and pelvis are tightly held. Martha offers Jack gentle resistance to establish a rocking from head to tail. Motivated by instinct, I have been working with passive manipulation while Jack is sleeping to free his cervical region. I see how Martha uses informed touch to stimulate the expression of a movement pattern that Jack is able to integrate more deeply. She offers a cushy endpoint to his nudging that allows him to find a movement sequence and connection from head to tail and back again. Jack begins to be able to move his head more comfortably up and down and right and left. He enjoys the sensation of Martha's resistance. Jack is not just moving; Jack is doing the moving. He is present, engaged and active. This change is remarkable.

Look before You Leap

In Bainbridge Cohen's model, connections through to the colliculi in the midbrain are established with the reach patterns of the head and tail. In infancy the reach of head and tail are reflexively connected to the senses for the purposes of taking in food and eliminating. Activities, such as nursing, that occur in a parasympathetic posture of increased flexion and lying in prone while experiencing gravity acting on the body (tonic lab reflex) tone the front of the body, supporting the further reach of the head and tail so that the senses can be directed in space.

Jack's perceptions and movement seem to be suspended in space. Martha supports Jack so that he can experience weight falling through his center of gravity and stimulates the sense of connection between his limbs and his center. He slowly begins to sense that he can use his center of gravity as a launching pad and support his senses by reaching his tail to make level changes. He becomes more aware of himself as an entity, moving and changing position in space. Martha is adept at helping Jack follow his curiosity and take in information without losing touch with who he is.

I see the importance of the place where a child developmentally links yielding and pushing to reaching and pulling, even at this basic spinal level. In the space between these actions, Jack begins to link the ability to attend to self and the ability to attend to the world. Rather than experience the world as a barrage of stimuli that he must defend himself from, he gradually begins to have the experience of himself acting on the world in a pleasurable way. He is linking sensory and motor acts in a new way. The cycle of yield and push, then reach and pull, is repeated in the progression through homologous movement (of two arms or two legs), homolateral movement (of the arm and leg on the same side), and contralateral movement (of the arm and leg on opposite sides).

Oakland, October 18, 1999

Martha holds Jack and helps him to reach with his head and eyes, taking clothes pins off a clothesline. She puts him down and encourages him to push with his legs while maintaining the reach of the gaze and the arm.

Baby Push-Ups—Upper before Lower
(and How About Those Elbows?)

"In homologous movements we develop symmetrical movements ... [we] differentiate the upper part of our bodies from the lower part of our bodies and gain the ability to act."[6]

As a toddler, Jack looked like a little linebacker—he held his arms up and close to the body. His arms seemed passive, like they didn't belong to him. His little baby fists couldn't open and take weight. His fine motor skills seemed to develop without gross-motor support. Pushing with the arms connects the arms to the back and feeds pushing with the legs.

Bainbridge Cohen's experiential research indicates that the medulla (part of the spinal cord) activates the upper extremity push, and the inferior peduncles (part of the cerebellum) activate the homologous push from the lower extremities that straightens the elbows and takes the vision to the horizon. Bainbridge Cohen says that all of the autistic children she has worked with skip the pattern of pushing with two legs. When they change levels from the belly to creeping, they flex at the hips before fully straightening the elbows, leaving them collapsed in the thoracic region and with the gaze still inward.

Martha has helped Jack to find his comfort lying on his belly, and he now has some sense that his arms and legs belong to him. She reminds him through touch and movement to feel the weight of his arms, pelvis, and legs to accomplish whatever he is attempting. She reminds him playfully of the early reflexes of flexor withdrawal and extensor thrust that support his volitional movement in the homologous push patterns. She reminds him of a centered place of rest and flexion to push out from.

Oakland, October 19, 1999

Again we work on the connection from the ground through the spine to the arms. Martha brings softness to Jack's belly and diaphragm. She works on maintaining flexion or getting up without overarching the spine. They play with brachiation patterns, hanging from the arms, and maintaining elongation through the cervical spine. They find yielding and recuperation.

Oakland, October 29, 1999

Jack is playing on the floor. He softens and allows—almost invites—Martha's touch now. He works through a head-push pattern (a birth pattern) while Martha offers support and gentle resistance. A common theme of Jack's when upset is "I'm stuck." Martha helps Jack to find the proprioception in the hip joints to push himself through with his legs. They work through the push patterns to connect the head to the spine and the limbs to the spine.

The Cloverleaf for Beginning Drivers: Homolateral Movement

In Bainbridge Cohen's model, as a baby begins to push with one arm and then another, he has moved from the cerebellum to the pons and is scanning across the pons. This weight shift allows a lovely lateral flexion in the spine and enough support through one side of the body to reach the gaze and the opposite arm toward a desired person or object. Sequencing the push of one arm and then the other takes the baby in circles or backward in space.

As weight shift and lateral flexion increase, the child is able to push with one leg at a time to move forward toward his desire. Bainbridge Cohen's research indicates that this homolateral push of the lower extremity tracks from the cerebellum forward to the pons of the same side, sweeps across the pons away from the midline, and loops back through the center of the cloverleaf, to the cerebellum on the opposite side. (If I draw this pattern starting in the center of the cloverleaf, the pattern renders diagonally intersecting figure eights.) With this movement, we begin to match our desire to what is available, and we "gain the ability to intend."[7]

The homolateral pattern is supported by ATNR (asymmetrical tonic neck reflex) and hand-to-mouth reflex. In this reflex pattern, when an infant turns her head to one side, the limbs on that side will extend (ATNR) or flex (hand-to-mouth reflex). Bette Lamont advises the stimulation and integration of these reflexes when children present with developmental delays and learning disabilities.

Maps of Perception and Movement from Neurodevelopmental Therapy

When Jack is four and a half we meet with Bette Lamont in Seattle for three appointments about a month apart. Lamont typically performs a thorough assessment of motor and sensory development, which includes mobility, language and manual competence, and visual, auditory, and tactile competence. Her testing of Jack reveals poor eye convergence, poor visual and auditory filtering skills, and hypersensitivity to touch. She observes poor midline awareness and a distortion of information across the corpus callosum (the membrane that separates the two halves of the brain), which she feels also leads to excessive impulsivity and learning difficulties. We discuss Jack's under- and oversensitivity to pain, heat, and cold. Bette feels that if these vital sensations are mute, we cannot bridge to the world. Motor indicators observed are wide base, toddler-like walking, toes turned in with some pronation of the right foot, impaired cortical opposition, and limited supination/pronation of the forearm.

Seattle, February 21, 2000

Bette clearly explains to me the sensory/motor basis for the specific delays in Jack and develops a program to follow routinely to treat these central nervous system problems at the level of the nervous system. The activities of crawling on the belly, creeping on all fours, ATNR, vestibular stimulation followed by bonding and cuddling, and oral stimulation all promote pons, cerebellum, and mid-brain maturity.

My kitchen at suppertime becomes the scene of Jack crawling over Mom and Dad and his two brothers. Jack's brothers egg him on in belly races and lure him with toys while I interrupt his preferred pattern of lifting his butt and only pushing with one leg. Pons and cerebellum

Homolateral belly crawling is hard for Jack. He is beginning to find the ability to soften into a C-curve of flexion, but the full emergence of his lumbar curve and hip extension will take time. The sacrum and coccyx at the back of the pelvis are key to mobilizing weight transference through the legs. Jack is rigid and held in this area. It is important to follow Jack's motivational cues and support his comfort while encouraging this pattern. Anything forced makes him feel out of control and brings up more resistance. Martha has shown me the importance of relationship in repatterning.

stimulation bring out a more emotional and demanding Jack. His anxiety is expressed in tantrums but his autistic meltdowns are few. I feel this is a necessary stage in his developing an emotional self and the potential to be in relationship. I am willing to open up those parts of Jack that are taxing to deal with. Jack is responding verbally to sensations of too hot, too cold, and hunger, and he is sharing his gaze in bonding and cuddling. Jack has also gained more tolerance for vestibular stimulation, such as rocking, swinging, and playing on his tummy on a gym ball.

Seattle, April 21, 2000

When Jack becomes anxious, Bette notices that his voice is very much like a birth cry in maturity. His common expression when anxious is "I'm stuck, help." Bette teaches me her version of the birth reflex patterns. Jack's crawling has improved, but he still has difficulty pushing with his right leg and foot. He still does not open his hands on the floor. Bette feels this inability to release is apparent in children with bonding difficulties.

Jack's dad, the actor, supports his language development. Jack's brothers take on his T-ball and basketball training and help Jack to be a kid, to joke and be sneaky. For an autistic child, learning to be devious is a celebrated milestone. My hands are learning to support and tone Jack's tissues. It becomes routine to work hands-on with Jack after cuddling him to sleep.

I study BMC, Laban, craniosacral therapy, and massage therapy. In June of 2000, Jack and I have the opportunity to venture to Massachusetts, to complete my somatic movement therapy training. Martha Eddy recommends that Jack and I see Bonnie Bainbridge Cohen.

We meet with Bonnie for a series of seven sessions. Jack's dad flies down to join us. Bonnie takes us deeper into the relationship between the body systems and developmental movement.

Multitasking and Patience

With the underlying push patterns in place and the head-tail reach active, a typically developing baby can reach the upper limbs in a given direction and push off. For this movement the baby returns to the cerebellum, specifically to the mid-cerebellar peduncles. If a baby has mastered the push of the arms, he can also use the reach pattern of the legs to locomote backward or to change levels by employing the superior cerebellar peduncles. This baby is already multitasking better than any Macintosh computer. There is a sophisticated level of sensory-motor integration and a concept of self and other present, as well as the beginnings of integrating social and emotional growth with sensory-motor systems.

Jack's nervous system is making connections too, but his development is still scattered. Now almost five, he can read at a third-grade level but has only recently mastered toilet training. His vocabulary is immense but social interaction is still overwhelming. New environments and making transitions tax Jack. Fortunately, he is a bundle of energy and curiosity and, despite his limitations, is highly motivated to explore.

Jack was introduced to gravity later than most children. His righting reactions and equilibrium responses that support reaching into space are still emerging. These are reflexive responses to moving off balance. As these responses emerge, Jack begins to feel more secure and confident moving through space. The playground offers opportunities to climb, slide, yield, push, reach, and pull. In the Canadian winter months my house becomes the playground, with gym balls in several rooms. Jumping, wrestling, ball throwing, and being on the floor are encouraged.

When working outside the window of opportunity afforded by the time frame of typical development, movement patterns integrate more slowly, and neurological success is more incremental. Bainbridge Cohen is expert at "following the child" and senses where Jack needs more foundational support to emerge. Jack is very comfortable with Bonnie. They play with various toys, the only rule being that he has to put one away before he gets another out. Bainbridge Cohen works through touch to balance his autonomic nervous system. She invites him to open his grasp and to carry his center over his legs. She also works hands-on with me to balance my autonomic system so that I can model this state of being for Jack.

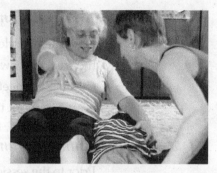

Bonnie Bainbridge Cohen and Jack wrestle and play.

Amherst, June 6, 2000

Bonnie Bainbridge Cohen's notes: "Jack is clearly an exceptionally bright child who needs help discovering himself and how to relate to others and move through the world. He and his mother related in an emotionally bonded and loving manner. This requires an unusual amount of trust for Jack, due to his disorientation in relation to himself and others. He also tried very hard to cooperate and trust me, even when he was experiencing great anxiety and emotional distress

After the session, I observe that Jack is softer and more comfortable. He offers hugs and his gaze is clear.

Bainbridge Cohen shows us how to help Jack by meeting him where he is without escalating his anxiety, so that he can experience working through things. Between sessions I notice more facial expression and eye contact to get my attention. Jack shows more ease with new situations. He responds emotionally and with an awareness of danger when I get upset with him about running ahead of us through the woods. Until this time he had not been able to understand this kind of cue.

Jack is more relaxed. A rhythm of play and rest starts to emerge. I notice more weight-sensing in his body. His back-and-forth conversation is clearer and more sustained. In a restaurant at lunch after one session, he spontaneously displays his feelings with lots of hugs and kisses. When we go to the beach for the weekend, Jack is very cautious and afraid for his dad, Trevor, when Trevor goes for a swim.

Amherst, June 9, 2000

Jack is less settled and focused. We are transitioning to go home from the weekend away. Jack tantrums about putting toys away at Bonnie's studio. She meets him where he is, without escalating his tantrum. He is able to work through and own his feelings without falling apart.

Amherst, June 12, 2000

Prior to the session, Jack's dad leaves to return to Canada. Jack expresses to me, "My heart is sad and I am mad," "Dad is lost," "Dad is disappeared," and he tries to hide and "wait to be found." Bainbridge Cohen's report describes her work with him:

> "Jack's sympathetic tone was heightened. After playing with a train he refused to put it away and went to get another toy. As previously, I then held him gently but firmly as he struggled and, hysterical, screamed 'I'm stuck, help me, let me go, please,' over and over. I, in turn, continued to respond by saying that he had a choice—he could cry, he could scream, he could be angry, he could be afraid, he could be stuck—but, when he wanted, he could put the train away and be unstuck and get down for another toy. While I still held him he picked up pieces of the train and scattered and threw them. At the height of his rage, he pushed up from the floor with extended elbows without flexing his hips first: a major neurological breakthrough. As the end of the session came I told him that it was time to go, that his mom and I would help him put the train away and he could borrow a bat, a ball, and T-ball stand to take home that night. When everything was put away he took the ball and bat and quietly walked out, calmly saying, 'Thank you, Bonnie.' And 'Good-bye.'"

After the session I sense the profundity of what Jack has just worked through. We are both tired and more at ease with one another.

Contralateral Movement

As Jack runs joyfully down a mountainside at full tilt in June of 2000, I see him reflexively move into a contralateral pattern, arms swinging, legs pumping, and I know a door has opened to the future possibility of mastering this pattern on level terrain. Creeping forward is initiated by reaching with one arm, and the ease of this pattern includes and depends on all previous patterns. We yield, we push off, and we reach and pull. Bainbridge Cohen postulates that the upper contralateral reach comes from the thalamus. In creeping, the child brings the limbs underneath midline.

In changing levels to standing, a typical infant uses a brachiation pattern, reaching and pulling with the arm while yielding and pushing with the leg. Bainbridge Cohen postulates that the tracks that support this pattern radiate from the thalamus through the basal ganglia. The infant practices a homolateral cruising pattern, usually side-stepping while holding on to furniture, taking neural development from the internal capsules of the ancient forebrain to the limits of the ancient forebrain. When a contralateral walk emerges, neurological connections are supported through the corona and radiate to the cortex. In contralateral movements we "gain the ability to integrate our attention, intention, and actions."

Amherst, June 13, 2000

Bonnie and Jack play on big riding cars. Jack is pushing well with his legs in a chase game. Bonnie follows, pushing her car, varying time and spatial direction. Jack begins to play with the surprise of confrontation and crashing and chasing her. He has no problem stopping, starting, anticipating, and changing direction. He later tantrums about putting a toy away. Bonnie holds him as he struggles and throws toys, but he doesn't say, "I'm stuck." Instead he says, "No, no way."

Bonnie writes about what transpires: "Jack then went through my arms as in a birthing movement out of my arms, extending his arms over his head and releasing his low brain/neck and atlanto-occipital joint, cerebellum, and pons."

Witnessing this is profound. I again understand the importance of not forcing or bringing up resistance, but meeting Jack where he is.

I hold a question: What supports relationship? I ask this question to determine where relationship is interrupted in autism.

Jack and I return to Amherst in the summer of 2001, 2002, and 2003 for my classes at The School for Body-Mind Centering and for his sessions with Bonnie, Lenore Grubinger, and Saliq Francis Savage. Between visits I work with Jack as both mom and therapist, finding the subtleties of the work that are shared with me. I bring the work into my teaching and choreography. We lure Martha Eddy to Canada to teach and do sessions.

The themes of development are overlapping, attesting to an agenda that emphasizes relationship. I begin to see that the emergence of autonomy is necessary for relationship, and that relationship is necessary for the emergence of autonomy.

An understanding of the Basic Neurological Patterns of movement endemic to the developmental process is valuable to anyone working with special-needs children. Jack has taught me a lot. This knowledge is even more valuable to those who daily see and work with young infants. Traditional milestones of movement are constellations of many incremental patterns. When we see the stars in the constellations and each nova of development, we are closer to helping children like Jack with more timely interventions.

With the support of an aide, Jack attends third grade at a school for gifted children. His abilities to tolerate change and to make transitions are greatly improved. He is beginning to negotiate the split between fantasy and reality, and he doesn't always like that he can't just invent reality. I watch Jack play with his dinosaurs. He crawls across the floor in a lovely contralateral pattern. He is linking the encyclopedia of dinosaur facts he has stored in his cortex to his remarkable creative abilities and, more importantly, to his own vitality and experience.

I have (exponentially) what I prayed for in those initial sessions with Martha. Jack can talk incessantly; he loves to argue, and with probing he will relate the complexities of third-grade social dynamics as he sees them. He has a few friends and a rival, who is teaching Jack about competition. Laura is very kind—not a very good speller, but that's okay. Jenni has three pet turtles, two tadpoles, and a leopard frog. Her mom works at the zoo. Tommy is always doing everything wrong. (He always beats Jack in foot races.)

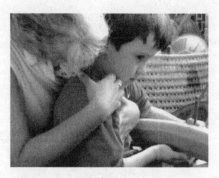

Bonnie Bainbridge Cohen and Jack.

Jack is becoming ever more aware of the people who constellate his world, as his interests shift from the ether to more earthly matters. Four years ago, when we first met with Martha, my one wish for Jack was that he could express his experience. I now encourage him to trust and empathize with others.

Twelve Visits to a BMC Playroom (excerpt)

~ **Lenore Grubinger,** USA (2000)

[Pseudonyms are used throughout.]

David Goldberg is a bright three-year-old boy who had a very difficult birth and severe health challenges at the start of his life. He spent his first twenty-seven days in the hospital. David and his parents initially came to my practice for families, based in Body-Mind Centering, in July 1999 when David was twenty-one months old. Other early-intervention providers had assessed him as "delayed," "uncooperative," and "possibly ADHD." He was one of the speediest, high-motor toddlers I had met. He registered so little sensation that, as he moved constantly— careening through space, falling often, and throwing things—he noticed almost none of the consequences of his actions. His warm nature and lust for life were evident, yet disorganization and discomfort were predominant in results of his efforts.

In the couple of years since we met, David has become significantly more organized and more comfortable. This is an informal report of the Body-Mind Centering part of his journey over that time, applied in my office through developmental movement therapy, and at home by his parents through specific touch practice, handling and care practice, and an enriched environment with suggested toys and play. Including his initial visit, David had ten visits over the course of six months, and his mothers had two sessions without him present. Following is an informal report of six of those visits.

(1)

7/12/99 RE: David Goldberg—Date of Birth: 10/10/97

David was twenty-one months old at the time of his initial visit. A local Western Massachusetts pediatrician referred David's parents to Bonnie Bainbridge Cohen, OTR, for Body-Mind Centering. Ms. Bainbridge Cohen, in turn, referred them to my practice.

David's Birth Health, Described by His Parents

David was one week late and stopped moving *in utero*. He was born by Cesarean section. He had a seizure right after birth. He was put on a respirator, receiving one hundred percent oxygen. He had very low blood sugar, low blood pressure, brain bleeds, and a liver infection. He was in the neonatal intensive care unit (NICU) for twenty-seven days.

Concerns Initially Listed by David's Parents

Arching back; occasional fevers; low tone; bowleggedness; bad eyes; stumbling; overactive; slurred and delayed speech; shy at times; biting/pinching; not listening; fighting diaper changes; not cuddly; limited and frequently interrupted sleep.

Initial Assessment

- Overall, David has achieved verticality and walking, yet his physiological flexion is profoundly weak as an underlying support. Concomitantly, his navel yielding response is also weak.
- Developmentally, David did not learn any homolateral push patterns from his arms or his legs. He found a way to pull to standing from sitting, then learned to walk forward. He did only a small amount of homolateral movements in cruising, and only to the right. His feet are inwardly rotated from his birth position and the lack of homolateral movement at the time the brain and body are expectant for it.
- Muscularly, David has low flexor tone and high extensor tone, throughout his body, particularly in his trunk.

- Structurally, he has extensor compression of the cervical and lumbar regions. His tibias are noticeably bowed.
- Organically, his digestive tube is low-toned, his liver and kidneys are pulled superiorly and right-rotated, and the motility of his esophagus is mildly reversed.
- Attentively, he does not align his body and his attention together at his midline. He is highly multi-focused, and moves from activity to activity at rapid-fire speed.
- Visually, he rarely focuses both his eyes forward for bilateral vision. His left eye is rotated to the left and appears to provide very little visual information to his brain. His right eye appears fully functioning. Testing is recommended.
- Auditorally, his hearing appears normal. Again, testing is recommended.
- Enterically, the lining of David's digestive tube appears irritated and mal-absorptive. Some of his frequent irritation and unfocused behavior appears initiated in his enteric nervous system.
- Autonomically, his sympathetic nervous system is over-active and his parasympathetic nervous system is under-active. He exhibits behaviors characteristic of someone chronically sleep-deprived. His appetite is described as small and very limited in range. He is lean for his age. He drinks copious amounts of water, asking repeatedly to have his bottle refilled. He often clamps down on the nipple of the bottle with his teeth and keeps it swinging there from his mouth as he moves about.
- Somatically, he is highly active in his motor nerves and dull in his sensory nerves. He is barely receiving sensory feedback of the consequences of his own motions, and much of the little feedback he does receive he is not processing, and therefore he does not respond to it. David often throws things, almost always over his head and behind himself, arching himself back with his extensors as he throws. People have to protect their head when playing with David.
- Reflexively, David's Moro reflex is unintegrated, activating often in

his movement. The asymmetrical tonic neck reflex (ATNR) and the hand-to-mouth reflex on the right side are over-active, and the left side under-active. This affects his postural tone in that he is markedly right-rotated from the head. This both causes and is caused by the weakness of his left eye, which also causes him to feel oriented in his head when it is right of midline. He has a rigid preference for holding his bottle in his right hand and turning his head and mouth to meet it, again causing and caused by the unintegrated ATNR and hand-to-mouth on the right side and the right-eye dominance.

- Verbally, he speaks only a few intelligible words, such as "pig" and "moo." He makes a few communicative repetitive sounds. The tone of his mouth is low; he drools easily.

- Behaviorally, he plays with driven intensity. He does smile, infrequently. He often does not respond to what someone says to him when he is engaged in an activity, although he appears to hear. He can respond if the timing of the remark is lined up with the flow of his attention.

- Musically, David immediately responds joyfully and kinesthetically to both recorded music and musical instruments.

- Sensorily and emotionally, David is bonded with his parents, whom he looks at and listens to. David is tactile-defensive, tolerating little touch initiated toward him, yet he will "touch-in" to his mothers' bodies at his own initiative for fleeting contact while he plays. He almost always makes physical contact with the back surface of his body rather than the front. He fusses, kicks, and tries to get away when placed on his back for a diaper change.

Initial Conclusions

Most characteristic of David is his absolute lust for life. He is a bundle of physical energy and curiosity. He is a warm boy who tries to connect with others despite his significant challenges. David has physiological and structural weaknesses that he was born with, and those he acquired from early stress, from side effects of his medications, recovery from procedures, and reflex imbalances and delays due to hospital position-ing. This large set of challenges invariably leads to high extensor tone, which is manifest in what has been described above.

David falls often, sometimes constantly, while he is moving about the playroom, and always to the side or the back, always in a pathway of extensor tone, never around his own center with the navel yielding reflex. Usually he moves sideways, not forward, even when his atten-tion is directed toward an object or activity in front of him.

To express most emotions, whether joy or stress, or simply in response to the pleasure of moving, David throws his head back. He does this with great intensity, usually falling without showing any pro-tective extension responses sideward or backward. He does have some occasional protective extension responses forward. In sitting or stand-ing, he holds his arms at rest posterior to the lateral line of his body.

His sensory nervous system is dull; David can "dismantle" a room in minutes but does not register that he has done so. Sometimes he seems to be trying to create sensations so he can experience them. This is paradoxically difficult for him because he fears even the slightest feeling of being physically trapped or restricted, yet he craves com-pression and bumps into everything in an attempt to get it.

Some of David's organs seem stressed, indicated structurally and digestively and by his tremendous thirst. His request for the bottle is to some degree an ordinary effort to self-comfort, yet it is so frequent as to perhaps reflect some imbalances he may have been born with and/or sustained due to high doses of antibiotics and other medications as a neonate.

Initial Recommendations

- Provide compression in flexion. Work with the physical and psy-chological dynamics of compression, recognizing how much David has "patterned" the adults around him not to touch him.
- Support David's parasympathetic tone, helping to direct the activity of his esophagus downward and toward gravity.

- Help David with navel yielding. This includes compression, with a specific focus on the front and middle of his body in relation to gravity.

- Cultivate David's sense of his midline through touch and play. Kiss his forehead, nose, mouth, and belly button. When handing him toys, be sure to do so below his eyes to his midline, to encourage the coordination of flexion with midline. Play games of moving toys, touch, and sound up and down the "zipper," or midline of his body, from forehead, nose, and mouth to sternum, navel, belly, and pubic bone.

- Lower your own sympathetic tone, your goal-oriented self, when playing with David. Embody a quality that can serve as a guide and model to help him lower his high sympathetic tone. Find your "here and now," parasympathetic self. Find your enjoyment of your child in the present, if possible. Become aware of your digestion, and release any tension you notice if you can. Remember that your body is in a gravitational field, and let yourself soften into the Earth a bit. Imagine your body organized around your navel. Find your midline, or "zipper." In your own way, feel the parental love in your heart and mind, and in your tissues as well.

- Provide play that involves using both hands at the same time to help David organize his gross motor play bilaterally. Try using a large ball. Help him relate his eyes with his hands. Again, explore embodying this yourself as you encourage it in him.

- Hand David his bottle and offer him toys to his left hand, the one he rarely uses to reach and grasp with. Twice a day, when you have his attention, offer something to his left hand while quickly and gently inhibiting his right arm. Do not force. Trying this is more important than if it "works."

- Verbally ask and articulate what David is doing, and what he has done after he has done it, to help him process his sensations. "David is riding the truck." "Did you throw the ball?" "You threw the ball!" "The ball you threw landed right here." "Where is the ball?" "Did it leave your hand?" "You are making the ball fly through the air!"

- In play, act out various animals and encourage him to do the same. Have some books and if possible hang some pictures of animals moving homologously, homolaterally, and contralaterally. Imitate them and let some games develop. Any game that gets David enjoying himself moving on his belly or on all fours is good for him, as it is never too late to activate the reflexes that support these positions, which improves body tone and posture overall. Lizard movements are a natural approach to stimulating better alignment in the ankle and foreleg, and the movement enhances the efficacy of shoe supports, splints, should his parents later choose to try these.

The above principles were discussed and practices explored in response to David's needs and activities during the session. David was able to sit and play with one toy, with adult involvement, for several minutes—something his mothers said he "never" did—while I did hands-on facilitation with his nervous system, digestive system, and muscle tone. Of all the above approaches, it was particularly the "mind" of the parasympathetic system, combined with compression and flexion, that brought David to a quiet, focused state.

(2)
7/20/99, Session with David's Parents, Angela and Becca

Following the initial visit, David's parents, Angela and Becca, had a session without him. At my recommendation they brought photos of David's life to date. There were pictures of his stay in the NICU, which helped them reflect on what they have all been through, and helped me to explain how deeply impacted he was by this experience and to point out a few of the "roots" of some of his current challenges.

We discussed Becca's and Angela's application of the suggestions from the initial visit. We reviewed those suggestions, and their successes and discouragement with them. We reviewed the organizational

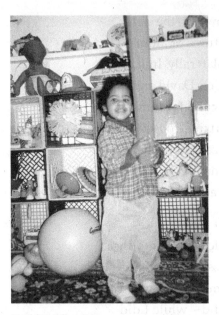

David Goldberg, at age twenty-eight months.

principles and practiced the techniques to apply at home.

I also recommended that David's parents do some lay research on probiotic supplementation, and suggested they speak to a professional nutritionist to whom I regularly refer families. I have seen several other children with post-antibiotic digestive irritation improve with a course of this supplementation. I asked them to let me know what they learn, and to keep careful records when they start this or any other medication or supplementation, of the products, the amount used, the results, and to bring this next time.

Supporting and modeling parasympathetic function for parents of a child who is intensely active during the day and sleeps little, with much need for attention during the night, can be difficult, sad, and ironic. David's parents have been far away from optimal states in their own rest and parasympathetic systems since David was born, due to high stress and ongoing sleep deprivation. Intellectual, physical, and emotional exploration was needed for them to learn about their own autonomic nervous systems, in order to support their confidence to help their son's parasympathetic/sympathetic balance.

(3)

10/16/99, Summary of David's Sessions (Five in All) Since His Initial Visit in July

Over the late summer and early fall, David made steady, noticeable progress. These five sessions built on the initial visit. As usual, I applied healing-touch techniques during play with David, and didactic and experiential work with his parents to help David increase:

• Parasympathetic rest, recuperation, and nourishment

- Navel yielding response
- Flexor tone of organs and muscles
- Bilateral use of arms and legs around midline
- Feedback between mouth, nose, eyes, ears, and the brain
- Tactile bonding in extension and flexion positions

I emphasized David's tremendous need for compression.

The gains from this were apparent. David's flexor tone and digestive organ tone improved; and overall, the relationship between his flexor and extensor muscle tone became more balanced. This was reflected in his play, which became more organized. His attention and visual focusing improved and his speech progressed. He more often chose bilateral, midline physical play with the objects in my playroom. While David remains a fast, busy, demanding child, his gains in organization and communication, as well as minor improvement in his sleep habits, and increased tolerance of diaper changing, allow family life to be a little less exhausting and more pleasurable.

David's sensory nervous system is continuing to myelinate. He is receiving more feedback from his own actions and the environment. He is still not processing the feedback well, in the sense that he does not use the information readily to inform his choices. This is a difficult phase in his healing because while his sensory processing is increased, his ability to respond to that increase is not yet skillful. We are still using touch, play, and verbal cueing to help him receive, process, and respond to his sensory experiences.

David continues to be more expressive in his sympathetic than his parasympathetic nervous system, which is manifest in part through his rapid multi-focused attention. We worked on helping David "stretch" whatever interest he is having, even if only for seconds or minutes longer. This is a clear way that adults can participate in David's play to help him.

David's less-than-optimal sensory processing and his underactive parasympathetic system are exacerbated by and exacerbating to his weak left eye. Because he does not make visual transitions well, he can be easily distracted when he is focusing or can easily lose his original intention when he is on his way from one activity to the next. We are working with this through visual tracking within play and through hands-on work.

I taught his parents a touch technique to gently support the function of the nerves of David's eyes. This is generally easiest to apply when he is playing with another person or involved with a toy on his own. The facilitating person's hands are placed as surreptitiously as possible on David's head, one near the eye and one near the back of the head on the same side as the eye. This stimulates the nerve fibers between the eye itself and the midbrain region, where the cell bodies for the visual nerves are located. Because some of these nerves go straight back while others cross the midbrain to the other side of the head, it is recommended to do this touch on each side of the head and then across, in an X, also on both sides. This technique can also be done when David is sleeping, if necessary, even with hands off the head but held very near, to affect the nerves without waking him.

David enjoys spinning himself, which he always does to his right. I recommended playing "spin" with him, first in his preferred direction to the right, and then spinning him to his left. When picking him up, bend his body first in the direction it goes most easily, and then gently bend him in the opposite direction. By doing this his spine can experience lateral curving, initiated by his head, in both directions. We focused on David's bowed legs, particularly his tibias. During each session, I did some hands-on bodywork with David's bones while he was playing, to lengthen and straighten the bones. He seems to like this work and will tolerate up to ten minutes of focused touch, often twice in one session. I have taught this type of touch to his parents and recommended that they practice it with David every day.

I recommended last time that they try a tricycle. Angela said she found one at a yard sale and reported that David really loves riding it in the house. The tricycle encourages the combined use of his muscular vitality with bilateral visual focusing, and simultaneous weight bearing into both his arms around midline. It is also potentially advantageous to the straightening of his tibias through compression into the compact bone while pedaling.

(4)
10/27/99, Observations Since Beginning to Work with David (Eight Visits Total to Date)

- David shows remarkable improvement today. He is at his organizational and communicative best since we started working together. I am delighted for him and his family. Overall his challenges are the same, yet subtler.
- David's vocabulary has increased twofold. He is now sounding the consonants b, k, m, and s. His other consonants are taking shape. He occasionally utters full sentences with meaningful intonation, although sometimes only a few of the words are decipherable. I recommended imitating the sound and rhythm of David's speech to engage him in "conversation."
- David's play is far more focused and occurs mostly in midline. He can now play for extended periods. Today he maintained the longest self-initiated focus since we began therapy—over twenty minutes. I worked with his mother and the family childcare provider while he played next to us in the playroom. He has begun to talk to himself while he plays, which is often a sign of feeling comfortable in one's organs.
- When David holds a book, he combines seeing and moving in such a way as to be "reading."
- David's sensory pathways receive more. He can take in far more information and processes more of the information that he takes in. His metabolic and motor rhythm speed is still much faster than average.
- David's left eye occasionally organizes with his right eye. His left eye functions in a limited way. Further bodywork to apply at home

for his eye was demonstrated and practiced. (David's parents pursue care for his vision with another provider, and I have not yet seen that report.)

- When David throws a ball backward over his head, his notice of what he has done and where the ball goes is significantly increased. His sensory pathways are continuing to heal and develop.
- David now has some fine motor activity in his play, whereas he had almost none when we met. At his own initiative, he successfully put basic puzzle pieces in their correct places without any difficulty or stress.
- At his most recent visit David sat in my lap of his own accord, for the first time. This compares with the first visit, when I was able to hold him near for a few seconds before he pushed away.
- David now shows an associated reaction in his left hand and in his mouth, as he is refining his fine motor abilities.

(5)

11/18/99, Progress Report

David is not doing as well today as his last appointment. He is "speeded up," moving recklessly about the playroom, dispersing most of the objects quickly, as he used to do often.

His parents and I discuss some contributing factors for his setback. He has grown a lot lately; he seems to be coming down with something; and he has still not adjusted to daylight savings time, so his sleep has been disturbed for three weeks.

We review the approaches we've been employing since we started, particularly the value of using one's own tone to help David with his tone. We practiced this while David played with a large plastic circle. Slowly and gently we sat closer to him to "contain" him with our bodies and our intention, while still giving him a lot of physical space and without changing quickly or intensely, so that he wouldn't feel trapped. He stepped inside the circle and enjoyed the combination of physical control that he maintained along with the support he got from us. He calmed down and got involved in some focused play, the first since he entered the office.

(6)

12/2/99, Summary and Recommendations

David has continued to proceed in a "two steps forward, one step back" rhythm. Some of this can be attributed to the energy needed to heal. That energy comes from the parasympathetic system. David's parasympathetic stores are low to begin with and are further depleted because he sleeps little and is digestively stressed. When he makes progress by using new neurological connections, David uses parasympathetic energy. This can mean that sometimes after a burst of improvement, he may be tired and poorly focused. This can appear to be regression. It's important to take the long-term perspective with David by understanding that lows, which come after a period of improvement, may actually be a time of parasympathetic rebuilding. It is also true that when he gets over-stimulated he behaves in older, more basic ways.

David can still get easily agitated and become multi-focused. Yet he and his parents have many more tools for rest and restoration. At times David cannot comply with his parents or other adults. As a newborn he learned to shut out the sensations he found intolerable. He is slowly repatterning this early survival response. I observe that he wants to participate and tries, sometimes without succeeding. His overall sense of satisfaction is likely lower than average. David's parents will be speaking with their pediatrician about possible next steps in medication.

Music is an area where David has shown some of the greatest satisfaction, and I strongly recommended building on this. A toddler music class without too much structure would be ideal. It would be optimal if the instructor were open to David's parents' recommendations as to how to help him focus, including knowledge that forcing David disrupts his focus. The teacher would need to be able to let

David's focus wander briefly at times, for his recuperation. Psychologically, David is becoming accustomed to being admonished for his physical actions. Music is an area where he stands to receive praise and hence a positive sense of himself.

Recalling how profoundly life-challenged David was at birth, and how he was further challenged by the aspects of the medicine and procedures that saved his life, can still be painful for Angela and Becca. And it is still hard for David at times to tolerate and process sensation. Yet it is through identification and interaction with David's challenges, with support for him and his parents, that he can heal neurological function and gain new abilities and more satisfying choices.

David has momentum in his healing. The elements of his healing process, such as the balance of flexor and extensor muscle tone, the function of his digestive tube, the feedback loop between his sensory and motor nerves, and visual convergence in midline, are all progressed enough so as to be mutually reinforcing. His mothers are much less anxious and far more confident in their understanding of how to help David. This is good for the whole family—back to the principle of a fuller parasympathetic foundation for all of them.

David's case is a testimony to the efficacy and cost-effectiveness of Body-Mind Centering. It did not require many sessions, nor cost much relative to his other health expenses, for this troubled boy to become dramatically healthier and for his parents to feel more positive and productively informed about life with their son. While David is unique, as is every child, the progression of his case is typical in my practice. A series of approximately four to twelve sessions, over several weeks or months, may provide marked enhancement of a child's developmental potential and well-being.

Playing Toward Healing: A Child-Parent Journey with Lyme Disease

~ **Gill Wright Miller**, USA (2001)

A Fire Island Drive

Some of the most pleasant memories I have of raising my four children center on time spent in an idyllic summer community on Fire Island, fifty miles due east of New York City. Every year since the late 1970s, I have taken my boys to the water for the summer. Water seems to have been borne into my psyche—perhaps out of need: I was raised in the middle of Ohio,

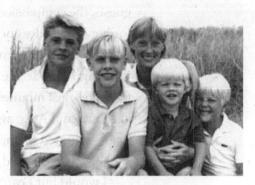

As an academic mother, I was able to take my boys to Fire Island every summer, where we reorganized around food, friends, and relationships.

where there is no water. I find myself "collecting" when I am near water. My fluids unite; they are not separated by content and function—blood, CSF, even discharge. I wanted to share this experience of collecting with my children. Each summer, on Fire Island, in the company of the sounds and smells of the ocean, we changed our patterns of relationship with ease.

I devoted the past twenty years to developing a department of dance with a liberal arts curriculum, experiential anatomy/kinesiology and movement analysis as its theoretical foundation. During the school year, I spent long days and many a night pursuing pedagogic and scholarly interests in the company of students awakening to somatic awareness. In contrast, during the summers at Fire Island my four children had my full attention; we would play, swim, beach, and read together, and I would cook for them as if they were precious company. My children came to anticipate the summers, most of all because the food, the friends, and new acquaintances were welcomed into our home.

Through our time on Fire Island, I developed an appreciation that my children did not interfere with my career, nor did they take me from important matters even in September through May. It was there I learned to offer to my children the generosity scraped together for guests, the compassion afforded close friends, and the respect reserved for honored colleagues.

Extending the summer as long as we could, one fall weekend ten years ago I made the ten-hour drive to Bay Shore, approaching the ferry dock just minutes ahead of the last boat to the island with Stewart, age nine, and Alex, age five, in tow. The children were restless and so I had separated them, putting Alex in the front seat of the car with me.

"Stewart?" I asked, "will you hand Alex a pillow?"

"I would but I can't move my arms," Stewart responded.

I was silently infuriated. We were running late for the ferry. I needed their cooperation to make this work.

"Stewart," I tried again, this time with impactive phrasing, as I carved in and out of traffic on the Southern State Parkway. "Please hand Alex a pillow. Now."

"I can't," he replied calmly.

I adjusted the rearview mirror to watch him defy me. Usually when I look at my children I can tell where their resistance is coming from. Something about their bodies reveals just how I can best meet undesirable behavior. I glanced at Stewart. He looked distorted. I couldn't read him. I left the request hanging in the air.

"When we get to the ferry," I explained to my little helpers, "jump out of the car as fast as you can. Stewart, grab Alex and wait for me by the boat. Do not get on it until I say so. I don't want you going over there without me. I did all the driving; I deserve to go too!" The boys understood my teasing. We all grinned.

Soon we pulled into the parking lot. "Are you guys ready?" I asked. I stepped on the brake, shifted into park, and squealed, "Go!" like a kindergarten teacher, every element of my body enthusiastic for the relay race that was just beginning.

"I can't move my legs," Stewart responded matter-of-factly.

We didn't have time for his game. I turned around to scold him and was shocked by what met me. Stewart looked like he had gained twenty pounds on his short nine-year-old frame. I felt suddenly alone, isolated with a sick child. Levering most of his weight, I rushed the boys onto the boat and sat with Stewart, investigating his body through my grip.

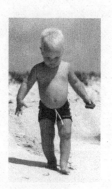

Little Stewart travels the beach at age two.

My mother used to hold me like this. Whenever I was off balance, she touched me. She seemed to travel deep into her recesses, deep into my bone marrow. Her simple action grabbed my attention, and, if we waited the ten seconds it took her breathing to settle into mine, she could diagnose me without effort. By example she taught me to meet my children in that same space—to sit with them and listen to the information transferring from them to me through touch rather than words or vision or intellect.

We arrived at our small Fire Island community thirty-five minutes later. Stewart and Alex climbed into our wagon and I pulled them to a friend's house. "What do you think this is?" I asked her. Person after person insisted I get Stewart to a doctor immediately. One neighbor, a doctor, wanted him life-flighted off the island to the emergency room. "If he continues to swell, it might interfere with his breathing," the doctor told me. What I heard was "He might die."

I looked at Stewart. I took his body into mine cell by cell. I felt mysteriously like Superman affixing his X-ray vision, only through touch rather than sight. "No," I said, "he's not in that kind of danger."

The next morning I took Stewart to the local physician, a volunteer who happened to be weekending in our community. He made several calls, quickly networking us to the Hospital for Special Surgery (HSS) in Manhattan. We ferried off the island and drove to HSS. When we arrived, Doctor Lehman met us and began asking some routine questions.

"What he has," I explained, "is exactly what his brother has. No one seems to know what it is, and the symptoms seem more abrupt and extreme in Stewart, but they have the same energy and exist with the same support in his body." Dr. Lehman scrutinized me thoroughly, giving me a look that revealed I was a Midwest alien. I ignored his look and continued, "If you can figure out what Stewart has, I'd like to have Matthew's pediatrician fax his records over here. Will you look at them too?"

With some reluctance, but because I had been brought to Dr. Lehman through a personal friend, he agreed to take a look. After receiving Matthew's records, he announced, "I can't make a diagnosis without seeing the child and running some tests, but these symptoms look like Lyme disease to me."

Lyme Disease Symptoms

I have heard that, second perhaps only to HIV, Lyme disease is the most terrifying condition prevalent in American society today. First, it is nearly impossible to spot or feel the tiny tick—much smaller than a dog tick— that is carried by deer and rodents, but also on foliage and pets, a tick that can also hide in carpets and curtains. Once attached to a body, deer ticks wander looking for safe havens: folds of the skin like underarms and between toes; dark, moist recesses like waists next to swimsuit waist-bands; and shifts in texture like hairlines at the back of the neck. "Hosts" carry on their daily routines without noticing they are carriers.

Lyme disease is terrifying because it can cause problems in the joints, nervous system, and heart. Lyme disease is terrifying because the medical community does not know how to cure it, only how to contain its symptoms. Lyme disease is terrifying because its symptoms are chameleon-like, shifting and changing within one person as well as from person to person. Further, many people hold the disease at bay for a year or more and then are suddenly compromised by its impulsive presence and vehemence.

One telltale symptom of Lyme disease has developed "rock star" media coverage: a bull's-eye-like rash may develop at the site of the tick bite. When it appears, this rash begins as a pimple-like spot and expands over the next few days into a purplish circle with a deep red rim up to six inches in diameter. Over the next several weeks it may grow as large as twenty inches across. Sometimes concentric rings appear within the original ring. After three or four weeks they may fade. Patients often describe this bull's-eye ring/rash as one that burns rather than itches. Yet this ring is not nearly as common as its absence, and none ever appeared on either of my children.

With or without this visual sign, the early stage of Lyme disease is often accompanied by a few days of flu-like symptoms: fatigue, chills, headache, stiff neck, backaches. Medical journals report that widespread muscle and joint aches, nausea and vomiting, swelling, sore throats, and conjunctivitis may also occur. These, of course, are periodic but common occurrences in some children and may well be dismissed as nothing serious when the symptoms readily resolve.

Weeks later, the child may experience extreme fatigue, prolonged bouts of arthritis, and severe neurological problems. One study indicated that the neurological symptoms most common in children with Lyme disease were non-descript headaches, sleep problems, and mood disturbances. But they could also develop the more alarming Bell's palsy, serious pain, or sensations of pricking, creeping, crawling skin; mental abnormalities; breathing difficulties; and kidney problems. Ultimately, Lyme disease has been held responsible for sensitivity to light, meningitis-like symptoms, seizures, or even comas. In one study of Lyme children, arthritic symptoms developed on an average of four full months after the disease had been diagnosed, indicating that earlier treatment had not halted it but rather allowed it to progress to a more advanced stage.

Living Unwittingly with Lyme

I don't recall whether or not, early on, my children had experienced the simpler flu-like symptoms. By the time I was alarmed, Matthew and Stewart were experiencing the appearance of severe joint swelling and pain in asymmetrically distributed joints. Matthew's symptoms first appeared one night when he and his next younger brother, Chris, were visiting their grandmother, the mother of their estranged father. The boys were never happy about going there, feeling somehow abandoned by and separated from their younger two brothers, who were of a different father. Matthew's form of objecting to visiting his father's family almost always appeared as illness of one sort or another. That Sunday night at his grandmother's, Matthew's left knee swelled to "unimaginable width" (his grandmother's description), and his fever rose to 103 degrees. By the time his grandmother telephoned me, Matthew was dragging his left leg with his arms and right foot and refused to get off the ground. "Honey," she said to me, "I really think he's very ill and you need to come get him immediately."

Frankly, I was annoyed. "Let me speak to him," I demanded.

Speaking with Matthew convinced me that I needed to go pick him up, although it did not convince me that he was desperately ill. Something hiding behind his voice begged me not to leave him in this place, and I responded from my heart rather than from any parental disciplinary center. When I arrived he surely looked relieved, but I noticed that his knee was red, swollen, and hot to the touch. I tried calling the pediatrician but got the answering service instead. Upon their advice, I agreed to take him to the emergency room. In part, my decision to go to the hospital was to teach Matthew once and for all that to call me away from the few activities I did for pleasure without him was not going to be taken lightly. He was nearly nine now, and he could survive for an evening with his brother and grandparents.

The other part of my decision was in response to the hidden voices.

After a short wait and a shorter diagnosis, the doctor called me out of the examining room. "We're going to admit him," he said unemotionally.

I was startled. "What's wrong with him?"

"We don't know, but he needs his knee drained and we need to watch him for several days." In the course of that week, the doctor announced that Matthew had some sort of infection in his joint, and there was concern about the infection crossing the growth plates. They were unclear what the cause was, but the doctor put him on an antibiotic and sent him home.

Matthew's symptoms appeared again and again, now in this joint, now in that one. It was always a synovial joint, never a fibrous or cartilaginous one. Usually it was a knee or an elbow that was affected; occasionally it was a shoulder. I started wondering about the nature of a joint cavity, obviously a comfortable home for this infection. What was the energy in this home—bony ends covered with cartilage, housed inside fluid-filled capsules? What in the membranes or the fluids was nourishing the infection? And what kind of vitality and support distinguished this from the nature of the cartilaginous joints?

The doctor was confused about what was happening in my little boy's body. The treatment was giving him immediate relief, but only briefly; the fear that the pain was surely going to return was overwhelming him. Matthew began to complain of headaches. I noticed that he stayed up all night, and he was developing a fondness for dark over light. Periodically his knee or elbow would flare up and his temperature would rise, and for those several days he was miserable. A doctor would drain his joints and give him amoxicillin or ampicillin. That brought him temporary relief. Then his back started to hurt and he lost his interest in walking, running, or getting up and down from chairs.

At this point, my read of Matthew was that the disease was spreading to his spinal column—vertebral or cavital, I did not know—and he was withdrawing from the world of his usual physical activities. I learned that the disease was in both his axial and his appendicular systems through observation of another trigger: when Matthew rounded a corner—say, in active pursuit of one of his younger brothers—he often ran into things and collapsed from lack of support. In response to this playful inattention, his joints were sure to heat up and swell, and he would be incapacitated for up to a week. Soon, Matthew learned not to play.

Working with a Preteen

I had started working with Matthew before the Lyme disease had been baptized with a Christian name. It was the fall he turned nine years old. In retrospect, working as we did was likely helpful for two reasons. First, I didn't meet with typical resistance to what appeared as a "new age" solution. No one knew what to do for Matthew, so my intuition had to be as good as anyone else's. Second, since I am not a medical doctor, working together allowed me to focus on Matthew's symptoms and their energies rather than on the chemistry of the body or the potential of invasive therapy.

In the earlier stages of the disease, over the course of several years, official diagnoses beyond "This is just the flu" or "He seems to have developed allergies" ranged from asymmetric juvenile arthritis to osteomyelitis. Through many hospital stays, Matthew had joints drained and drugs prescribed; he endured many neurological work-ups; and he underwent an operation to remove a mysterious tumor—what I now think might have been swollen lymph glands.

My pediatrician, who considered me slightly atypical, knew to resist over-drugging my children. I trusted Larry Heiny from the first moment he sat on the floor to examine Matthew as an infant. At the time, he was not my regular pediatrician, but he substituted one morning and I switched to him immediately. I had rarely brought my children to him for treatment beyond the yearly check-up required by the public school; nonetheless, somehow I had conveyed to him, even in those brief visits, that I was less interested in a quick fix and more interested in long-range solutions. We developed a relationship that allowed him to perform the memorized "speechlettes" at each stage of my children's growth, and allowed me space to work with my own children using alternative methods.

Mother-instinct encourages me to coach my children back to wellness through eating well, sleeping more, and communing with their cells through touch. I have come to believe that not only is movement vital to health, but that age- and activity-appropriate movement is essential to healing for all people. If it is true that at conception the cell holds all the information necessary for both form and function of the future individual, and if it is true that the fetus's biological survival depends on individualized movement for differentiation of sensory, perceptual, and psychological development, then by extension it must also be true that eight- and nine-year-olds—and later, teenagers—need to engage in personalized movement to continue evolving and to differentiate from one another. My nine-year-old was witnessing his peers moving in certain ways: neighborhood basketball, team soccer, tennis, and sailing at the beach. Not to be engaged in those activities put him at a disadvantage vis-à-vis perception, learning, and development. Here I had a boy who was expected by his family, his peers and their parents, and his teachers and school administrators to be physically active. His choice not to participate was often chalked up to a personal lack of motivation or self-discipline—in short, a lack of respectable (or in our neighborhood, "normal") behavior. Few people stopped to consider the fact that Matt was unable to participate in these activities without the anticipation of pain, and that the very anticipation taught him to avoid the engagement. The lack of engagement subsequently taught him to defend himself, usually verbally, against others who perceived him as lazy. The cycle was inexhaustible.

In starting to work with Matthew, the question I asked myself was this: What would re-engage this child from the beginnings of the movement patterns to his current age? And what might age-appropriate equivalents of the developmental movement sequence look like for a nine-year-old boy?

My intuition was to have conversations with multiple systems at once. Matthew described his joints as painful and his bones as unreliable, so I left any appendicular skeletal work for him to determine, as a situation demanded. I turned my focus instead to his fluids. Fluids change easily, it seems, and they mediate health and sickness, death and rebirth. For some reason the circulatory system was obviously off balance, maybe even interrupted somehow. His synovial fluid was also obviously affected. But if all fluids actually had a "sameness," wouldn't contacting one help to shift another?

My first efforts were geared toward stimulating the spinal fluids and not letting the flow bog down. My image was of a rushing stream, clean and flowing, as opposed to a stagnant, mosquito-laden pond. Matthew was afraid of rapid movement, so in order to get the blood pumping around and through the system I had to dream of another way to encourage quick aerobic combinations that specifically involved dropping and lifting his head. We started playing games that involved climbing on the furniture—using the bunk bed sideboards as uneven parallel bars, swinging and wrapping ourselves around the edges, trying to get from one surface to another without ever touching the ground. In these exercises we could investigate math problems like adding up distances, measuring the time it took us to get from one place to another, and then hiding answers that could only be retrieved with successful journeys from dresser to bed to blanket chest. We used this format to make a game of cleaning the room, picking up dirty laundry along our journeys, replacing shoes in closets, and grabbing pillows with our teeth. The idea was to use the body in extreme ways—dipping and lifting the head, turning upside down as much as possible, flipping around crossbars and occasionally falling to the plush carpet below, scrambling quickly to get off the ground before the other one noticed. These activities promoted blood flow but avoided most sudden contact from external moving objects, like balls or other people. In this pursuit, Matthew's keenness was challenged and his muscles were active. Further, he was competing against a thirty-one-year-old gymnast mother so he was not at all sure to win!

One of the benefits of this game was the sophisticated and complex mouthing and spinal patterning Matthew was called to engage in. He had been both breast- and bottle-fed. I imagined that, buried in his consciousness, he had adequate experiences of searching, fending, and personal power, but that "knowing" had faded in the face of his

more recent and more compelling experiences. I assumed his "searching and fending" skills were sleeping and needed to be reawakened.
For his part, he loved that we were doing something he was rarely
allowed to do on his own. Roughhousing on furniture surfaces was
not "sport" at our house; it was grounds for a "time-out." So breaking
the rules was attractive to him. Playing this game seemed like a good
way to begin.

I worked with Matt's back and spinal area in more passive ways as
well. The relief he experienced in elongating from C6/7 to under his
scapula and then out and down allowed Matthew to stop focusing on
the tender areas and imagine them much longer in space. (I am repeating his ten-year-old language here.) He breathed more spontaneously
when we played, and he didn't experience the punitive joint response
he had when he would come bounding around a corner, laughing and
lunging at one of his brothers.

The elongating work felt to me like parting curtains, like drawing
space for the spine to do what it had to do. It felt to Matthew like a
free backrub; he would lie still for hours, and in that process he began
communicating with me, describing what he felt like being trapped
inside his own container.

I started thinking about birthing and rebirthing, about expulsion
from the womb. We developed a second game that we played at the
dance studio where I worked. Wrapped up in newspapers that were
held together using a sealing tape dispenser, Matthew was tucked up
as tiny as he could be. We pretended he was a present—like that new
puppy every boy wants to receive on Christmas morning—and he had
to be perfectly silent and still while I wrapped, lest the grouchy parents
came stumbling down the stairs to see what Santa had left under the
tree. Then suddenly he burst out of the paper, surprising me with his
recuperative energy and his glee.

Later the "womb" was made out of small blankets and, later still,
larger and heavier ones. Here he was curled up next to the wall, sometimes on his back with legs folded on top, other times on his shins with

his spine curved protectively over his legs. Once he had the hang of exploding out of the paper and blankets, I joined Matthew in his game. We pushed ourselves out of the womb, off the wall, creating a clear competitive effort at twisting and soaring. This was an act of will—of demanding that we leave the wall, going faster and farther each time. We announced Matthew's arrival with sound and surprise.

Eventually, we came to the game with "weapons" to defend our records, trying to surprise each other with just how clever we could be. We discovered that certain fabrics slid farther, certain floor surfaces were slicker, certain clothing items (like belts) impeded speed. Wax paper, trays, blankets: anything was fair game. And the measuring got creative. Resist, rebel, surrender, cooperate: whatever would get the best score. The game always seemed to end in gentle roughhousing— laughing, hugging, exhausted.

As Matthew got older we worked with cerebrospinal fluid and sensation. He continued to talk about "feeling outside his body," and I heard that as desiring integration. Indeed, most all coordination had diminished substantially. I created two movement games. First, I worked with his spine by manually folding and unfolding his back. My image was of "sloppy somersaulting." Beginning on the floor, I grounded my feet next to his, giving him something to push against, then I grabbed his hands, pulling his body up and over his secured feet. Placing his hands on the floor, I rushed around him, tucking his head under from thoracic to cervical to top of the head, then picked up his rising hips, smoothing his spine under so that it didn't slam to the floor, encouraging sensation from head back toward tail in an inverted position. Once the center of weight and gravity met, I had to rush quickly to his legs, stroking them down the posterior surface, flexing them at the hips, folding them at the knees, and reaching for his head to stay "connected" spatially to his knees in order to keep the roll going. Sideways, forward, backward— any and all directions of the body were part of this traveling sequence, as long as we kept progressing across the studio floor. His body was big now; this manipulation was sloppy and awkward and silly.

We continued rolling around the studio floor, taking on yield-and-push patterns and reach-and-pull patterns. But instead of my moving his passive body, like in the sloppy somersaults, in this exercise Matthew moved himself and competed against me. The object was to continue moving forward spatially. No matter what part of the body was in front, the rest had to move to it, rather than drawing limbs into the center or using more familiar patterns. Up over our hips, dragging our weight to our feet, sliding our bodies sagittally forward, only to learn that reaching with our hands meant having to creep our bodies forward toward our fingertips by pushing with our toes, we learned to mediate how far from center we extended. The farther we reached, the more peripheral the initiation of the next movement had to be.

Because of Matthew's age and my determination to keep him interested, there were prizes ranging from ice cream cones to rented videos and sleepovers with friends. This game playing was decidedly competitive—I made our work a game, and the desire to win kept Matthew playing. His pleasure was immense and, whatever our work was doing physically, it was countering the severe mistrust Matthew was developing of his body. In retrospect, I doubt it was his mother he was competing against; I believe he recognized that he was actually preparing to meet his friends. But healing was not coming fast enough.

An Angry Teenager

By the time Matt was in his mid-teens, he was making decisions for himself that fell outside the choices I would have made for him. At age fourteen he was staying up later, barely able to roll out of bed in the morning, and he was smoking. He was avoiding school with a myriad of excuses and failing miserably, with a nonchalance that an academic mother found baffling. He was mistrustful, surly, and arrogantly yet powerfully intellectual with superior verbal debating skills.

At sixteen, he dropped out of high school in response to a plagiarism charge on a paper in English class. While he was innocent of the

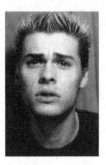

Matthew's appearance as a teenager grew angry and sullen.

charge and the school agents (teacher, principal, and superintendent) were sorely inadequate in their processing of any evidence, Matthew didn't yet have experience enough to realize that not all of life is fair or just, and that sometimes one proves innocence over time and through other assignments. This young boy fell into quite a bit of casual drug use; he hated the world and his inability to participate in it with the power he wanted to exert; he was angry with himself. For two years, Matt holed up in the unfinished cellar of our 1840 home. Stored there was every textbook his parents had purchased in college, and while avoiding the light, he read everything he could get his hands on to pass the time.

When his younger brother Stewart exhibited symptoms of swelling and immobility in the car ride from Ohio to Fire Island, after Stewart was transported to HSS and routed through a maze of red tape via personal friendships and networking, after our pediatrician sent Dr. Lehman the paper diagnoses and we returned to Ohio to run a simple battery of blood tests on Matthew, it was confirmed that Matthew did, indeed, have Lyme disease. Late that autumn, the two boys and I drove to Stony Brook, New York, for treatment at the Center for Infectious Disease at Stony Brook University's Medical Center.

Getting Help

After an exhausting twelve-hour car ride through a rare 1989 November blizzard, we arrived at the Stony Brook Center only to find that the doctor scheduled to see us was not in; we were told we would have to reschedule. Stunned, I was hardly able to speak for myself. After many tries I sat down, needing time to think through what I could do here. A woman sitting in the waiting area read my face and immediately walked to the reception desk. "This woman has driven many hours through dangerous snow to get here," she reported as if she knew me, rather than having simply overheard my pleas. "She is worried about her children and she is in no position to fight for herself. You *must* find a doctor who can see her children, and you must do it now." She moved closer to the reception desk, raising instead of lowering her voice. "Now!" she screamed. "Take care of her now!"

The receptionist tried to explain that she could not invoke a doctor's presence, but my ally would not let up. "Are you a mother?" she asked the receptionist rhetorically. "Do you have any idea what this woman is feeling? She needs your support, not your excuses."

Eventually, the receptionist called in another doctor. He arrived an hour later, examined the boys, and started them on a program of intravenous antibiotics. My nameless friend waited with me.

Before she left the waiting room, the woman revealed that she had a daughter who had died recently of cancer. When doctors and hospitals were unsympathetic to her needs as the mother, an anonymous woman had "spoken" for her, had fought for this mother's right to have medical information spelled out in a clearer fashion, in a way she could understand while under duress. Once the lay interpretation was secured, the woman said to my new friend, "You don't owe me anything. You owe a debt to all those who care for the world. When you see a mother in need of your strength, you must repay my help by helping someone else. You will know when it is your turn, because you will be unable to stop yourself from participating." My friend and ally turned to me. "I expect the same of you," she said. "Use your skills, your training, your job, your friends, whatever it takes. Listen for your turn." Then she vanished.

Awaken the Sleeping Child

At age eighteen, in the Center for Infectious Disease at Stony Brook, Matthew was given intravenous doses of ceftriaxone, a drug normally administered for the sexually transmitted diseases chancroid and gonorrhea. According to the Atlanta-based Centers for Disease Control and Prevention, it is also the drug of choice for Lyme disease. As reported in the *Journal of the American Medical Association* (Feb. 24, 1993):

"Long-term use of the antibiotic ceftriaxone by people infected with or suspected of being infected with Lyme disease may cause biliary (gall bladder) complications." The journal goes on to say that occasionally taking this drug induces diarrhea, nausea, vomiting, abdominal discomfort, headache, rashes, liver disruption, or dizziness. Matthew and Stewart experienced none of these.

Stewart responded like a child with a sore throat who has been given amoxicillin or ampicillin—that pink chalky liquid which is administered for ten days. After twenty-four hours, there seems to be marked improvement. After a few days, the patient feels fine, and the caretaker has to remind him to take his medicine. Stewart returned to his bouncy self, full of energy and orneriness toward his younger brother. His remaining symptom rested in his skin: it retained an extreme sensitivity to the sun, and burns and peels even when protected under high levels of sunscreen and layers of clothing.

Matthew was slower to recover. His symptoms subsided immediately, never to return. There was no swelling, no achy joints, and we were both surprised at his gawky but merely eight-year-old coordination in mundane tasks. Yet the psychological damage was severe. Living inside a diseased container had shaped his image of himself, and he was not as quick to reshape that image.

A little more than a year after treatment, Matthew moved to New York City. There he found new friends, talked people into letting him stay with them rent-free, and eventually got a job in a record store. He donned black leather and piercings and designer-colored hair. He developed a sickly gray look as the foundation for an aggressive and angry demeanor. He was barely recognizable to a Midwestern family.

A year later, he found a way to approach his father and me about shifting his environment. Matthew asked about college and reluctantly agreed to a trip across Ohio looking at schools with his next-younger brother, Chris. Not expecting to find anything interesting in Ohio, he was startled to find Antioch College in Yellow Springs to his liking. Starting with the admissions interview (where he challenged the counselor to accept or deny him on the spot, too impatient and unsure to wait for committee consideration), Matthew set an early pattern of resisting, procrastinating, and arguing with teachers there. But eventually he recovered from the psychological imprint of the Lyme disease and graduated at the top of his class, fluent in a second language and fascinated by trends in the global economy. Within a few short years he had developed a marvelous game of tennis, he learned to kayak, and he subscribed to and used a gym. In short, he found a passionate physical body anxious to learn, respond, and grow.

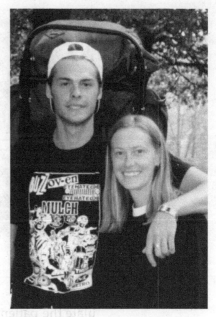

Here Matthew is pictured going off to college. In the family, we affectionately call this his "First Day of School" picture.

I experienced Matthew's healing as the conception of a new creation. We consider the time from the ceftriaxone to his graduation from college as one long, seven-year gestation. He was testing his new body, a body dismissed as healed by the medical community. Since that graduation day, he has made progress in stages. An infant, a toddler, a boy, and now a thriving twenty-seven-year-old man, he is healthy, happy, and living and working in Germany as a financial analyst for a major company. No longer fearful of rapid movement, he is confident, athletic, and strong.

I feel my primary responsibility is as a mother. When I agreed with my body to bear children, I also accepted the challenge of fending for them while they were learning to fend for themselves. As a parent, I want to embody respect for my children's individual journeys while guiding them with my knowledge of life's challenges and the body's capacity. Neither Chris (my second son) nor Alex (my fourth son) seemed ever to have contracted Lyme disease, in spite of the similarities of their playful summers at Fire Island. Yet Stewart has battled repetitions of Lyme's symptoms twice since his Stony Brook treatment, and there is no way of knowing whether the antibiotic treatment was not as successful for him as for his older brother or if he has been re-infected.

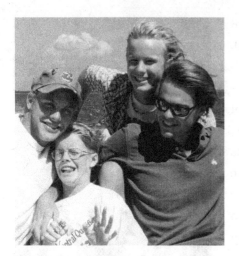

As a family, we continue to return to Fire Island summer after summer for renewal.

Nevertheless, his coordination was not impaired. He is an actor, a dancer, a singer, a beautifully physical twenty-year-old living in Switzerland while he studies and snowboards.

Matthew's journey illustrated how the body *is* mind and vice versa. There is no distinction. He was healed only when his bodymind was healed. My pediatrician insisted that the drug "pushed" his system in a beneficial direction. Yet it was the developmental movement work that kept Matthew learning while his neurological system was "sleeping." The experience, he claimed, reminded him of talking to someone in a coma: although there are varied results, in some cases it seems to stimulate the patient even when we cannot see the immediate results of that stimulation. I am reminded of Bonnie's wind and sand comment.[1] Here, the playing we did when he was not able to progress consciously along a developmental path maintained in place a foundation for fast-tracking once the antibiotic contained the bacterium. To have treated him with one but not the other would have left him, simply, imbalanced, unwhole.

For me, our journey taught me something of patience—that the seeds I plant may take time to grow, and I am not to lose faith as their roots are developing underground. This lesson applies to my children and also to my students at the university. I learned that I do not know what impact my actions will have in a later situation. But I do know that generosity, compassion, and respect are seldom misplaced, and I have every reason to embrace and practice these moments, as they may well be returned to the world in tangible ways through those whose journeys I have been honored to share.

Clara: A Case Study

~ **Naomi Duveen,** The Netherlands (2008)

With thanks to my daughter Djuna for her help with language.

"Clara" is ten years old. She has a long and thin body, long arms and legs, and a soft voice. She often sits with her feet close together. Her presence has a light quality like that of the craniosacral fluid (CSF). As a baby, Clara had a stroke. It happened when she was very young, soon after her birth. It caused a lot of fluid on her brain. Although she has worked with several therapists over the years, including a Bobath therapist and a physiotherapist, Clara still holds her head tilted to the right. Her mother thinks that social contact, especially with children, will be easier for Clara if she can hold her head upright.

I will only have a few sessions with Clara, so I must gather as much information as I can as quickly as possible.

First Session

When we meet, my first priority is establishing a relationship with Clara. Instead of focusing on "the problem," I am interested in learning about Clara's experience. I wonder with her if she knows why she has come to see me. I ask her about her brothers and sisters. As I am asking these questions, I worry a bit that I may be making the process too conscious for her, evoking the cortex when where I really want to go in the session is toward lower brain functions. But I discover that it is not easy for Clara to find words for what she knows. She knows how many brothers and sisters she has, but she cannot tell me. Her mother has to help her. I wonder if our work together might help her find a way to word her inner experience so that it can come out into the world.

The physiotherapist Clara had worked with recommended that she practice keeping her head upright while looking at herself in the mirror. This exercise called on Clara to use her cortex to maintain the upright head posture. I notice that Clara is able to keep her head upright when she concentrates on it, but as soon as she loses her focus, her head tilts to the right again. I am reminded of Bonnie Bainbridge Cohen's words: "The nervous system cannot do what it does not know. It can only register." Trying to access head righting through the cortex isn't working. I wonder if exploring earlier patterns might help Clara find and maintain this position on her own.

I notice that Clara's feet are everted. She stands with her weight more on the outside of the foot and her arches turned upward. I start to work with her right foot. I touch and brush the skin on both the top and the bottom of her foot. I brush the outside edges of her feet so her toes spread out, drawing her foot more into inversion, and I let her draw the outline of her foot. Then I ask her how her right foot feels compared to the left. She responds that she doesn't understand what I am saying. I suggest to her that she can feel her own body. She responds very concretely; she begins to touch her foot. I realize suddenly that I will have to choose my words very carefully with her.

I then explain to Clara that she can experience her body from within as well as from without, and I suggest that she close her eyes. She tells me then that her right foot feels touched and the other doesn't. I am very moved by her response. I realize that this is totally new for her, the experience of paying attention to her bodily sensations, experiencing her body, and learning to embody herself. Afterwards she sits on the floor with her feet parallel, silent and with her eyes closed.

Clara exhibits a very strong extension pattern. Her mother tells me that Clara didn't have much tone after her birth. She has some flexion now, but the two patterns are not in balance. When Clara is on all fours, her coccyx points almost to the ceiling. She has a strong break in her lumbar area where she divides her body into upper and lower halves.

I want Clara to lie down on a large ball so that she can experience more frontal tone but this makes her feel nauseated. I find a smaller ball and have her push homologously through hands and feet while I press on her coccyx with my hand, directing it downward. I then invite Clara to lie down on her right side to continue our work with flexion and extension. I ask her to push with two feet against me so she can unfold into full extension. I notice that she pushes strongly with her legs, but there is little connection to the upper body. I ask her mother to help me so I can work with my hands to wake up the connections between her head and arms. Her arms have particularly low tone and are not very present.

Next I am curious about Clara's sideways movement. I check her Galant and abdominal reflexes; the movement is a bit stiff and unnatural, especially on the right. I ask Clara to lie on her stomach on the floor. I make contact with her organs, especially her lungs, because I have noticed that her right shoulder rides higher than the left. I gently hold and shake her organs. She tells me that she experiences a tickling in her left shoulder and that this area feels strange. I reassure her that learning new things often feels a bit unfamiliar in the beginning but that this soon disappears.

At the end of the session she gets up quite quickly and picks up a children's magazine. To my surprise, she sits on a chair and reads with her head held upright.

Second Session

I check to see how Clara stands on one leg. To keep her balance she tilts the pelvic half of the raised leg. She has a strong protective stepping reflex, forward and to the side, but she has no sense of this reflex going backwards. I have to catch her to prevent her from falling.

I am drawn to work with navel radiation, an early movement pattern.

In this pattern, which develops *in utero*, the navel holds the center for six encircling "limbs"—two arms, two legs, the head, and the tail. From the moment the fetus develops its umbilical cord, s/he folds and unfolds these limbs around the navel center. The limbs are connected to the center, and the center to the limbs. Later in life one can use body memory to reestablish this connection. Because Clara's upper body/lower body separation is so stark, I see that she needs to experience a more integrated whole-body pattern in order to find her way back to connection.

With Clara on her back, I work with cellular touch. Her cells react almost immediately. I touch her cellularly at the navel and move my hands toward her fingers, then touch her fingers and trace the pathway back toward the navel. I ask her which direction feels more comfortable to her. For most limbs she prefers being touched from center to periphery, though on her arms she favors touch from periphery to center.

I shift Clara to the ball to work further with navel radiation. However, it is clear that Clara doesn't have enough flexor tone yet. The strong upward direction of her coccyx and the break in her lumbar show me that having her on her front, with support only on her belly, is not really a good idea. I feel a bit lost about what Clara needs and what I can offer her.

Third Session

Clara's mother tells me that she notices more rest in Clara's body and more grounding. Clara herself answers my question about how she experiences the sessions with *"leuk"* which means "nice." I ask her to tell me more about what is nice for her, and she says she likes the sea star, an image for her that comes from the navel radiation work.

According to our original plan, this would have been our last session. I notice that there is a sense of "waiting for change" in the room. I respond to this by doing the opposite, going back to what we know. I return to our low brain work, making contact with Clara's navel area, front and back, for a long time. I can feel Clara's breath coming deep into her belly. I take all the time I need to stay there and to touch her six limbs again. I take more and more time. Then I ask Clara to lie first on her right then on her left side in flexion, and I invite her to push with her legs and turn onto her stomach. The old pattern reappears. She lies crooked, with her upper body to the left. I bring her back into flexion and ask her to start the movement with her navel area instead of moving her legs first.

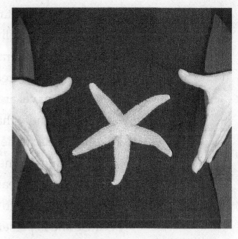

A sea star embodies the notion of center to periphery and periphery to center.

And there it is! Both her mother and I see with surprise what Clara has done. Her body is full and present from belly to arms and head. Completely connected, center to periphery and periphery to center, Clara lies on her stomach.

Fourth Session

When Clara enters the room, the way she walks is striking. She walks almost on her toes, as though she is pulling herself up from the earth. Her steps are tiny and quick and her body looks rigid. I ask Clara what she has done in school, and she tells me that she and her classmates have drawn pictures of an oak. I am pleasantly surprised because I realize that I can use this image of the big tree.

I am wanting to help Clara find connections in her body as well as presence and ease in her movement. Standing and walking upright are complicated for Clara. So I begin again with her lying on her belly. I use touch, imagination, and later on, somatization. I touch her to bring awareness to specific parts of her body. First I touch her feet and legs. Using the image of the tree trunk, I ask her how high the trunk is. She points to her shoulders. I ask her to imagine that the branches and leaves are her arms and head. I ask her about the colors of the tree. As she answers, I notice that Clara has a vivid imagination.

I make firm contact with Clara with a bloodful touch, accessing my own organs and cellular presence. Then I ask her where this tree likes to be touched. Clara enters the somatization easily. She is very clear about what the "tree" wants. She likes my hand on her lower back, then on the navel area (for quite a long time), and then on her occiput. She lets me know that this helps both parts feel connected and strong. Together we scan her whole body, checking what feels connected and what doesn't. At one point she mentions that the strength in her "tree trunk" has disappeared a bit. I touch her legs but she stops me, saying that she wants me to touch her feet instead. I like this part of the session because she is present and so clear. Compared to the first session, she is able to tune in to her bodily experience in a direct way.

We work with homologous push of the lower limbs with Clara both supine and on her belly. I have her push with her feet against my sitting body so she can move herself through space. I have her push into extension and back into flexion. She feels strong and connected.

I ask Clara if I can take some pictures of her. She tells me that it is OK as long as her face does not show and she doesn't look like a "patient." She offers to work on the sea star for the photo. So we do.

At the end I ask Clara to stand upright. But again, standing gives her too much information, and her old patterns reemerge. It is obvious that for her, transformation happens closer to the floor.

We shake hands to say goodbye. As we touch I notice that Clara's hand has a light, CSF quality, and her arm does not feel connected to the rest of her body. I remind Clara of the images of the tree and the sea star. I feel a shift, and then suddenly I can feel her feet while holding her hand. I can feel my own feet as well.

Dragon Riding through the Abyss

～ **Karin Spitfire,** USA (1999)

I was thirty-four years old and exploring the nervous system in a class
during my first year of the Body-Mind Centering training. The instructor was using Aikido to challenge us with the fighting sticks. This was
not the first time I had used my body as the anchor and projected my
mind. I was already greatly skilled at leaving my body pinned on the
bed and floating away. This was, however, my first experience of "separating" by conscious choice.

> *The Aikido teacher instructs me:*
> *Walk straight at*
> *His*
> *Red oak fighting stick,*
> *Send fully to*
> *Him,*
> *My energy/intention*
> *Move aside*
> *My body*
> *Away from*
> *His*
> *Lowering the boom.*

In Body-Mind Centering we are trying to embody, and thus to understand and dialogue with, the various tissues of the body. We do this
through movement, bringing our awareness to be within the consciousness of the tissue we are embodying, and acting from it.

183

Trauma is a perceived life-threatening experience. Trauma affects all the tissues in the body as well as the psyche. It is a whole-body, whole-person event. This whole-body response happens quickly and automatically. Current research, both empirical and experiential, identifies different aspects of the trauma matrix. In this essay, I will focus on the nervous system response.

In the nervous system's spectrum of options for survival, there·are two body/mind separations that are inverse opposites. One is an empowered decision to learn; it requires staying in the body. The other is a next-to-last automatic physiological choice of a person in a powerless, life-threatening circumstance (the last being coma); it requires leaving the body. This latter choice is a response to trauma.

The nervous system is a complex relay course of messages, "processing centers," and responses. Information from the external environment (the world) and the internal environment (the body—that is, the organs, glands, and muscles) travels to the central nervous system (the spinal cord and brain) to be processed. A response is then sent from the central nervous system back to the world through the body environments. This describes the basic sensory-processing-motor "loop."

The kind of information coming into the central nervous system determines where in the spinal cord and brain the "data" get interpreted. For example, when the doctor taps your knee, the sensation goes only as far as the spinal cord to get processed, and the motor response comes back immediately. While related messages may eventually reach your brain, causing you to register consciously that the knee kicked—that is, you saw it and you felt it—and while your brain may think, "Oh good, I'm healthy," all this processing takes place long after the tap and response.

The central nervous system has a hierarchy of need in relationship to where the first step in information-processing happens and from where a response is sent. In a highly simplified description of functions and locations, the spinal cord receives and responds to reflexes. The brain stem processes and translates vital signs, such as heart rate and breath rate, and such actions as coughing, swallowing, and gagging. Moving up the brain stem, we have sense interpretation. The diencephalon responds to the autonomic nervous system and to bodily states such as hunger, rage, and thirst. Finally, the highest region of the brain, the cerebrum (the thought and language center) responds to all sensory input on interpretive and motoric bases. While the lower regions of the central nervous system respond to what is primary and vital, the cerebrum—which has the capacity for selective interpretation—can choose the words to write this sentence and direct the motor activity of my hand, as well as "process" my experience of trauma after the fact.

The information from the *outer environment* comes into the body through the somatic nervous system, which brings sensation in from the skin and skeletal muscles and returns impulses to these same areas. These nervous system responses are under our conscious control. We direct our muscles to stand when the judge enters the room, raise an arm to ask a question, and so forth.

The information that comes from the *inner environment* of the body and then goes back into the body travels through the autonomic nervous system. This system is essential to the vital (life-dependent) functions of our internal organs. The autonomic nervous system, as a whole, acts without need of our conscious thought. For example, we do not have to send a message consciously and continuously to our heart for it to beat. However, the rate of the heart's beat can be affected and modulated by conscious activities such as (but not limited to) meditation and yoga. The autonomic nervous system's primary job is to maintain balance and homeostasis.

The autonomic nervous system is composed of the sympathetic and parasympathetic nervous systems. These two operate continually to balance one another. The sympathetic nervous system is about action and harnessing the body's resources to mobilize for that action. It is commonly referred to as the "fight-or-flight" nervous system. The parasympathetic nervous system, on the other hand, induces relaxation and digestion. It also has an extreme state, which is less recognized. This state is called "freeze."[1]

In that moment with the Aikido instructor, I was able to move my nervous system out of its freeze pattern and into fight. The experience of staying in my body and consciously sending my mind via my intention during a simulated attack precipitated a colossal realignment of my nervous system. After my first turn with the master, I was quite agitated—I felt I had been too nervous to really do it. I got back in line. I repeated the exercise. I remember the room, peripherally, as being chaotic—some people were re-forming a circle, others were getting sticks, others were milling around. I tried to sit down. Enormous energy, however, was rising in me. I tried to calm myself. It was like trying to slow an active volcano with speed bumps. At every bump, I felt a pulling in my tissues—a burning, tugging sensation. At some point, I thought, "Why keep this down?" Suddenly I was on my feet, yelling, "I want to *kill him!*"

The master handed me one of the pair of red oak sticks and instructed me how to alternate sides in meeting hers and how to do the rhythm of it. We proceeded to do the sympathetic nervous system stick "exercise," with me screaming bloody murder, then retreating and cowering, and then returning. The sticks cracked against each other. The volcano had erupted.

The sticks lay cracked on the floor as the class moved on to play a parasympathetic game of Nerfball. I felt a lightness and clarity in myself that I had never before experienced. I had moved from "fight" to a body state I did not recognize and could not name. I had moved from the trauma response of "this is a life-and-death crisis" into a physiological state most people call "living."

Most of us have experienced a "simple" shock of one kind or another.[2] For example, a short while ago a physically active and well-loved man in my community dropped dead of a massive heart attack. "What a shock!" was the universal response to the news. Shock feels as if every-thing stops—the conversation stops, the flow of the day stops, and the body stops. Most, if not all, of the tissues of the body are affected by shock. The breath, blood, and cellular movements all stop action, and there is a gap in nervous system processing. Then there's a little kick-start, a shake, and usually either an emotion will start flowing, evi-denced by tears or anger, or there will be a numbing feeling of denial. The process continues to alternate between numbing and expressing as we grieve, mourn, and finally come to accept the experience. The nervous system is integrating the experience as the body releases the news, bit by bit—as the emotions flow and the reality of that which overwhelmed us is processed.

If the shock is traumatic—that is, life-threatening—this basic pattern still operates, but the impact on the body and the psyche is greater and the process more involved. In an overwhelming trauma, some of the body processes do not simply stop momentarily; they can turn off or even "reverse," as the autonomic nervous system's "survival" pattern is activated.[3]

The reversal is a pattern that needs further explanation. In a trau-matic or life-threatening event, the sensory ganglia entering the spinal cord are overwhelmed by too much information. In that moment, only that which is absolutely necessary for the organism's survival gets processed, and the autonomic fight-or-flight or freeze responses get activated. The rest of the input from the event is received but cannot be processed. The body is first and foremost responding to the threat to life. It is not concerned with the color of the attacker's shirt or even whether the experience is scary—these aspects of the reality of the trauma get stored. Such details and feelings will sit in the association neurons (the neurons between sensory input and motor action) or in the synaptic gaps (the spaces between one neuron and the next).

The trauma can be powerful and overwhelming enough to change the polarization of the sensory neuron, causing the input to "reverse" its direction of movement. When this happens, the input enters the spinal cord through a collateral motor neuron that connects the sensory ganglia to the motor ganglia. It then synapses with the autonomic nervous system to be carried to and held as memories in the organs and body tissues.

Typically, the autonomic nervous system's survival pattern activates a massive fight-or-flight response. All the body's resources—including blood, muscles, hormones, and blood-sugar stores—immediately focus either on moving the endangered self out and away from the situation or on fighting vehemently to survive. Peripheral life activities, such as digestion, shut down at this time. If, on the other hand, we are completely powerless in the situation, the autonomic nervous system resorts to freeze. Freeze occurs when flight is impossible and fight is deemed to be useless, when the only option open is conserving all our energy and waiting for the danger to pass.

In freezing, two constellations of body activities occur simultaneously and to varying degrees. First, the cell membranes change permeability and cellular metabolism shifts; fluids reverse or go into a holding pattern; organs slow their rhythmic movement; and breathing becomes shallow to the point of taking in just enough oxygen to stay alive. Second, because of the reversal in the nervous system, all the adrenaline and energy that would be used to fight or flee is fed back into the body. For instance, someone who has been in a car accident might go into a freeze response. If that person's body knows how to unlock the freeze and it is acceptable behavior to the person and to those in his environment, he may be able to feel and express the fears and grief in a relatively short time—say, in one month to one year.

When the trauma is both severe and unresolved, for example due to its social awkwardness, there can be a disassociation—the "spirit" or mind can leave the body and watch from the ceiling, go down the road, or create a fantasy world until it is okay to come "home." For example, for survivors of child abuse, the "incident" is unspeakable and the context for expression is unsafe. It's likely that the power of the incoming energy of the fight-or-flight response, which "should" be motoring out, in part enables the disassociation. Disassociation causes a gap in processing the trauma—in connecting with self, feelings, others, spirit, or community. Coming home, thawing out, and connecting through the gap can take a few months, a year, or fifty years, given the trauma (or traumas) and the context.

While waiting to be integrated through the nervous system, the aftermath of this unresolved trauma lives in the body as unprocessed information. As a traumatized person is waiting to thaw, the nervous system continues to act as if that person is in a life-threatening situation. During this time, two contradictory extremes are functioning in the body. In order for the body to stay alive, the sympathetic and parasympathetic states must balance. We call this homeostasis. In this case, both states are extreme. The emotional symptoms of post-traumatic stress disorder (PTSD) have been widely described as alternating between numb and agitated, depressed and enraged. These swings reflect the body's internal state: some parts are numb while the rest is in high gear. Survivors exist on a continuum of these extremes—some live more on the depressive/numb side, others on the "acting-out" side—until the "thawing," the integration process, occurs.

Survivors find all kinds of creative ways to live with this balance, functioning amazingly well in more situations than not. However, this "stuck-in-extremes" response to trauma takes an inordinate amount of energy to maintain, and it affects all the body's tissues as well as the psyche. In coping with these extremes the whole system simply begins to wear out. This response to trauma often results in many of the autoimmune diseases we see today, including chronic fatigue, fibromyalgia, and allergies, as well as many forms of addiction as the survivor attempts to medicate and modulate.

Each survivor develops a unique nervous-system route for managing the world around and over the frozen material of trauma. Previous to the events described earlier, in which my nervous system began its releases, I had often characterized my understanding of life and my thinking process as "inside out and backward, the way a shirt comes out if you pull it off from the bottom with crossed arms." Also, before these releases, many actions that seemed risky for me necessitated what felt like leaping across the Grand Canyon. After the stick fight, I was able to track the path of my sensory-motor loop through the spinal cord as an opened-ended figure eight with a leap at the end. The feeling of this was around and out through fear, powered by fight energy, which enabled me to actually speak and follow through on my intention. This path was a way of motoring in spite of the nervous-system reversal and the gap in processing. It accounted for the fact that, despite being a survivor, I had been doing a lot of fighting and acting out. After the Aikido fight scene with the BMC instructor, action on my own behalf became a direct route in and out—a shorter, simpler, and less intense path.

Integration or "thawing out" means several things. Overall, it is many completions of the sensory-motor loop—the cycle of information/sensation coming in, nervous system processing, and the response or motoring out. In a kind of hierarchy of resolution, consciousness (spirit) first returns to the body. Next, the tissues and fluids that shut down (or froze) get reactivated. Then the fight-or-flight energy that was focused inward finds a motoric resolution outward from the body. The information that was stored in the body—the details and emotions, the horror, the anger, the loss—now has time to get processed, expressed, and integrated. Finally, the survivor comes to terms with the crack that now exists in his/her world.

All of this is predicated on some reestablishment of safety and trust. The process is not orderly. It is time-consuming and fraught with difficulty, primarily because when the spirit reconnects or "re-associates" with the body, it reenters at the nexus from which it left, which was a state of shock. So the whole process of nervous-system reversal can easily be re-triggered by the shock. Also, as life-threatening situations are terrifying by definition, experiencing any of the fear one did not feel initially, when the survival mechanism kicked in, can also set the cycle off again.

The experiences in Body-Mind Centering classes described earlier precipitated my nervous system's release of freeze into fight or flight, and then into a new and totally unfamiliar perceptual state. These releases provided the means for a clearing, a changing of the nervous-system pattern, a new routing. Some may see these experiences as cathartic acts, and that they were. They were not, however, a reinforcement or reenactment of the trauma, nor did they set off a physiological recycling of the PTSD pattern. The reasons for this are fourfold.

First, as the completion of the sensory-motor loop, these experiences allowed for a different outcome. They opened a different door, rather than repressing (again) or recycling the energetic forces that came up. Expression of feelings is one completion of the sensory-motor loop. Such energy often got repressed because I did not have a previous experience of taking the energy into a resolving motoric action, and so did not have a track for resolution already laid down in my nervous system. Without this motor pathway I did not know how to complete the loop; I had to do something new in a very scary context. Also, this energy was so big that it was rare that the people around me knew how to respond to, support, or demonstrate a different motor expression.

Second, focusing on using the fighting sticks kept me present in my body, as did negotiating the run. I had to direct my motor response. I could not go into a blind rage, an out-of-my-body rage, because I had to pay attention. I went instead into a righteous anger, an anger that claimed "I have a right to save and defend myself with all I have!"

Third, these experiences were not induced; the energy arose organically from the environment. I was recognized as being angry in one situation and scared in another, and was invited to express. I was witnessed in that expression and supported in the follow-through. As I was actively engaged in my Body-Mind Centering studies, an investigative process that both teaches and requires the development of an internal witness, the focus was on the learning and not on the trauma—not on either holding it down or letting it go. The focus was on something for my life, something positive, something I desired, rather than on my oppressive history. Ironically, under those circumstances my nervous system's expression could then come out.

Finally, in both situations there was a large group present to hold the intensity of the release. The large group of witnesses or "container-holders" allowed for an enormous amount of safety.

My first experience of being "in my body" had occurred a few years earlier during an organ exploration, also in a Body-Mind Centering class. We were lying on the floor and the instruction was to breathe into our pelvis. I said to the teacher, "When I do that my gut turns and my legs shake...."

"Run," she said. So I ran and ran and ran.

The Aikido confrontation was the second major event of my long journey through all the tissues of my body, through the release, the un-patterning, of trauma. In that string of moments, rather than feeling I was behind a video camera watching myself, I moved my nervous system from freeze into flight. Opening a new pathway is the inherent difference between a flashback or reenactment and a release. It is my experience that when a flashback/memory occurs and the expression can be rerouted, the flashback does not come back. It is resolved. Since I have learned how and when it is possible to motor out the terror or rage and to move through the normal progression of feelings of fear, anger, sadness, and relief, the visceral, present-moment intensity—the "I feel like it is happening now" of a flashback/memory—has not returned. It is no small feat to clear a flashback/body memory from the body tissues and to move into the higher nervous system for that processing and integration. To this I say, "Hallelujah!"

Of Many Minds

~ **Ellen Barlow,** USA (2009)

Body Reactions, Body Costs

An intention is set. The scene unfolds. I change my mind and do for another what I had planned on asking her to do for herself. I am stooping down, moving the heavy object, and as the discord dawns on me, I am turning to rise and … my back "goes out." Mild shock, pain, and then the trumping mindset takes charge: the show must go on. It'll be OK.

Later, the pain gets louder. It will dominate my awareness, impede my movement function. The symptom, back pain, rules. It will be hours later before I remember: Oh, that betrayal, a plan override, my change of mind at the last second that did not sit well with the internal well-being meter.

It will be a few days of repair and return to structural integrity. Such a quick loss of the intention to take care of myself while working with others!

A Conversation

I say:

In current health education terms, my story is a teaching in (how not to and) how to positively impact my own health behavior. Positively impact = listen, negotiate, and heed cognitive~emotional~physical guidance in relation to the demands of the environment, then, motor plan accordingly; health behavior = do the right thing on my own behalf.

In health education research, awareness of bodymind interaction before, during, or after a somatic disruption of equilibrium is not exactly a hot topic. However, learning self-care skills certainly is.

Science says:

A psychoneuroendocrinoimmunologist might tell me what part of my brain shut down so as not to carry through on my intention of self-care. Having demonstrated "cross talk" between body systems, their science will trace the brain-body process.

A mental health clinician hearing my story could diagnose me with a "somatization disorder." I am presenting with a somatic complaint, assessed to be psychogenic in origin. Her field's clinical research is based in psychophysiology, the term currently preferred to psychosomatic.

I say:

I'll agree with both. These specialized lenses illustrate something of my experience. But there's more.

Integrated Routes

I will say to the psychoneuroendocrinoimmunologist that in addition to my story demonstrating a brain-body process (your language), or conflicting thoughts and emotions tripping off low back dysfunction (my language), I have a predisposing physical condition: a weak structural link in those precise vertebral segments. An old injury.

I will say to the mental health professional: My back goes out when my physical conditioning is not sufficient to sustain physical stresses, or because unconscious, unmediated emotion and thoughts divert attention to this weak link. Either way, my body directs the healing process.

It could be said that I approach my back health from the continuous loop of Brain~Mind~Body ("top–down") and Body~Mind~Brain ("bottom–up") systems, which act in concert with environmental input.[1]

I went into somatic work because I hungered for a more holistic perspective on bodymind interaction, functional movement, and the art of movement than what medical or physical therapy or psychological education was offering. I wanted to be part of a worldview that would land us in our bodies, cultures, communities, and environment as nature, art, and spirit. (Art and spirit deserve a discussion beyond the scope of this article.) From a health care perspective, I wanted to apply body awareness in a wellness model.

Lost and Found Threads/Modern Reweaving

In health care, science is charged with establishing the primary warp and weft of progress in our social fabric when it comes to understanding and positively impacting bodymind interaction and health behavior. Thank goodness, scientific convention can be forever reviewed, renewed, and rewoven. Too bad valuable threads have been downgraded into obscurity.

It is unfortunate that the words "somatic" and "psychosomatic" became primarily associated with pathology in the last century. It was also unfortunate that the field of Psychosomatic Medicine was not able to realize its vision in the U.S.: for the merger of mind and body to become an integral part of every medical specialty. Instead the field, formalized in 1939, rose and then fell, according to historian Theodore M. Brown, fragmenting into reductionist approaches, sub-specializations, and separate "schools," never to become the unifying force for a biopsychosocial model the founders espoused.[2]

Yet look at what the fields of Somatic Psychology and Body-Oriented Psychotherapy are offering now, picking up dropped threads of soma-centered research initiated mid-twentieth century, such as physiologically-oriented psychosomatic studies, organismic physiology and the social sciences, while weaving in the biological bases of consciousness itself.[3] And what collaborations might be possible between biomedical and/or behavioral health research scientists and practitioners of Body-Mind Centering?

We explore "how the mind is expressed in the body through movement"[4] and apply phenomenological research in how this somatic intelligence positively modifies experience and behavior. We interweave philosophical and aesthetic and scientific theories like twine, playing around the edges of the social fabric. We could use researchers' help in designing and conducting the kinds of studies that would test the efficacy of our best practices as applied in a wellness model.

Wellness: Agreement and No Agreement

Everybody seems to agree: the wellness model should be established across all health disciplines. Whether one is living more fully in the presence of a disability, learning/choosing healthy behaviors to prevent illness or injury, or generally improving quality of life, we as health workers can all support and represent the ideas of well-being, well-functioning, well-relating, well-feeling, well-thinking, well-giving/receiving, well-living, and well-dying.

However, while "perhaps 50% of the most common causes of death in this country are related to modifiable behaviors,"[5] everybody does not agree on an applied biopsychosocialspiritual model of health (care), let alone access to basic health care as a human right, which would confirm the worth of wellness for all human beings.

Collaboration

Body-Mind Centering best practices could be of use in health care beyond the current scope. Some of our best practices yield external behavioral change, and others yield perceived internal-state changes that in turn, we believe, positively affect all levels of function and expression.

What would we want to "test"? In a conversation with a freshly minted graduate of Georgetown University, MA in Physiology, versed in the latest mindbody medicine and biomedical research (which is growing at record speed), I learned that perception occurs in the brain.

When I told this woman that BMC posits that direct perception is (in) the mind of the body systems and cellular consciousness, she said she hadn't been taught that in graduate school; rather, she learned that perception happens only in the brain.

Which of our theories, which of our practices would we want to explore with research scientists? We'd need to risk truth(s) we hold to be self-evident, our hunches that our belief systems sometimes register as doctrine.

Cognitive Models: The Brain~Mind~Body and Body~Mind~Brain

Numerous models from various fields intellectually support as well as challenge the model developed by Body-Mind Centering practitioners.

American academician and researcher James Giordano, PhD, MPhil, makes the case for a comprehensive model where he would include both Brain~Mind~Body ("top–down") and Body~Mind~Brain ("bottom–up") systems that act in concert with environmental input. He advocates using the tilde symbol (~) to represent complementarities.[6] BMC might bring new breadth, depth, and meaning to his "bottom–up"/"body informing the brain" construct.

Norwegian researcher Rita Agdal, MA, has studied the use of Complementary and Alternative Medicine (CAM) as it leads to more diverse perceptions of the body and the ensuing relatedness to perceptions of illness, health, and risk. She presents five models wherein the body is described as a machine, a plumbing system, an energy field, a computer, or part of a wireless network.[7] While a Body-Mind Centering perspective would see the merit of each model, we would not settle for any one of them alone.

The ideas of others help us to identify and extend our own. In my case I would include John Sarno's work with Tension Myositis Syndrome, John Gardner's theory of Multiple Intelligence, The New Cosmology philosophy of Brian Swimme and Thomas Berry in the tradition of Pierre Teilhard de Chardin, E.O. Wilson's concept of Consilience, and many more.

Not So Fast, Oh My Aching Back

Back to my story again. I fell from a cliff while rock climbing when I was nineteen, sustaining multiple injuries to my spine, ankles, and feet. After recovering, I maintained my health with yoga, well-chosen body-based therapies, and then the self-care practices of Body-Mind Centering.

Years later, after almost twenty years of no back pain, back pain returned as if a sleeping giant had remembered his power to bodily capture and completely dominate my attention. Thereafter, when I did not heed somatic signals of emotional~cognitive~physical discord and probe them, back pain seemed to just sit right down, brood, and take me over. When I engaged body-based rebalancing acts I could get relief, yet no resolution. Eventually, physical wellness would be re-established. Or a benevolent, skilled, body-based practitioner could tap the healing instinct and voila, my symptoms would resolve—what a gift, yet what a mystery. And that was OK, until I realized I wanted to know why my back kept "going out."

Not until I learned to identify what was setting off the pain syndrome in/around the weak link in my spine could I pause the automatic tripping of the switch. Sometimes it's a quick, electrical, turn-on-a-dime, saving-grace reorientation. Sometimes it feels like a slow-motion waterwheel churning water one way, then reversing its weighted direction, dragging to a halt, digging in to a complete stop, making an about-face and releasing its force to move flow the opposite way. Oh, freedom! Then I can use my skilled body awareness and movement knowledge to reorganize and recondition myself back onto a functional track. It's personal, each time.

And, as I said earlier, being a member of "the bad back club" (a friendly term I use with clients) provides me with teachings, whether

I like it or not. At times I've blessed, at times cursed my situation while waiting for my disc to talk with my ligaments to talk with the digestive system to talk with the vagus nerve to talk with the thoracic diaphragm to talk with the crura to talk with the bodies of the vertebrae to talk with the muscles to talk with the motor nerves to talk with the sensory nerves to talk with my heart to talk to my brain, so that my cortex and limbic system can say: hello, can we stop this spiral, sweetheart? Let's hear what needs are vying for attention; let's let up this mute bodily strain; let's reunite. "Be nice" (to oneself), as a friend used to say. Then, after a spell—seconds, minutes, hours, or days—back on the road again.

A Shooting Smile

~ **Piera Nina Teatini**, Italy (2001)

Introduction on Tiptoes

Northampton, Massachusetts, August 1994. I remember Bonnie Bainbridge Cohen, the founder of Body-Mind Centering, giving a speech at the graduation ceremony that crowned what, for our class of eighty-some people, had been an intense, demanding, rewarding four years of training. Bonnie's speech was simple in structure, far-reaching in meaning. It was a hymn of gratitude to a whole lot of people whom she called her teachers. All she did for twenty chanting minutes was say their names, plus one or two sentences that conveyed the gist of their gift to her. Among those teachers were listed, in continuity with her more formally appointed trainers and mentors, Cohen's clients.

I have chosen to tell Monica's story because she's the client and person from whom I have learned the most in all the years I've been working as a Body-Mind Centering practitioner. She taught me not only about the marvels and intricacies of the body-mind-soul-spirit continuum, but also about some of my lifelong, cherished themes: the life of complex systems, the web-like matrix of patterns and patterning, riding entropy backwards, and beauty.

I see beauty in how deeply she has identified with her natural drive toward unfolding, despite life-threatening challenges, and in the relentless courage she displays in dealing with her condition—the magnitude of either being such that I sometimes would like to disappear as a doer and let her story speak for itself.

However, since I will never disappear as a sentient agent, in the choices I've made as a practitioner and those I'm going to make as a narrator, let me clarify my own background just a little more. A Body-Mind Centering practitioner since 1994 and a Neuro-Linguistic Programming trainer[1] since 1992, I integrate the two streams through a deeply felt affiliation with Arnold Mindell's Process Work[2] and an extensive connection to what goes under the vast umbrella of Systemics.[3] What I love in all these disciplines, each with its particular emphasis, is the subtlety they're after in exploring how body, mind, soul, and spirit more than interconnect—how they literally become one another.

What I especially love in the BMC approach is manifold. In alchemical terms, BMC balances the ascending (from matter to spirit) and the descending (from spirit to matter) paths. It balances East and West— accessing states of consciousness akin to meditation, yoga, and mystical experiences, yet talking "Westernese," operating on anatomical, physiological, and kinesiological maps of stark precision and taking advantage of the latest scientific discoveries. It is excruciatingly specific in making contact with body structures, while simultaneously utilizing a broad focus in embracing the whole person with their history, context, idiosyncrasies, and predilections, all of which are meaningful both in assessing and assisting their process.

So I will tell Monica's history in some detail not because I worship biographies, as if the past were the direct cause of our present. What was is surely traceable in what is, but so is what will be, at least in the form of seed, inclination, potential, and dream. I'm relating her wanderings and discoveries because I would like to recreate for readers the tone of her aliveness, which is ultimately what I'm following in each session and hope to be serving overall. And because anything that I say about Monica's interactions with other body-based methods will reflect my BMC filters.

Of all the awareness training I've encountered, BMC is the one that has best emphasized not mixing up the visible with the superficial. The surface that shows itself to our perception can lead us to unsuspected depths, in the wake of Norman Maclean's words: "All there is to thinking is to see something noticeable that makes you see something you hadn't noticed before, that makes you see something that isn't even visible." And, as an agent of fathoming, our touch is even more potent than our eyesight. So much power, I feel the need of a sobering disclaimer. All that I know is for me just the tip of a temporary iceberg, shaped by the flow of seasons, the motion of sea currents, the geological events that have molded a certain area, and so many other co-influences, from fleeting to enduring, I cannot number or name. Every sentence I will write is an act of here-and-now knowingness, raising many more questions than it answers, embedded in so much not-knowing that it awakens awe in me, respect, and a desire to be silent even while I speak.

Disappear I shall not—I'll try to type on tiptoes.

The Landscape

Everybody is unique, yet some bodies are more unique than others.

Monica was born in 1972 to a working-class Italian family, temporarily dwelling in Caracas, Venezuela, but originally from Parma, a serene but lively town of central northern Italy. It's the place where they would hastily fly back when, at age seven months, the previously healthy, jovial baby started to swell all over the mandibular area, for no apparent reason and to the bewilderment of the local doctor. Following the advice of her MD uncle, Monica's parents took her to the main hospital in Bologna, the capital of the region. There and then she was put in the hands of a renowned pediatric surgeon who diagnosed an internal lymphoangioma and decided to operate immediately, to prevent the swelling from developing any further and possibly hemorrhaging.

What is an angioma? It is an abnormal proliferation of capillaries. It comes in different forms, the most common being the quite harmless birthmark. What lay behind the surface of Monica's baby face, however, was of an unfortunately different kind: it was a cavernous haemoangioma, deep and wide, fanning from the sublingual area out to both ears. Treating it required a surgical technology called embolization, which the doctor didn't know how to perform because he simply didn't know it existed. (This was thirty years ago.) So when the baby started to bleed alarmingly under his blade, he had no choice but to cut and carve out tissue layer after tissue layer, until he had removed parts of a few facial muscles and nerves, split the tongue in two, performed a permanent tracheotomy, and closed Monica's left carotid artery. And this was just the beginning.

Monica is now twenty-eight, and she comes across to me as a sensual, creative, spirited young woman who dances, paints professionally, and has plans for the future and a penchant for laughing. She lives with the support of her mother and sister (the father fled back to Venezuela soon after her first surgery, and died of a heart attack in 1989), plus a disability pension from the state—the money graciously accepted, the label of disabled graciously dismissed. When we met, after twenty-some operations, Monica had no teeth; two stumps of a mandible connected by a rib taken from her left side (after two other grafts from her iliac crests had been rejected); a steel tracheotomy plaque at the base of the neck, whose hole she shuts with a finger to be able to speak with a muffled, lispy voice; both carotids closed; a deep and intricate web of scars in the whole area defined by her ears, neck, and the tentative chin; more scars on her back and pelvis resulting from the bone transplants; several cranial and facial nerves and upper body muscles severed; and a portion of her trapezius displaced and taken across the front of the neck to attach to the opposite stump of mandible. Due to trauma, amputation, and the subsequent loss of neuromuscular function, both voluntary and reflexive, until last year she could not close her eyelids, and she cannot smile.

A Developmental Perspective

Yet, because Monica has all it takes to make the reality she envisions real—an instinctive certainty that decisions do make a difference, that free will exists—all the major turning points in her life have resulted from choices she made at the exact point in time when she felt like making them. What was crucial in the whole process was the attitude of her mother, who knew that the technical help they could get was somehow peripheral to their true core developmental consultant—her daughter herself.

A general principle of BMC is "support precedes movement." If a given movement is not present, look for the stability that, once awakened or restored, allows the desired mobility to arise spontaneously. It could mean going back in the developmental sequence to find the gaps, the steps the child couldn't take, the areas in which she wasn't able to mature, and complete the process in the here and now. Or it could mean finding places where ease and vigor are well settled and harnessing their help; or teaching principles of functional intelligence that help the body release stress and reach elegance. It can also mean holding a psychological space that does to all of the above what the right climate does for a piece of land—provide the right context for thriving and fertility. Faith without naïveté has been the support that preceded all of Monica's movements and helped her overcome the sense of being a victim of circumstances. She states with serene ruthlessness that for her, a necessity is never an infliction. It's the inner decision that something must be done to meet what one is initially subjected to, thereby overturning the initial impression of being at the effect of terms outside one's control. She says: "What I've inherited from my family is a total trust in natural processes, the sensuous, sensible life of animals, plants, bodies. It was and is the preverbal source of my instinctive strength, of the courage to cast my heart beyond the obstacle, knowing the rest, somehow, will follow."

Inner World, Outer World

As a child, Monica didn't go to school. She did play as any other child, but she was quite shy and withdrawn because she didn't like the questions other kids would ask, like "How can you eat and drink with a mouth like that?" Innocent questions in and of themselves, but they addressed the oddness of her condition, which for her wasn't a condition at all, but simply her normality as she had always known it. After that first operation, at age ten months, she spent six full months at the hospital—there she learned how to walk and speak, and that eating was something you did through a tube. In her childhood she was also generally clumsy and self-conscious, so she spent most of her time painting and drawing, especially animals, but didn't know how to read or write until the age of eleven—exactly when her first battery of operations ended to give way to another phase of her life, and another battery of operations.

By the end of her ninth year, Monica had had another fifteen surgeries by the hand of professor X. What he basically kept doing was cutting out angiomatic tissues that would subsequently regrow. It was only in 1982 that, as Monica says, her body decided: enough!

An acute appendicitis required her immediate transference to the pediatric department of another hospital, where professor Y led a team of bright young doctors, among whom there was a woman who became and remains to this day Monica's medical reference point. At that time Monica had her original mandible and teeth, but they ached almost constantly, the tissue was so swollen she couldn't close her mouth, she couldn't breathe except through the vent in her trachea, and the angioma had surfaced to the chin level, where it looked like a bruise. Professor Y tried to operate but soon had to face the evidence that he couldn't do anything. More: Monica was mistakenly given an overdose of anesthesia that not only sent her into a nearly fatal bradycardia, but overloaded her nervous system in such a way that she had hallucinations and color misperceptions for about a year.

On the other hand, some of those young doctors knew that in Nancy, in the North of France, one of the most advanced maxillofacial departments in Europe was run by doctor Z and his team. Monica and her mother went there immediately and she stayed for extensive periods of time, spanning an arc of ten years during which she underwent another ten or more operations. Thinking back, what Monica remembers with fondness and great respect is precisely the team approach to her issues: a maxillofacial surgeon, a neurologist, a neurosurgeon, an odontoiatric surgeon, and a pediatric microsurgery doctor were all present to assist. The drawback is that neither she nor her family have been precisely informed about the details of what they did, and to this day Monica is still trying to obtain her clinical records from the hospital, which will help greatly in the present process of surgical reconstruction.

All the while, Monica kept drawing animals, and even though she was shy about playing with other kids, she did play with animals in the courtyard. But animals also meant and provided something more profound to her growing bodymind: while she usually kept very quiet and didn't move a lot out of whim or intention, she enjoyed immensely "playing animals." She would identify with a chosen creature, most often a dog, then move and sound like that beast for hours, both outdoors and at home. She was so good at barking that on one occasion a neighbor approached her mother, reminding her that keeping dogs was forbidden by the flat's rules. At which her mother replied, without a shade of embarrassment, "It's not a pet, it's my daughter."

By doing that within the protective framework of child's play, Monica could practice avenues of movement, accessing reflexes and nervous system pathways that allowed her to come to bipedal maturity in spite of her initial physical impairments. This illustrates an important developmental principle that BMC reinforces: ontogeny recapitulates phylogeny.[4] While animals, in drawing and moving and sounding, made up her elective world, Monica didn't feel any inclination to learn how to read and write. But around age eleven, Monica simply decided that now she wanted to acquire the usual kid's endowment of school material, and she did so in a comparatively short time, with the help of two private teachers.

See Me, Feel Me, Touch Me, Move Me

At age eighteen Monica was ready to study by herself, face the "real" school system, and she decided that her focus would be art. She took an evening course, not because of any residual shyness, but precisely the opposite—now her daytime hours were devoted to a passion that had grown in the past couple of years, which was going to make her cover a lot of ground with grace, speed, and power. Monica had started to dance.

It's amazing that Monica's drive to dance had begun during the second round of surgical operations, in some sense the most devastating, that ended with the displacement of her trapezius. It began by a God-driven mistake: her mother wanted to take her to see some cartoons, but they entered the wrong movie theater and found themselves looking at *Grease* instead. Lightning bolt. Monica thought "I like this," and the mantra kept buzzing in her system until, stoked also by *Fame* a little later, it became a decision and an opportunity.

At that time in Italy, it seemed that if you wanted to move your body to music in an organized way, you were bound to choose between ballet and jazz dance. But, fortunately, there were niches where the ruling paradigm wasn't an obsession for flawless technique and stage performance. Monica discovered right there in Parma a woman who offered contemporary dance classes open also to disabled—or better, differently-abled people—not simply out of an ideal of political correctness. She didn't make those differences matter that much—in her mind, she was offering dance classes for human beings, and that class welcomed among others a slightly scoliotic woman, a red-haired boy, a short lady, a Down's syndrome girl, two very muscular dance maniacs, and Monica. Patronizing was blissfully absent, and Monica moved her first dance steps with the awareness that moving with finesse and pleasure was, albeit difficult at times, available to each and every body.

The first difficulties she had to take care of were very basic: her feet, her balance. Her body had refrained from active movements for such a long time, except for a few bike rides and the animal journeys, that at first while she believed she was performing a given movement, to her amazement and distress she found her body doing something else. But Monica says, "I just wanted to dance," and that unbending desire fueled the exercise and practice that repatterned her body until she did dance, and danced beautifully.

Once again it seemed like Monica was giving flesh and bones to the old adage "Don't take no for an answer." Doctors had repeatedly predicted that she would never do this or that, and repeatedly she had proved those predictions wrong. So when her teacher said, "Fine, if you want to dance for your own development and entertainment, be my guest, but you'll never be able to make a profession out of it," Monica didn't swallow the gloomy, precooked perspective, nor did she overreact. She just knew it was another "no" she was going to belie, even though she didn't know how, yet. Not out of stubbornness or defiance, she wants to make clear, but simply because her path was dictated by her inner truth.

Just Keep Moving

Monica admits that the "no" of that teacher was particularly hard to process, like a gong banging in her head for a long time, coupled by the evidence that she couldn't yet perform so many "normal" movements, such as lifting her arms above shoulder level. But her body was aware that bodies have "3,500 billions of possibilities," to quote her rough and spontaneous estimate. As we've seen already, she perceives necessity as the mother of invention rather than limitation, an attitude that allowed her to keep, in BMC terms, a cortical image of her goal— a movie or a picture of herself dancing freely—which gave her lower brain centers, and hence her body, the clarity of intent and the perceptual space required to orient and adjust itself toward the desired outcome. Rather than a proof on behalf of telekinesis (the ability to move matter with the power of thought), it is evidence of what Candace Pert elucidates in her Molecules of Emotion. Within the complex, systemic chemical lab that our body is, there's no thought without molecule—and molecules, veritable building units of ours, messengers of intention and template effectors, come in geysers and whirls and tidal waves that interact, organize, and eventually stabilize themselves into cells, and tissues, and organs, and muscles, and....

One major aspect Monica had to take care of was the radical image change brought forth by the displacement of the trapezius. Since her first operation Monica has always worn a white elastic gauze around her jaw and head, to keep a piece of cloth right below her mouth to absorb the free flow of saliva. This shroud hides from view most of the evidence of her condition. But her neck is bare, and accepting the sight of this odd muscle, bulging and looking like a crossover meatloaf, was a tough psychological ordeal. Monica says it took five years to digest it, the same amount of time it took to complete her art schooling. After that, she allowed herself one full year to rest from any activity except dancing. Then she took painting at the Academy of Fine Arts of Milan, and at the same time started to study with Luisa Casiraghi a combination of Aikido and contemporary dance.

The work they did together was of great significance—for the first time, the importance of perception and subjective reality were directly addressed and woven into the fabric of Monica's conscious experience. It was also through Luisa's seminars that Monica came in touch with Laura Banfi, a Feldenkrais practitioner and a pioneer of Contact Improvisation in Italy. For Monica, entering the world of Contact Improvisation was a revelation. She thought, "This is the language that can integrate everything I've done so far." What impressed her with a novel impetus of recognition was the free, dynamic, constantly negotiated relationship between form and spontaneity. She feels it echoes and mirrors the life-long mixed blessing of her condition—form is not there to constrain you, but to stimulate you to find unexpected ways of expressing your core. After a few years, Aikido and dance passed the baton altogether to Contact Improvisation, which Monica is still fully involved in. And that's what became a thread in the tapestry of Monica's story.

A Fall to Rise Up To

We met in October 1998: Monica had come to a seminar I was co-teaching with Laura Banfi at her center, called "Il Cortile." Laura had previously invited Monica to attend for free the Feldenkrais classes that were taking place right before the Contact classes. Monica says her bones are very grateful to the Feldenkrais teaching—and by that she means something we can relate to from a BMC perspective, in which the mind of the skeletal system is one of clarity, structure, leverage. Monica recalls how, as she discovered the reality of her skeleton and the power of the muscles that moved it through space, coordinated by the patterning of her nervous system, her days became gradually much more structured, organized, and efficient.

The seminar was a mainly-for-dancers weekend combining BMC and Contact principles, all revolving around gravity and antigravity. Our flyer showed a sketch of a brisk angel by Paul Klee, and a quote from G.K. Chesterton: "Angels can fly because they take themselves lightly." The BMC part was based on organ support, yield and push, and tensegrity concepts.

Organ support is something I learned, before BMC, from my grandmother. When I occasionally refused to come to dinner because I was too engrossed in my playing, she commented, "An empty sack cannot stand," implying that in order to continue with renewed vigor, I had to fill my inside to support my outer expression. Organs are the warm, cozy home of our inner sense of fullness, intrinsically expanding in three dimensions regardless of gravity, an expansion that reverberates through cellular resonance and tissular communication to the periphery of the system, sustaining all limbs (head included) to move in an effortlessly buoyant way. Yield and push is, more than a pattern, a metapattern—an attitude of relating to gravity that goes into it so fully (the yield phase) it can't help but emerge to the other side, antigravity (the push phase). Like Antheus, the giant who reenergized himself touching ground, the more we receive the pull toward the center of the Earth like a mutual embrace rather than a collapse, the more it becomes an embodied stability baseline from which we can propel ourselves into space with sustained thrust.

The word "tensegrity" was coined by the designer, architect, and genius Buckminster Fuller, known for (among other achievements) "inventing" the geodesic dome—those huge round things that look like a giant half-soccer ball, created by juxtaposed hexagons and pentagons. The term suggests a dynamic relationship between the solid and the tensile elements of any structure that results in a natural predisposition toward uprightness. In bodily terms, instead of imagining ourselves like houses made of concrete with legs as pillars and bones as rigid buttresses trying to withstand the compression of our weight, we can access the resiliency provided to our skeletal scaffolding by the ligaments and the more elastin-endowed fibers of our connective tissue; this lets us experience a springing, skybound tendency. If you can picture one of those toys made of sticks and rubber bands that, whenever squeezed and released simply bounces back to its original shape, you can imagine how elastic your movements, how Pink Panther-ish your gait can become.

Monica was thrilled by the concepts presented in the workshop. What delighted her most, she said, was how specific and differentiated BMC work could be. Being able to name, awaken, and activate body structure after body structure, from system (organs as a whole) to molecule (finding the elastin-mediated rebound effect), opened a window on a landscape that matched Monica's intuitive estimate of the endless possibilities that consciousness-endowed flesh is heir to.

Meeting Place

A glimpse through that opening, and Monica was ready to jump across it. We started to meet regularly, with a rhythm of about one session of one hour and fifteen minutes every three weeks. She didn't come to see me with the idea of "going to therapy": amazing as it may seem, she has never had psychotherapy. Life, she says, provides what she needed to develop, and that was all.

An ideal match with my own stance. I have never thoroughly liked the word *therapy*—a rejection not based on its original meaning, which comes from a Greek root signifying "to accompany, to care for, to serve," but for some of the implications that have developed around the concept of therapy that seem to reinforce a "one up, one down" relationship between the appointed "therapist" and the appointed "client." I prefer to view myself as a coach, dedicated to the revealing and honing of what is already present, albeit in potential, in the system wanting to take advantage of my person and expertise. In BMC lore, all we do is "Give the body a place to change its mind." Also, following the work of Arnold Mindell and Bradford Keeney, I tend to view the therapeutic relationship as a spiral dance where, with different roles, therapist and client cooperate to bring forth the unfolding of both parties. Keeney writes in his seminal book *The Aesthetics of Change* that clients offer their symptoms as stimuli for the development that the therapist must experience in order to create the right intervention. In this way, he simply states, as the therapist treats the client, the client treats the therapist—recalling the speech of Bainbridge Cohen's mentioned at the outset of this article, where she calls her clients her teachers.

But I'm keenly aware of another recursive leap. As the dyad treats itself, it treats the field it dwells in. How many times have we seen in our practices the reflection of cultural, social, sexual, and political issues translated into the suffering of bodies and souls? How much of Monica's pain comes from the concepts of ability, disability, even kissability that our culture reveres as non-negotiable truths? It all depends on the perceptual boundaries we create whenever we decide to take into account a system as such. What if, as Arnold Mindell points out, the system is more global than we might have thought? What if the whole world needed you (or me) to have, process, solve this problem and thereby facilitate other people's sorting out the same kind of stuff? Such virtual questions are always lying actively dormant in me, real questions for us to ponder, whose answers lie in dialogue—one of the reasons why it is so important, for me, to share our stories, on paper or any how.

Getting Along

Monica came looking for something. She was aware that dancing alone wasn't going to, in her words, "solve my physical problems." While both dancing and Feldenkrais classes were providing for her a group context that was a playful springboard to overcome her self-consciousness, she missed the directness, concentration, and intimacy of a one-to-one relationship.

The first thing we did was to touch, feel, trace, name. Her body expressed a clear intent of recovery through a sea of confusion—both being there on understandable grounds. By then her configuration of nerves, muscles, and bones was so peculiar that it matched no existing anatomical map—an uncharted territory that also posed a tricky puzzle to the would-be explorers as to what could be the appropriate means of investigation. She declared her first goal: to lift her arms above shoulder level. So we looked for organ support: intact lungs and bronchi, the memory of a healthy trachea, the pleasure of an elastic, contractile esophagus, and gland support, especially thymus and pituitary for a proud lightness—all places where untapped strength was waiting to be awakened. (Gland support works in a way that is similar to the organs, with a much more vibrational, ringing, and concentrated feel.) At the end of that first session she was overjoyed to see her arms rising about an inch higher, but most of all feeling for the first time in years open, loose, and full in her previously tight and collapsed thoracic inlet.

So far the methodology we had applied was so basic that I could rely on its effectiveness. Even given that the situation was much more difficult than what I had encountered up to then, I was confident the basic BMC approaches would work, though I could not have imagined the response would be so immediate. Soon to come were more events equally basic, in BMC understanding, but not as predictable from my still-a-sister-of-two-doctors-and-daughter-of-Western-culture perspective.

I wish I could draw the scars between Monica's ears and neck. Reddish purple and deep, each of them wider than a finger and dented on both sides, bearing the mark of the original stitches, they randomly crisscross the whole area—the missing tissue between neck and mandible the size of a huge tangerine to the left, of an orange to the right. The left side, however, presented itself as more flaccid and lifeless, the left cheek cold and drooping. In the second session, she said right away that the nerves there had been severed, and I detected the unmistakable hue of resignation in her voice. I said, "Remember how your trachea recalled itself intact? Shall we remind your nerve of its original pathway?"

We did. First we played with reflexes—oral rooting above all, the reflex that brings a baby's mouth to the nipple when its cheek is lightly stroked.[5] Then we followed the nerve's trail hands-on with a, if I may say so, "mind of conductivity." It responded after three or four minutes: Monica felt something resembling an electric shock discharging from the temporal area down to the mandible, and a faint buzzing afterward that lasted for a while. I was the first to be surprised. Later Monica's friends asked if she had had surgery to lift her cheek—recovery of tissue tone being the substantiation of what had transpired underneath. As a cameo of cosmic jest, Monica called me to announce this news the morning after I had dreamed she was smiling. I told her. She was silent for a second then replied, "Now I know I can, and I feel I will."

Between those sessions and now many things have come along. Monica would introduce a theme of her choice, let's say "arms," "shoulders," "hips," "head," "perform a vertical," "lightness and direction," and allot the topic a number of sessions that she felt was right. Then we would clean and cook and season the given theme in a number of ways, some suggested by the classical BMC tradition, some dictated by the ruling zeitgeist, demanding complementary approaches, a pinch of common sense, and loads of creativity on both parts.

On the fifth and sixth sessions, for example, we addressed directly the muscles of the rotator cuff, to help her raise her arms even higher. It was for her a great solace to understand how so many of us, even having all the proper muscles in the proper places, use them in such a way as to move inelegantly, inefficiently, even to the extent of hurting ourselves. Two main discoveries for her: one, how the tiny, deep, smart, and cooperative muscles can help greatly the big muscles' job; and two, how the muscles usually deemed to be antagonistic to a given movement actually increase its efficiency, accuracy, and grace if they actively elongate while the agonists shorten—both underpinnings of the BMC principle called muscle coupling.

At the next session Monica said her muscles and bones were having a polemic relationship. They didn't really see each other's intelligence, let alone purpose and right to be there. The muscles wanted to move, she said, and the bones wanted to stay where they were. She claimed she was frustrated and stuck, but she also was so lively, spunky, and childlike in the way she acted, while recounting each contender's point of view, that I decided to opt for a more narrative way into the issue. We followed loosely the NLP technique called a "visual squash," aimed at integrating two aspects of a person that may initially seem to be in opposition. A visual squash draws a lot on the imagination of the person, who lets the unconscious have its say by giving each "part" the status of a full-blooded character, with its own personality, assets, and shortcomings. The crucial point is usually when, after the characters have acknowledged each other and introduced themselves, they disclose the positive intention they hold on behalf of their host. The simple recognition of pursuing a common goal of a higher value than petty difference is already a mighty way to recover wholeness, beyond "parts" and eventually beyond partitions. So we got in touch with her deeply buried bones, and at first a cranky old guy showed up, who seemed to be there only to sabotage her moving on; the muscles, however, felt bloodful and ready for action, with a certain mindless feel to them, and they metaphorized themselves into a youth who wouldn't even talk. As the work proceeded, it was clear how these two chaps actually were there to collaborate and help Monica find a way of going into the world that was neither reckless nor braked, and the brief dance that she did at the end of the session showed how a new physical quality had accordingly emerged from that symbolic union.

From that session on, Monica developed a personal rhythm, according to which every four or five "bodily sessions" she would, directly or indirectly, ask for a more "imaginative and verbal" session. What has been really exciting for me is that the latter have always found a seamless transition into the active involvement of space, movement, and body awareness. One important realization that gelled for Monica, thanks to the overlapping waves of bodywork and reflective practice, has been how what she's learned all her life is by default idiosyncratic in form but universal in value. In this respect she's not "different" from other humans.

A few examples out of a lot: One time we were addressing the flexibility and selective permeability of her cell membranes, and after about twenty minutes the smell in the room changed while she started to feel a little spaced out and dizzy, even though she was lying down. We started to wonder what that might be, until she blurted out, "Anesthesia!" She had a little shudder then felt like she was releasing from the inside of her cells residues of the twenty-odd narcoses she had experienced on the surgery table. She then started to devote much more attention to ecological issues and the presence of other chemical intakes in food, drinks, air, understanding how intensely toxins coming from the external environment can affect our internal one, and for how long.

Many times we toyed with mouthing, one of the first developmental patterns that highlights the mouth as the primary focus of action, perception, and interaction. After allowing herself to reexplore her heavily sanitized and taboo oral area, on the basis of her own fresh perceiving she felt how important it is for everyone to play and give oneself pleasure, improvise with one's desire and curiosity regardless of social, cultural, medical should and should nots. Many times we plunged in somatized seawaters, with navel radiation taking the lead in connecting her center with all her extremities: arms, legs, head, and our reminiscence of tail, the coccyx. There she found out that by reestablishing the lower-body-to-umbilicus link she would instantly effect the analogous connection in the upper body, and she grasped how body intelligence is non-local in nature. So her path is similar to every other soul's, and yet she knows she has to honor the difference in her perceiving to fulfill her artist's call and pursue her destiny, the concrete expression of which—pictures, paintings, dances—becomes the means of sharing.

Surprises Are Bite-Sized Mysteries

Destiny is a big word I'm usually shy to use, but Monica's story is big. One time we devoted a whole session to connecting more firmly and fluidly trunk and head, working mainly on spinal and pre-spinal movements. She fluctuated between the undulations of her soft spinal cord, proceeded to gradually bring a sense of firm continuity to her vertebral column, then ended the session by sounding from and through her thyroid gland, to enliven the front side of the neck and bask in its rounded amplitude. She went home and talked to her sister about the sensations she had felt, and her sister reminded her of something stunning that came back to Monica in a flash after years of oblivion. As a kid she used to "see" this little character, a tiny venerable lady that dwelled in her throat but would appear anywhere anytime, to be her companion and advisor on all sorts of things, with a humorous and naughty flair. Monica was perfectly conscious of the different nature of "reality" that this vision had (compared to a cupboard, a cat, a kid), yet she trusted their relationship as a source of wisdom. For this woman called herself Vita, "life" in Italian, and to Monica it was just matter-of-fact that she was privy to some secrets about how life should be dealt with. She appeared when Monica was around five, stayed with her until age eleven or so, then stepped back into the mists of her unconscious until that evening. Monica is not prone to speculating on this story: she feels lucky not to have been deemed psychotic by her mom and sister, who knew about it (in any case, her post-anesthesia hallucinations were totally different from this), and she is very happy to have retrieved the memory of that private counselor who was so literally and comfortably at home in the abyss of her wounded throat. While Monica says this her eyes are smiling a slightly impish Mona Lisa smile.

Do all of our wounds hide a blessing in disguise? If we don't give in to despair, that's how it seems. I personally feel that despair has its place as well within the human palette—a place I'm glad I've visited, I hate to indulge in. One time I asked Monica about a shift I had been perceiving in her approach to our work, and she answered, "Sure, there's been a shift. The turning point? I decided to change language. I used to speak of my body in terms of 'problems,' a habit that led me into hounding myself to exhaustion to 'fix the wrong thing.' Both Laura and you have helped me to reorient my attention away from catastrophe and toward accomplishment—not through a meek, old, boring 'think positive,' but thanks to the bold creativity-fostering assumption that any problem is included in a larger space, where the solution is to be found. Like in a Contact Improvisation duet, it's the interaction between problem and outcome within the possibility-laden wide-open space that creates the healing. So I've gently disposed of hounding, not because that has become the bad thing now, but because I'm more interested in an ongoing process of dialogue and discovery. Who is this never-totally-known myself, in shape, feeling, mind-state? This 'myself' is my treasure hunt. And since the beginning, I don't know what the next clue will be, I only know it will be there, and now I reckon every clue a treasure in itself."

And how her unruly blood could be a treasure has been one of the latest clues that life has bestowed upon Monica's willingness to become who she is. One early spring day Monica came with a different smell, a more emotional aura: she was menstruating, and for the first time she spoke of her monthly flow, which was floodlike and lasted seven to eight days. It was big news—a topic so deeply feminine, somehow unrelated to "the issue" yet so primordially linked to blood as an archetype, hence leading back to the angioma. We started to spin and weave threads of her story that had never come up before: how she would experience sudden explosions of emotions, fits of ravenous eating, wild uncontrollable blushing as a response to just a hint of psychological challenge. Then we glided into hands-on tracking, sensing, feeling the blood flow and its routes.

It seemed so simple, so ready, so easy that I was hesitant to tell Monica what I was feeling. I asked her open questions instead, as neutral as possible, and she candidly confirmed what almost sounds banal: her capillaries, all of them, felt like an overcrowded anthill, buzzing and bustling with uncoordinated activity, whereas larger vessels and especially the deep veins were half asleep, stagnant, as if in stand-by. But when questioned with genuine care, they leaped forefront as if they had been looking forward to it for a long time, retrieving their job of keeping the blood in its bed going toward the center, pulsing toward the periphery. The physiological transformation helped Monica to find a healthy balance between holding and letting go, of still choosing while accepting, that resulted in an effective repatterning of her menstrual cycle. In turn, this has led her to reframe the whole meaning of the monthly bloodshed in a way that's more in tune with ancestral wisdom, where menstruation is seen as a source of purification, its blood a fertilizer.

After a while Monica discovered a welcome side effect. Up to then, the angioma under her tongue was still bleeding occasionally, almost always while she was menstruating. It required constant laser therapy and preoccupied monitoring, with the possibility of having to take away some more of Monica's tongue with sorry consequences on her ability to speak, let alone to hope. But since that session, also thanks to the herbs prescribed by another woman doctor who specializes in Chinese medicine, that bleeding has come to an almost complete stop.

Monica, stop she won't. One of the latest layers of our work has been regaining the motility and mobility of her cranial bones, which were suffering from the surgeries as well as from having worn the elastic band for twenty-eight years. The first time we ventured there, following the cerebrospinal fluid rhythm, she said it was a revolution. The world was different, the connection with self, others, goals more direct through a clearer use of the special senses; since then, her eyes have become brighter, more defined in focus and color, and the mind of definition has started to manifest on other levels. She's lost weight, and her femininity in full bloom is now enjoying more visibility, raising themes related to "how to find a bodymindsoul mate" that, again, are uniquely shaped for her but also quite common to any pulsing heart. What she's come up with recently is the awareness that her deviations from the ruling paradigm of sexual desirability could work as a draconian but effective means of discriminating between people who come to tease versus genuinely interested folks. It opened her to a higher degree of risk-taking and intimacy with people, with a new willingness to be asked about her life. She now says, "Instead of digging a moat, I realize how what I've been through can bring me closer to the people I care for, and who care for me—snug is the air when we share our sap."

What Time Is It?

Monica is coming out. The first and very well-received public exhibition of her art took place in October 2000. It's titled "Il Corno d'Argento," the Silver Horn that is her tracheotomy cannule poetically transfigured. It showed photographs of the scars on her back, slightly colored by hand and magnified to the extent of looking like landscapes. The light is normal indoor light, the film is for outdoors, so the result is both eerie and warm, like reportage from a planet very far away yet uncannily familiar. She's now considering how to take the idea further, to include some dance improvisation with those landscapes as background scenes.

Coming out, revelation, exhibition, definition, reconstruction. One time last year, right before a session, I sat on the floor musing, "There's something subtle, almost sizzling in the field around her—I bet something's up," when she hurried in and, at top excitement, told me she had just found through the Internet a Scottish surgeon specializing in the maxillofacial reconstruction of people who've suffered severe trauma and injury. In fact, as I was reviewing these lines, the lines of Monica's history and anatomy were being shifted quite a bit. She had recently undergone a thirteen-hour-long operation in Bearsden, Scotland, in which three thin sections of her right fibula have been removed and transplanted, joined by a silver plaque, to eventually become her new mandible. The bone graft is being supported by a vascular transplant to provide it with the necessary blood supply, and while exploring the inside of the neck they've also used small segments of venous vessels to restore a few closed arteries, even if they could no longer find the internal jugulars—they've probably atrophied. A small deviation of a few muscles and tendons, the masseters for sure, probably the ptery-goids as well, will serve as a sling between the orbicularis oris and the temporalis muscles, to endow the reconstructed mandible with a higher degree of functionality, whose extent is, as of now, hard to predict. What remains of her tongue has been brought slightly forward, to ensure a better articulation of language. She's also received the first of many-to-come skin transplants, to help integrate the new structure, the content, by giving more sense of continuity to the outer surface, the container. I haven't seen her yet, and she still talks almost unintelligibly over the phone, but she sent me a long fax full of tips and ideas and sparks. She reports how the biggest hardship has been a prolonged infection, as having open fronts simultaneously in her mouth, neck, and leg made her vulnerable to streptococci and bacilli. Of all the English she's learned while she was there, she especially fancies the expression that in her clinical records describes the procedure used for a large part of the oper-ation: "dynamic reanimations."

One of the last times we met, she said to me: "To rebuild myself, I had to go further and further away from the narrow province of Parma." Due to a slip of tongue on her part or a slip of ear on mine, I heard "the province of Karma" instead. I told her; we laughed—confident that a time will come when we'll also smile together, on this and more.

Carrying the Message

~ **Kate Tarlow Morgan,** USA (1993)

*This thing that is so much mine and yet so mysteriously and
sometimes—always in the end—our most redoubtable antagonist, is
the most urgent, the most constant and the most variable thing
imaginable: for it carries within it all constancy and all variation.*

—Paul Valery[1]

Cenesthesia

In 1794, Johann Christian Reil coined the two complementary terms
"gemeingefuhl" or "general sensibility" and "cenesthesia," defined as
"the vital sense" or "the undifferentiated complex of organic sensations
by which one is aware of the body and bodily conditions."[2] The cen-
esthetic ability of the body was one of three that informed the soul,
according to Johann Christian Reil, anatomist and psychiatrist of the
early nineteenth century. First was "external sensation" or the perception of the outside world through the senses. Second was "internal
sense," otherwise called "the organ of the soul," where the abilities of
imagination, judgment, and consciousness were housed.[3] The third
was this "vital sense" otherwise named "cenesthesia."

In the second half of the nineteenth century, the evolutionists incorporated Reil's second principle, "cenesthesia" by calling it "the primary
body sense."[4] And, in spite of the classic dichotomies of external and
internal perception or the body-mind split, it was still maintained, on
a practical level, that "mental life was determined by sensory activity."[5]
Even in the 1890s, Theodule Ribot wrote in his *Diseases of Personality*

that personality varied as organic (physical) sensations varied. Therefore, the unity of the ego was intrinsically dependent on both consciousness and physiology. And the unconscious, as it was then perceived, continued to find its origin in the life of the body.

Ironically, this viewpoint locked the psyche inside the realm of medicine. Jean-Martin Charcot's "Theatre of Hysteria" was essentially a scientific laboratory that measured and recorded human examples of psychic pain (female, in particular). The search for a cure for "madness" was dangerously reductive and biologically determinist. By 1900, Freud had clearly opposed such an approach. He maintained that while mental suffering may express itself through the body, it was ultimately linked, in origin, to the psychic process alone. This groundbreaking paradigm shift relocated the unconscious by assigning it the task of being "custodian of language and the producer of palimpsests or puzzles that were then open to being deciphered."[6] In other words, it was from within the mechanism of human language-making that the life of the body could be tapped and understood.

But this new approach did something else. It also removed psychic healing from the world of science (medical) and placed it in the world of symbols (metaphor and metonymy). Freud maintained that what he was doing was an art, not a science; and by this, he was engaging in *a hermeneutical system*.[7] "Hermeneutics" has been the word traditionally used to describe the study of the early theologians who, in the process of reading the Bible, would explore the origin of the Bible's authorship and historic meaning. The dictionary defines this as "the unfolding of the signification or interpretation." But if we examine the root of the word we find that it derives from the name of Hermes, Greek messenger of the Olympians and also the god of invention, eloquence, and cunning. Thus, implied in the study of hermeneutics is the conveyance of new meaning as well as the possibility of deception.

By the first quarter of the twentieth century the interpretation of the truths of the unconscious, with its labyrinthine potential for creativity and obfuscation, became the project of Psychoanalysis. The systematic investigation of body-feeling and body-movement, as it related to personality and personal history, had become a serious hermeneutical pursuit. By this time there were very few clinicians who believed that the body could be a direct source of psychic suffering. Rather, the body was a Hermes *carrying the message.*

Nevertheless, there persisted an interest in methods for "reading" the body in the psychotherapeutic situation. Sandor Firenczi (1916) observed the expressive body movements as they occurred in the psychoanalytic session. Allport and Vernon (1933) studied human movement style as a reflection of personality. Wilhelm Reich (1933) made his "character analysis" based on scanning the physical self in musculature, posture, gait, gesture, and breathing. Deutsch, Mahler (1940s), and Lowen (1950s) all looked at body movement in relation to development and psychoanalytic principles. Warren Lamb's "posture-gesture-merging" (1960s) was a technique for observing movement style and integration with emotional states. And in the 1970s, Judith Kestenberg was using Laban Movement Analysis with a psychoanalytic grid to examine early childhood and mother/child interaction.[8]

Current with these personality/body language therapies were the developmental movement theorists of which Arnold Gesell (1934) was one. He viewed the human infant as a "growing action system" whose specifically sequenced movements led to the infant's ability to function in the world both cognitively and spatially. Later, Piaget's views held that the foundations of intelligence were unconditionally supported by the type and manner of a child's motor development. It was D.W. Winnicott, both pediatrician and psychoanalyst, who coined the term "good holding/bad holding" in the effort to educate parents on the importance of a child experiencing a healthy developmental history.

This single idea linking movement with knowledge is what Bonnie Bainbridge Cohen has based her developmental movement work on for the past twenty-five years. Her work comes at the end of a century-long interest in the impact of motor development on both cognition and emotion. Eileen Heaney, a student of Cohen's work, has said, "The infant must move or act on his world in order to know it."[9] Bainbridge Cohen and others are interested in the fact that the first pair of cranial nerves to myelinate in the fetus is the vestibular nerves, which assist with the orientation of the body in space. Therefore, movement is a primary "sense" of the caliber of Reil's "gemeingefuhl" and "cenesthesia."

The progression of human movement development includes the Basic Neurological Patterns (BNP) along with reflexes, righting reactions, and equilibrium responses. These patterns and responses occur in overlapping waves.[10] Earlier patterns provide a solid base for later ones and, once established, are subsumed into higher levels of movement ability and increasingly complex physical and mental tasks. Patterns and reflexes that are weak or missing often correspond to a weakness in motoric and/or cognitive skills. When these early patterns are strengthened or re-stimulated by hands-on facilitation through the developmental work, these skills can be improved as well as aid a deeper integration of the body as a whole.

What propels growth and development is a fundamental desire to move. After all, it is from the sheer act of moving that the baby finds ways to interact with people and with objects in space. This is learning at its very base. Therefore, what we think and perceive is tied up with the history of our body's movement-sense (sensation) and our body's body-feeling (cenesthesia). This means each human carries a signature corresponding to the history of their unique developmental experience.

Developmental movement ties into the therapeutic, then, in its ability to facilitate both repatterning at the motoric level and re-collecting at the level of the psyche. When people are touched, they feel something and they are moved. When they move, they are moved to remember. Therefore, the hermeneutic purpose of developmental movement is, like psychoanalysis, to follow along a personalized path of interpretation in reference to one's own story. In the case of developmental movement repatterning, the story begins at the level of the Basic Neurological Patterns and reflexes as they present themselves in or out of sequence.

But the Hermes in the work is the message that these patterns carry for each and every one of us.

As a Body-Mind Centering practitioner, my work with friend and client Camilla focused on the rediscovery of her development. This is the story of a pursuit for meaning from this orientation. We worked together for six years.

Camilla began as a Starfish.

Good Holding

From the first session, November 24, 1986, I wrote:

Working with the Starfish Pattern: She tended to use her head first. I initiated awareness of her feet. I noticed a weakness in feet/ankles. Weakness in flexion.

"Weakness of flexion" was a body clue to Camilla's psychophysical history. Physiological flexion develops first, during the last trimester of in-uterine life. It develops as the infant's size increases in relationship to the uterus and its boundaries are more defined. It is the process by which the flexor muscles on the front of the body increase their tone so that the infant's total body is curled into a flexion posture.[11]

This early flexion reflex is reflected strongly in the nursing pattern of early infancy as the baby is cradled in the mother's arms and curled in to face the breast. Flexion also encourages a fairly pronounced internal focus, as the baby takes in the milk and digests it. Complementary to this internal digestive state is a loading of the parasympathetic nervous system, which brings on a sense of calm, and normal sleep rhythms.

The extension reflex also develops *in utero*, but a little later. It is associated with the extensor muscles on the back of the body that encourage the infant to open, reach, and stretch—a reflex that is very useful during the birthing process. Conversely to flexion, the extension reflex encourages outer focus and loads the sympathetic nervous system, which contributes to physical activity upon and within the environment.

Using the developmental movement template, I was able to focus on strengthening Camilla's flexion and extension patterning. She seemed at once sleepy (parasympathetic) and high-strung (sympathetic), and without the support of a balance between the two. The fact that Camilla was weak in these patterns was an indicator that she may have suffered from "bad holding" or a difficult intrauterine experience. We worked with this by allowing her body to, literally, go into flexion: curling up and being held within clear physical boundaries. We called this "cradling" and we worked with this for three years.

The developmental significance of the "cradling" is discussed at length by D.W. Winnicott, pediatrician and psychoanalyst, in his address to doctors in 1964. He states, "The prototype of all infant care is holding."[12] It is, in fact, the holding and handling that lays the ground for the "integration of the self, the psyche dwelling in the body, and object relating."[13] The cradling that occurs between the nursing couple (infant and feeder) is also the prototype for what the child will expect from a safe environment that facilitates his/her growth. According to Winnicott, "safe holding" has much to do with secure and steady support of the head. Subsequent studies expand this view to secure and steady support from head to toe. Premature babies, as well as infants in non-Western cultures, often benefit greatly from the technique of "swaddling" precisely because of the tight fit of the clothing wrapped around the entire body. The "tight fit" reestablishes the tight fit of the last month *in utero*. It is this tight fit that stimulates flexion.[14]

In the case of unsafe or "bad holding" (as Winnicott would call it), the infant is stimulated to respond prematurely with the Moro reflex. Moro is caused by "a sudden change in the position of the head in relation to the trunk (about 30 degrees), a sudden noise, or a sudden movement of the supporting surface."[15] It happens in two stages. First, the infant will arch and extend its back, abduct its arms, extend to the side, open its hands. Second, it will curl or flex its spine, adduct its arms, and close its hands. It is the experience of the first stage of Moro that Winnicott assigns to "bad holding" and it is the movement-pattern that expresses surprise or fear—a position I often saw Camilla take.

According to Winnicott, were a baby to speak at the moment of such failure to be held safely, it would say:

Here I was, enjoying a continuity of being. I had not thought as to the appropriate diagram for myself, but it could have been a circle ... Suddenly, two terrible things happened; the continuity of my going on being, which is all I have at the present of personal integration, was interrupted, and it was interrupted by my having to be in two parts, a body and a head. The new diagram that I was suddenly forced to make of myself was one of two uncon-nected circles instead of the one circle that I didn't even have to know about before this awful thing happened.[16]

In terms of the infant's psychic relationship to the physical environment, Winnicott was mostly concerned with this first half of the Moro reflex. The second stage of the Moro resolves the "unconnected circles" by an embrace. The second stage reintegrates the head and body through flexion—retrieving "center" by curling back in, bringing arms to midline, and closing the hands in a grasp.

The Moro allows the infant to symmetrically widen through its upper trunk and upper limbs and to recover with an embrace. Phylo-genetically, this may be seen as a protective mechanism. A primate infant, when startled by sudden noise or movement of its mother, will open up to embrace more firmly its mother as she moves quickly through space. In order to fully embrace, one needs to first open oneself to width. The Moro is the precursor of all opening and closing move-ments of the upper torso and upper limbs in the horizontal plane. It also helps balance muscle tone on the front and back of the body.[17]

The total Moro pattern, a strong reflex in the first three months of life, allows for a spectrum of responses to the world and to the mother—from the widening of surprise to the narrowing of the embrace. Camilla was reeducating herself in this important ability to embrace, to reach, to grasp, to pull, and to hold on.

In Bonnie Bainbridge Cohen's work, the four developmental stages of yield, push, reach, and pull are woven together, sequentially, during the growth of the human infant. These principles continue to function in the adult body for balance, strength, and skill. I found, in searching for Camilla's reach (extension), that we tapped into her potential to yield (flexion). And it was in her yielding into the good holding, the safe rocking, that Camilla began to rediscover her reach. In March of 1988, I wrote:

Camilla is uncomfortable with "reaching." At a specific distance, the discomfort begins. She feels more comfortable being in a smaller kinesphere and relating to her own body.

It was in the area of what I was calling "the middle range" in relating to others that Camilla became anxious, dizzy, disoriented. We worked with this by my positioning myself in relation to her within this middle range. We arranged tasks such as passing a cup back and forth, stopping at arm's length, and discussing the uncomfortable feeling in relation to reaching for it. We discovered that "reaching" threw her off-balance, both at the level of the physical and at the level of her sense of self. She didn't feel safe.

It was around this time that Camilla's mother paid a visit to the house with Camilla's older sister and baby son. Camilla's mother sat in a rocking chair, holding the little boy. Camilla observed that her mother was rocking the child in a very fast, jagged rhythm. She wanted to take the child out of her mother's arms because it reminded her of the awkwardness and arhythmy of her early holding memories.

It was at this point that we expanded the reaching experiments to Camilla reaching for me, instead of an object. In May of 1988, I wrote:

I feel a strong feeling of compassion in witnessing Camilla reach for me, my hands, and my face. Sometimes her sense of discovery in the process of her healing is almost too poignant for me to bear.

I continued to hold Camilla, to wrap her up in blankets, and to follow her in search for a rocking rhythm that would be soothing. The rocking she found seemed to be the old rhythm of her cradle, not her mother. It was a medium tempo, soft and even. So I took this rhythm into my body and reflected it back to her through the hold. I now know that for Camilla, the "embodiment" came first. Then came her story.

She had memories of her mother: a painful nursing pattern; an unevenness in the way she had been cradled; and a strong sense-memory of having gagged on bitter-tasting milk. Later, Camilla reflected that in the 1950s it was the rare mother who nursed her child. However, the recommendation to cease drinking alcohol was not offered until later decades. It was not necessary to establish proof beyond a reasonable doubt that her mother's milk was bitter. What was important was establishing ownership of an implicit knowledge that was stored *in the body*, and manifesting with psychic origin.

The significance of reliving the holding (physically) and recognizing what the holding meant seemed an extremely important process for Camilla to go through. During this time I came across a chapter in Claude Levi-Strauss' *Structural Anthropology* (1958) entitled "The Effectiveness of Symbols." In it he discussed the results obtained by a psychoanalyst, M.A. Schehaye, while treating a case of schizophrenia that was considered incurable.

Schehaye became aware that speech, no matter how symbolic it might be, still could not penetrate beyond the conscious mind, and that she could reach deeply buried complexes only through acts. Thus to resolve a weaning complex, the analyst must assume a maternal role, carried out not by a literal reproduction of the appropriate behavior but by means of actions which are, as it were, discontinuous, each symbolizing a fundamental element of the situation—for instance, putting the cheek of the patient in contact with the breast of the analyst. The symbolic load of such acts qualifies them as a language. Actually, the therapist holds a dialogue with the patient, not through the spoken word, but by concrete actions, that is, genuine rites that penetrate the screen of consciousness to carry their message directly to the unconscious.[18]

Here is an example of the importance of the "presence" of the therapist. This passage helped me see the way in which Camilla and I were able to create a space in which there was not only the "naming" of an experience but also the "embodiment" of that experience. This process lies on an interesting trajectory to psychoanalysis, where the "embodiment" might also be seen as "the symptom" and is bypassed by and through the talking cure only. In my Body-Mind Centering, the symptom is acted out, as in the anthropologist's rite, through the Basic Neurological Patterns and reflexes that not only house the building blocks for survival, but also for memory.

Looking in the Mirror

As Camilla's "rocking" rhythm persisted, her speech increased. She came to me with more stories and more dreams. Then one day, I don't remember exactly when, the rocking stopped. I had written:

It was a beautiful, cool day and so we decided to go out to the park. She climbed up and down the jungle gym, practicing her step-ups and step-downs in attempts to challenge her dizziness. At some point, I met her hands, and we moved slowly face to face, in the rhythm that she likes to repeat. We talked about "rhythm." About the rhythms she used to use in her choreographic phrases—a kind of repetitive tapping thing she does, 1, 2, 3, before she moves forward or back. This rhythm is so powerful that I find it has infiltrated into my dance. And, I still have the rhythm with me now. We discussed the layers of communication that can occur between two people, two lovers, the touch of men she has known, but I brought the discussion back to our face-to-face dance and asked her how it felt. She answered, "It feels like you are very much with me, like you do what I do."

We were in a new stage. We were no longer in the "good holding" stage. Now, we were "looking in the mirror." What was interesting was that Camilla had used the rhythm of her cradle to carry her into this new place. She was facing me, reaching out, and making steps.

But she had to do this *with me* in order to truly feel herself. Before, I had been the cradle; now, I was the mirror. D.W. Winnicott writes:

"The self finds itself naturally placed in the body, but may in certain circumstances become disassociated from the body or the body from it. The self essentially recognizes itself in the eyes and facial expression of the mother and in the mirror that can come to represent the mother's face. Eventually the self arrives at a significant relationship between the child and the sum of the identifications that become organized in the shape of an internal psychic living reality."[19]

Perhaps, at this point, I had become the mother's face. Or, I provided the important physical feedback needed for Camilla to trust her own reflection. My work was to understand the effectiveness of the holding: to acknowledge her rhythm and have it guide our work together.

During this time, we developed a little saying—"two steps forward, one step back," a saying that represented both her old "rocking" rhythm *and* her healing process, for with every change for the better, she would have a backlash. The "one step back" also held for her the significance of remembering things. In her "recovery" and her moving forward, Camilla was also going back. Uncovering the past.

Section Three
Applying Body-Mind Centering:
A Presence Across Practices

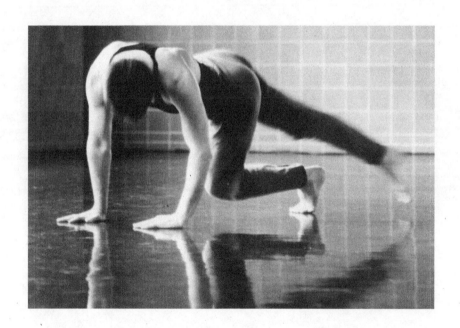

Norming and Difference: A Teacher's Guide

～ **Karin Spitfire**, USA (1999)

The information below may serve as a baseline for experiencing something new. While the author talks about group dynamics and serving as the "holder of the space" (here called "teacher"), the message may serve equally well when applied to learning new things oneself. Her message: Imagine being generous and kind as you approach new material in an unfamiliar way.

Group dynamics underlie the presentation and absorption of material in any educational setting. How these dynamics are attended to varies according to the values and goals of each setting. In experiential somatic education, we create a laboratory environment in which each student is using her- or himself and other members of the class as learning "tools." Therefore it is vital that teachers are skilled in working not only with the educational material but with group dynamics as well. Issues of safety, empowerment, and bonding and differentiation are at play and need to be recognized. Awareness of each of these dynamics goes a long way toward helping facilitate the "groupness" of your students while maintaining the class flow and structure and the enjoyment of "covering the material."

This article presents some suggestions and perspectives on how to work with the group dynamic of bonding or "norming" while at the same time acknowledging and supporting the many real kinds of differences among people. The first section suggests ways of widening our awareness of the group dynamic, and the second section offers ways of increasing our comfort level with "differences," thereby becoming able to hold the differences within the whole.

Regardless of our own personal views of difference—and of our experience of Body-Mind Centering, which encourages and teaches respect for differences—the group dynamic of establishing a covert normative behavior is, simply, normative behavior. It does not matter who the group is, what each individual's self-perception is, or what the group perception and purpose are; groups do this. Norming places some students on the edge, allocating them to the stature of "odd person out" and thus accentuating and aggravating differences that already carry loaded cultural connotations. When well facilitated, this process of bonding while holding differences can advance a surprising new learning experience for everyone.

The "Norm" Arena

By acknowledging from the start that all groups find a way to norm, the dynamic will not take you by surprise, either personally or in terms of preparation. In fact, part of your preparation is to acknowledge the fact that, as the teacher, you have a great deal of influence on how the group norm develops and how it handles differences. This is true even if you perceive your own teaching style to be one of adapting to the group norm rather than directing it. How you "role model" in your responses to the differences becomes a significant part of the norm. This means that you must invest in and learn about your own response to difference: When have you been in the norm? When have you been on the edge? What are your usual responses in each position? When you are in the norm do you take the role of mediator, or are you a champion for the underdog? Do you take a "let's get on with the material" stance? Are you apathetic about differences, or are you an interested member of the group, able to participate and allow the "other" point of view to get time and attention?

When you are on the edge, does it feel comfortable or familiar? Is it part of your long-term self-perception to be the different one, or is this a new spot for you? How do you feel about being different: ashamed? proud? arrogant? or able to stay self-assured, recognizing the dynamic and not taking it personally? Do you feel able to participate and learn in either position, or does being in one or the other group stop your process?

The dynamic between the norm and individuals falling to the edge of the norm creates a tension in the group. Those who fall within the center of the norm will not often experience the tension or perceive that they are creating the norm; they see themselves as simply acting as individuals, i.e., being "themselves." Those who fall to the edge will more often perceive the tension and more often take it personally. The challenge for the teacher is utilizing this tension between the norm and the differences, turning the results of that tension into learning opportunities rather than problems.

The Approach: Balance and Timing

Balancing your allocation of time and energy in the group so that the needs of all are attended to, whether in the norm or on the fringe, is one way you allow the tension to be dynamic rather than polarizing. This is tricky, of course. More typically, the norm—being the majority—will get more of your time. A group can muster tolerance and acceptance of differences for quite a while, as long as the oddballs don't take up too much time or force the issue of their difference. When the latter happens, it is often perceived by those in the norm as a request for special attention by those on the edge or as a request that is not to the point of the group. It is tough to get the group norm to recognize its dominance in taking time and energy, because it is not one person but many contributing to the dynamic. The normative group expects more time and expects the ones who are different to accept it, rather than expecting itself to tolerate and move toward the individuals on the fringe.

As a teacher, it is often more comfortable to stick with the norm because that group makes progress through the material being explored and taught. However, not acknowledging or facilitating the group in a way that gives time and attention to the needs of those on the fringe will eventually backfire.

Typing and Addressing Differences in Learning Styles

There are many ways to balance time and energy distribution that you can employ as a teacher. One way to balance overall participation in the group class is to use a variety of teaching tactics aimed at different learning styles that are almost always present. Auditory and visual styles are most often used in traditional education; the kinesthetic learners are, by and large, left out. In Body-Mind Centering classes, we emphasize the kinesthetic, with auditory as the second-level emphasis and visual the third. Certainly, many of us have reacted joyfully to this change in the balance of methodologies.

However, in any group of BMC students, the people who have traditionally been in the norm on the normative/difference scale in most educational settings will likely be the oddballs. This can cause interesting reactions. Other sets of differences that are generally present in any group are the introvert/extrovert, the verbal/nonverbal, and the cognitive/intuitive.

Varying the teaching methods within a class stretches everyone, including the teacher. When you vary the ways that you ask for group responses to explorations, it allows those with "differences" to have room within the class structure and lessens the tension. Some examples of the variations I use are verbal approaches, which include talking, free writes, and poetry. Talking responses can take many forms, for example, by inviting the class to speak right from where each person is in the room, keeping eyes closed and from the place of individual experience; this option is in contrast to having everyone re-gather before talking. Another talking response is to have one student teach the class what she or he just learned. Non-verbal responses include drawing, moving, and pantomime.

In working with differences that emerge in a group setting, my effort is to hold the space large enough to allow for and foster those differences. I work to keep the tension dynamic by holding the form of the class wide enough that the differences fall inside my form without throwing the class for a loop. This means I work to maintain my center as well as the whole, letting the differences be beautiful, amusing, creative, interesting, and not threatening to my authority, my self-concept, or my "control" of the class.

Learning this takes practice. Often, one or two students will have an integrating style that appears as a drop-dead *non sequitur* to what is currently being taught or discussed in the group—for example, a response to or question about material presented three days previous. Another may bring in points of reference that are completely out of the perceived group context, perhaps references to esoteric astrological data, physics, a television program, music theory, athletic strength training, or global politics. When this activity occurs, I will often leave the space for comments but not engage further, letting the other class members seek out the person later, maybe for lunch together or what have you. With the former, the student who brings up the *non sequitur*, I will often engage the question or comment, encouraging the group to respond as well and using the opportunity to integrate material. I do this because attending to this student often brings out students who are silent within the norm but feel they are "not getting it" or are uncomfortable asking for time and attention. This can help keep the norm from becoming concretized and break up cliques in a large group.

Differentiating Learning Needs from Psychological Needs

Not all differences, however, are the same. It is important to try to differentiate between and to balance learning needs and personal needs.

Watching how group members relate to being "in" or "out," you can recognize that a student may be choosing one or another position as a strategy (consciously or unconsciously) for getting personal needs met. If those needs are overplayed, it becomes beyond the capacity of the class to meet them. That "beyond capacity" boundary is an interplay of many factors, including school policy and stated learning goals, but first and foremost it has to do with your tolerance and capacity as a teacher (which goes back to knowing yourself well and how you are any given day).

For example, in terms of a student's personal needs, someone in the normative group might demand a lot of group time by repeatedly asking questions in order to garner attention, rather than out of an actual desire to understand the material in greater depth. Such a person is regarded as normative because she sticks to the material; but continually answering this person leaves less room for others to ask questions or express themselves. A fringe person can also be demanding or charming and persuasive enough to repeatedly pull the group's time and energy.

It's possible that people are more attached to the role they play in the group than they are interested in understanding the material. In these cases, while you may recognize the need, you do not usually want to address the personal dynamic directly in a class (as this realm is not the stated class material). I often choose to address these covert needs with a different kind of directness. After I have allowed ample time for others or myself to answer questions or respond to comments that seem to be coming from the need for attention, I will then say something along the lines of "I am going to let that question [or comment] sit in the group and go on to ..." or take other people's comments on the material.

A powerful personality can also lead a group into a norm that many aren't interested in. This happens because some people fall into the normative group by silence rather than by participation. For example, if a "talking head" is dominating class with interesting comments but the group consists mostly of movers, after an exploration you can ask the group to "demonstrate their learning in movement." This will often raise a chorus of "Let's keep varying the ways we express the result of our explorations." Switching styles will often bring out the quiet ones or otherwise turn the tide of the norm.

Differentiating Cultural and Sociological Factors

These are but a few of the dynamics of the push-pull of differences and norming that occur, but many other factors—in addition to learning styles, personal needs, and the individual's response to groupness—affect what "differences" emerge in a group. These begin with big ones such as race, class, gender, sexual preference, and culture and go to the particulars of personal, family, and contextual histories; trauma; age; values; language; and mental and physical health and capabilities. The responses to these kinds of differences that are modeled in our melting-pot culture are not very helpful. We have been taught to hide our cultural heritages in order to "pass" when possible, but gender and race are birthrights that cannot be hidden. We are taught to view the tension that differences create within a group as negative, often approaching scary. Differences, when acknowledged, have been looked upon as shameful, inferior, or at best something to tolerate. Hardly ever is difference seen as something to embrace, celebrate, learn from, and utilize. If we are to embrace differences, we must practice and expand upon our internal tolerance for conflict and tension and face the fears that difference or conflict bring up. We must also develop our curiosity about realities and value systems different from our own.

With these kinds of differences, the students on the edge can bring in vital perspectives that may become fertile learning experiences even though they might also "stray from the material." When this happens I participate, but I also see myself as the "facilitator." I monitor the level of anxiety as it arises—both within the group and in me—that "we are not covering the material." How far this goes depends on the context of the class itself: whether it is within SBMC (The School for

Body-Mind Centering) or in another school or in my own studio, and how the course content itself was advertised. It also depends on the maturity of the group. Often I will eventually re-commandeer the class, to make the point of making a clear choice about what we are doing and giving options as to how the questions could be explored with the material at hand. Sometimes the group consensus is to carry on; sometimes it is to return to the material. I will do my best to keep the group out of what I find to be the most dreaded and most energy-sapping "non-material" of all: taking all the time to decide if we are going to go in this way or return to the syllabus for the day, and thereby doing neither. This is where I, as a teacher, claim the role of moderator, group facilitator, and sometimes of decision maker, so that we all don't flop around like fish out of water and eventually expire.

Embracing Differences: A Methodology

The methodology of Body-Mind Centering taught me a great deal about embracing differences, whether created by group dynamics or inherent. Some examples are obvious: everyone's tibia resembles the one in the anatomy book, but the tibia is also different in each person. Everyone's facial bones have the same name but certainly we don't all look alike, although when presented with folks from another race or ethnic background we have to learn to notice the specificity within the general, to hone our perception of differences—in much the same way we can within whatever group we are accustomed to.

Using the facial bones as an obvious place to see differences among the "sameness," I often ask a group of students why we should expect the tibia, the organs, and the arrangement of any part of any one human's body to exactly match the textbooks. In BMC, we learn to see and work with what other professionals would call "anomalies" from the point of view of the person we are working with. We learn that problems in learning and in processing, for example, are not the child's "problem" but our own inability to find a way to engage them, to enter with them into their makeup. And then we seek to learn how to do just that. While a group setting creates a tension with the Body-Mind Centering approach we use to work with an individual, it also gives us an opportunity to apply these skills within a group. The BMC approach to "material," to the body, gives us many doorways into learning to work in a group with differences, pluralism, and multi-culturalism.

One of my favorite examples of learning to hold and appreciate difference and the central point of view of anyone coming from his or her own reality is the organs. Each organ is vital; we cannot live without them. Of course, we can now transplant some, we can have substitutes (such as colon bags), and it seems we can live without the spleen. But each organ's function is critical to the homeostasis of the body. When studying a particular organ, it is easy to say that that organ (the heart, for example) is the most important organ of the body. Just as when we work with the kidney, and we can say that *it* is the most important organ of the body.

From this point of view, each organ, each self is central, the most vital. To each and every one of us, on a most basic level, this is true of ourselves. The organs cooperate, balance, dance, support, and create tension among one another, in the whole. This is where I place each student: the most important, to themselves, in the whole. I work to make the whole big and wide enough so that each organ has room to move, has space to perform its vital function, and to balance with the others.

Those of us who have studied BMC can attest to the fact that our malleable differences show up in a process we call "switching from one system to another." Learning all of the systems (skeletal, muscular, organs, nervous system, fluid systems, etc.) with one group demonstrated that some people had facility and ease in some systems—they were the "normative" center—but in other systems these same people would all of a sudden become dumb, perplexed, and needy. Sometimes it was not that they did not "get" the system, but instead they were so strong in the system that they identified it as themselves rather than as an extractable quality. The opposite extreme was also present for those of us who really didn't get it. Here we experienced the dynamic of the group mind and staying in one system long enough to prove its mettle as a technique, because with the force field of the whole class in one system the sense/feel of it is usually transferred to every last one of us. The latter is an example of where the people with the "difference" have the opportunity to gently merge themselves into the norm and not only get the material, but process their experience of starting as an "outsider" and then moving toward center.

Utilizing BMC principles and combining the BMC approach to the individual with the recognition of group dynamics and our own response to these dynamics gives us a great baseline for working with differences creatively while teaching.

Postscript: For more discussion about differences, I recommend reading from feminist authors who have long been up front and struggling with these dynamics. Specifically I would recommend *Borderlands* by Gloria Anzuldua, *From Margin to Center* by bell hooks, and most especially the essays in *Sister Outsider* by Audre Lourde.

Postmodernism, Body-Mind Centering, and the Academy

~ **Gill Wright Miller,** USA (2005)

The healing effect of [BMC] work resembles the transmission of non-linguistic messages. It arises from a combination of touch, intrinsic movement, and the therapist responding naturally to her clients and providing them with new matrices of behavior.

—Richard Grossinger, *Planet Medicine: Modalities*

Before I knew what the label meant, I was already living my life with the conviction of a card-carrying postmodern feminist. Then I met Body-Mind Centering. I had been exposed to the somatic practice in the 1970s but destiny brought me to a 1994 workshop offering a survey of seven systems. As other scholars were claiming, BMC consisted of "a uniquely sophisticated way of teaching people how to direct their awareness into experiences of the most intricate recesses of the body" since this work included "remarkable healing of trauma" and "dazzling states of consciousness,"[1] but I felt that BMC often replicated, explained, and articulated things I had learned at the hands of my mother and had experienced in an active pursuit of postmodern feminist philosophy in action. For the first, as a child, I had been the fortunate recipient of hands-on work. For the second, as an adult, I had witnessed philosophers *talking* about ways of perceiving the world, BMC practitioners *doing* it.

From the moment of my birth my mother cuddled me up in her arms and felt how I was. She counted my fingers and toes with the surface of her skin. She calmed me with her embrace, carrying me with her breathing until I matched her gentle rhythms. She made up games for me with fabrics because, as she told me, colors have quiet vibrations, and textures express passionate responses. When I was sick she spent the day next to me, her soft, thin hands gently wrapped around my forearm, journeying inside me through her mind until she identified the place of discomfort and eased us, together, into another direction. She taught me to do this by saying, "It's like undoing a tight knot: work with it patiently until it is loosened and falls to earth ready for another encounter." I was not asked to imagine myself as the string, the knot, or the one untying it; I was all of them and none of them until our work together made space for me to feel better. My mother was my first "body-mind centering" teacher.

My responsive act to this convergence was a fairly straightforward revision of the anatomy course I had taught as a science for more than a decade. My intrigue to honor bodywork, however, began to bubble out into my feminist theory courses (like "Issues in Feminism" and "Women and the Arts"). Finally, this new form of sensing and feeling made its way into every segment of every course, including "Research Methods." Here I will share the adventures of a non-practitioner of incorporating BMC in the academy, specifically into dance and women's studies curricula. My intention is to show that BMC is not just a fancy New Age container and its contents, but in fact an approach to unraveling/performing life itself, and thus applicable to any endeavor.

Body-Mind Centering is both a cognitive and an experiential journey for understanding how the mind expresses itself through the body in motion.[2] In the many complex aspects of Body-Mind Centering—its teachings, its writings, its rich resources developed by and with the support of the philosophy and teaching of Bonnie Bainbridge Cohen—there is a versatile and comprehensive template for understanding even our most intricate nuances as individual people. Entangled in the healing and consciousness it purports, the study of BMC holds sacred moments of example for us as we work to make sense of our environment and our place within it, and as such, teaches us to honor and respect differences.

Difference, and most especially gender difference, is the central theme of my teaching, my student advising, and my administrative tasks.[3] I have learned to presume that the inventive work in each of these three arenas is contained by the same root system (a fear of women's expressive power) and bursts from the same seed (the centrality of women's bodies) while flourishing with the same support (celebration in connection) and against the same resistance (a version of dual-systems competition[4]). BMC both frames and gives language to the structure of gender/difference in society, the boundaries that limit gendered behavior in its many nuances, and the fluidity of gender definitions, as I perceive them in myself and in my students.

The pedagogical approach described by postmodernist/post-structuralist[5] philosophies makes clear a kinship with both the structures and patterns of BMC as well as BMC's teaching approaches. Consequently this kinship illustrates how the study of this somatic practice serves not just as preparation for practitioners, but in fact as preparation for understanding one's self in multiple relationships—the same mission a liberal arts college takes as its dictate. I am positing that the fleeting multi-speak of postmodernism captures perfectly the nature of BMC, and that since postmodernism is one prevailing approach in the academy right now, BMC can be expected to thrive there, acting as a cutting-edge example of embodied learning. In an era when most mainstream subjects are beginning to embrace experiential and service-learning components, Body-Mind Centering can illustrate the *how* and *why* of the academy's liberal arts mission.

Postmodernism's Multi-Speak: A Philosophical Frame for Pedagogy

In the academic dance world, the term *postmodern* has (retained) little meaning beyond a chronological reference to an era.[6] This unfortunate lack sits somewhere between ignorance and naiveté, between literalism and sloppiness, on the part of students of cultural analysis. In my considered opinion, *postmodernism* refers to a questioning of rational human progress, universal standards and values, and singular truths that were the fundamental assumptions of the Western Enlightenment period.[7] Marked in its earliest days (especially in the 1960s) by an epochal shift in consciousness that was accompanied or supported by technology, it was postmodernism that made global boundaries irrelevant and demanded

Born at home in New Orleans, the second of five girls, my mother was the daughter of an architect and a painter who met in the Armed Services just preceding World War I. In her twenties and thirties, she became the mother of six and caretaker of eight, experiencing her adult life in the sighted world of an upper middle-class suburb. She had been born albino—porcelain-skinned, white haired, with transparent lavender eyes. Culturally blind her whole life, she never took her turn at neighborhood carpool, read my homework for corrections, or let me spend the night outside of her earshot.[18] Instead, she offered me different parental gifts. She read me through her touch, taught me to tend to my own children though my cells and intuition, and embodied the importance of valuing those who are "different." This is the history I take into my teaching career in the academy.

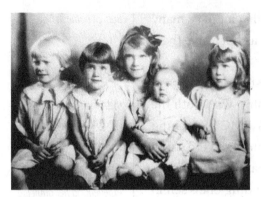

Unable to rely on her vision, Gill's mother developed her understanding of touch and intuition to augment what she knew about the people around her. Seen here in 1928, she sits (far left) for a family portrait with her four sisters.

reconciliation with electronics. This version of cyborg mentality necessitated that we travel both farther from and closer to the body: "farther" due to the fact that technology's mechanized disembodiment entices us to separate phenomenologically; "closer" due to the fact that the same technology beckons us toward understandings heretofore unconsidered by raw, unaided perception.

Both the label and the concept of "postmodernism" are difficult to wrestle still; what is consistently evident as we try to pin them down is an oxymoronic moving about/shifting/reorganizing. Postmodernism claims that we are simultaneously never really grasping the whole picture and always grasping too much of it, always really too close and too far away, concurrently myopic and hyperopic. To contend with this, we must fragment and localize

*1. One dimension of postmodernism is the identification of a **decentered subject**. While postmodernists claim that in any instance any of us may privilege one character or more over others, nevertheless there is no "core" character that—underneath all the charade or façade—is who we "really" are. We are all these characters all the time: both story and shadow in multiple dimensions. A decentering of the subject allows us to reevaluate what we conceived of as fact, and thereby we recalculate its value. Considering new facts/values provides for us the template for asking different kinds of questions—questions that direct us to redefine what we know—and for creating, exposing, and altering subtexts. Reversing considerations based on a temporarily imagined, newly "centered" subject is precisely what encourages us to decenter it again and again. Postmodernists would argue in favor of each person performing as open, plural, diverse, and different; postmodernists celebrate identity as shifting and dancing around the physiological/emotive/sexualized body. They recognize and contend openly with an abject body.[17]*

information in order to reconstruct a larger picture. Because of this "back and forth" movement inherent in the work of postmodernism, we can never be static.

BMC promotes getting in touch with ourselves in much the same way. When Bonnie Bainbridge Cohen says embodiment is a kind of "separating out," that to know ourselves is to know what is not ourselves, that it is essential in sensing to reach a point where we can let go of that sensing, we are subjected to a similar postmodern "moving about." BMC works with confusions to create healing, with individuals to create vast human understanding, with grasping in order to let go.

Postmodernism, like BMC's developmental movement concepts, is not simply a chronological step progressing linearly, one step at a time, in succession. Instead it is a narrative that defies current modern political power by (1) redefining identity (proposing there is no "real" self at the core and that each of us is always and only performing an aspect of our constantly shifting selves); (2) redefining the characteristics and definitions (proposing language as an ideological tool that can contain or expand our understandings); (3) redefining epistemology (proposing that there is no Universal Truth); and (4) redefining ontology (proposing that our ideology determines what we perceive as fact and value but that neither is stationary). Finally, postmodernism claims that (5) these ways of perceiving ourselves as participants in the world and of perceiving the world around us are subject to and never free from powerful and multidirectional political influences.[8] Within the recesses of these philosophical pinnings is the work of BMC, not only as practitioners might *practice* it, but also as they might *imagine* it.

Postmodern Teaching in the Academy

The most traditional direction for this essay to take would be to articulate (through examples) strong and direct parallels between

Twenty years after being introduced to Bonnie's work through my college modern dance teacher, I found my way to BMC in a seventy-five-person workshop in Massachusetts. After one of her extraordinary demonstrations, Bonnie reported matter-of-factly, "Colors give off vibrations." Although I didn't move in my physical space, I removed myself the way we do when someone whispers to us in a lecture hall, shifting my attention sideways. The people around me receded, became small and fuzzy. The room's light and coloring changed. I actively focused on listening to/hearing voices from afar. No one else knew the secret my mother and I shared: that colors could be sensed in ways other than through sight.[19] My mother's voice and presence merged with Bonnie's.

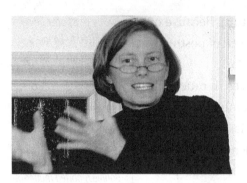

Miller notes that our own early developmental journeys are prototypes in the acquisition of anything new, including skills as researchers. She challenges her students to participate actively and examine newly noticed boundaries when meeting/ embodying new information.

five of the overlapping dimensions of postmodernism (listed above) and the teachings of BMC, or at the very least between these five areas and the work of practitioners, illustrating (as case studies) exactly how Body-Mind Centering works in separate individual instances. From these examples we could expect to sketch out theories about how the practices of postmodernism and BMC advance understandings of each other.

I would like to proceed in a different direction here for three reasons. First, I trust the readership to have a fairly thorough knowledge of BMC and to have digested this description of postmodernism (or to have traveled to the sidebar for more detailed explanation). Therefore I trust the readers are able to see their own parallels in their personal professional work. Second, I am not a certified Body-Mind Centering practitioner and would hesitate to speak as if I knew that work intimately. It is true that, over my ten years as a teacher of experiential anatomy, I have worked with many "clients" in the guise of "student" and "colleague," but I do not focus my time and effort in the daily being and doing of BMC work. Finally, I do not teach BMC; it teaches me.

It is this last statement that I want to explore more fully. The ways in which I use my BMC training are more abstract than the "traditional" interpretation of practitioner/client bodywork. Body-Mind Centering has provided vital and invigorating mind-shifts for me as a professor. In the spirit of that reorganizing, I offer below one postmodern example of the many ways I practice BMC while teaching both dance theory and feminist theory at a liberal arts college. This is a story about the "Alphabet of Perceiving" and teaching embodied research.

The class is called "Cultural Studies in Dance: Beyond Traditional Boundaries." It is a 300-level honors seminar offered to a maximum of sixteen students meeting twice a week for two hours each time. Each candidate must be enrolled in the honors program and have satisfied one of two other criteria to be admitted to this course: (1) declared a fine- or performing-arts major or minor (art, cinema, dance, music, theatre), or (2) have completed Women's Studies 101: Issues in Feminism. The prerequisites imply that the student is a capable academician and has identified some ongoing relationship (whether as a practitioner or theorist) with the arts or has confronted race/class/gender constructions in at least one basic class.

As is customary in the academy on the first day of class, students expect to receive a syllabus to assess their responsibilities. This document serves as a contract between the teacher and student. It also signals those students who would prefer not fulfilling their side of the contract, as they may drop the course within the first ten class days of the semester at no penalty. But on this first day, instead of a detailed syllabus these students are asked to pick a card from a Euchre deck and find teams by making a hand.[9] Initially they want to know if I mean those students holding the jacks are the leaders—all trump makes a strong hand? I explain that

2. *A second dimension of postmodernism is **anti-essentialism**, rejecting the notion that "at the core" of a subject there is something that "has to be here," something specific that makes it "itself." Anti-essentialism allows us to reevaluate and assign interpretation, realizing that neither concepts nor words have stable and fixed meanings. The essentialist, on the contrary, assumes that understandings are unchangeable because they are part of the definition not related to interpretation, thus rendering persons powerless to change them. While modernists tend to compare life's events to idealized performances available only in their imaginations, postmodernists would say concepts refer to what those in power want them to refer to, and the meaning is due to the structures of power that hold the meaning stable in one place or another.*

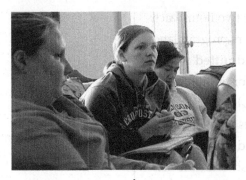

The students in "Cultural Studies in Dance: Beyond Traditional Boundaries" are assumed to be capable academicians who have identified some ongoing relationship with the arts. Varying levels of postural tone express the anxiety and anticipation that is palpable in the first class meeting.

their mission is to introduce themselves by naming their card, find out what each other person was dealt, and negotiate four teams such that each person is included and valuable. The criteria for a "good" hand depends, of course, on what is trump—which is, as yet, undeclared. Immediately they seek information about each other's "beings," since they don't know what the team will be responsible for "doing." We talk a bit about the process of finding teammates in terms of bonding and defending. We recognize that unnamed information puts each of us in a precarious situation as we seek advantages. We have our first experience of power submerged in "silent majority" politics. The students are confused as to why we are doing this.

The homework assignment has two parts. First, they have to meet in the newly defined teams and decide what the course title could possibly mean. What is "culture"? Whose "tradition" is referred to in the title? Do the socialist dances of the 1930s in Amer-

3. *A third dimension of postmodernism,* ***anti-foundationalist epistemology,*** *creates new political space for bodily-kinesthetic inquiries and knowledge—perhaps in reaction to the previously exclusive (rational) natural sciences and (logocentric) humanities. "Epistemology" (the study of knowledge) evaluates sources of evidence and methods of inquiry, seeking criteria for justifying beliefs and claims. Where previously invisible power structures determined what constitutes legitimate knowledge, postmodernists claim that concrete non-ultimates housed inside ourselves, in our own bodies, shed small and specific rays of meaning about socially prescribed ways of moving both inside and outside of "trained" movement techniques. They shy away from attempting to illuminate the "whole" world in order to convince us of its actuality/reality. In fact, feminist epistemologists such as Lorraine Code argue that embodiment is not incidental but indeed constitutive of both subjectivity in research and cognitive possibilities.*

ica read somehow as "less than" Martha Graham's and Doris Humphrey's work? How has the Judson Church era been revisioned as "high art" in concert dance? What in ourselves do we have to reevaluate to consider African-American fraternity step dancing as legitimate art? Where do mosh pits fit in?

Second, each team has to find a common interest in their interpretation of the title and decrease the scope in order to create a presentation about their common interest. In a future class, their peers are to learn from them what their choice of dance form looks like, how to move it, and whose politics it serves in which culture. At the same time, the presentation must illustrate what they already know about writing, public speaking, and numeracy (the three areas of general-education concern at my institution). This first assignment serves to identify a baseline for research and presentational technology, to share physical examples (whether these are participatory or through digital or video media), and to stay abreast of the race/class/gender implications in their presentations. I speak briefly about container, contents, and communication. They have one week.

I conduct the second class of the week for them in an effort to give them time to work together and to model one way of sharing. At this second class we begin with a circle and learn that silence is as commanding as the spoken word, so deafening is the hush that falls over the room as our body language designates the start. I talk about a ground of being, a cellular awareness, a respect for the boundaries that both separate us and connect us, and about the differentiation of cells, illustrating for us that we are here together all "alike" in a way but equally programmed for difference. Our focus migrates to the shared journey for the semester. I assure them we will grow/develop/mature into personalized roles as the semester, the school year, the college experience— indeed, life itself—proceeds. Before we learn to investigate, to explore, to debate, and to perform for each other, we practice

Recently, I read something Bonnie said about her own life story: "[It was] the extraordinary being natural, and therefore things other people considered miraculous or impossible never were impossible for me. [...] That's where the circus influence came in–it gave me the sense of possibility."[20] While I appear to be a part of a clearly defined mainstream (I inhabit all the cultural identity-makers except gender), I have never doubted that I was different somehow, due in large part to my upbringing by a woman whose "normalcy" was constantly challenged. She passed to me her greatest gift of seeing within, accessed through intuition and touch. I inherited from her a sense of possibility.

breathing together. We will do this every class to honor this will to grow. They realize from these first two classes that they must bring their active, alive, alert bodies to class. They are nervous; I am nervous. We survive the first moment.

The task in this second class is to engender an embodied trust. I am introducing language (both vocabulary and ways of speaking) that will help us build community. I explain to them something of the "building blocks" inherent in our journey: that the introductory class was about postural tone, the meeting in teams about physiological flexion and extension, and this one is the first of several about the primitive reactions, righting reflexes, and equilibrium responses that will allow us to push and yield and reach and pull on understandings, topics, each other with confidence and care. That form of transpiration is what this class will explore. We will call it "research."

We start with primitive reactions—spinal and low-brain work that is intended to develop pathways for expression. I call these "knee-jerk reactions" to something someone believes, says, or does.

4. *A fourth dimension of postmodernism is the idea of* **world-making ontology.** *Ontology attempts to articulate a theory of reality: What exists? How do those things exist? What is the relationship between and among them that sustains their existence? If, as modernists hold, there can be no meaningful world outside or preceding the linguists and the social realm, and that the disclosure of meaning will change with changes in these realms, then in the midst of language and social practice as the formulator/revealer of both world "fact" and "value," body knowledge itself comes into question. Postmodernists would argue that there is, absolutely, "meaning" pre-linguistically and nonverbally. Second, this nonverbal communication continues post-language acquisition and maintains its meaning-making both with and against the support of the social realm. Language is coupled with social practices (including what is loosely known as "body language") for fact/value building.*

We give ourselves and each other full permission to be neonates: untrained. We accommodate responses and look for modulators, shadows. We laugh. I talk about feminist theory and feminist methodology. We seek ethnographic research possibilities, locations where we might become participant/observers and submerge ourselves in experience more than a handful of times over the course of the semester. I share my hope that once primitive reactions have been developed and integrated they will proceed with all their explorations through embodied learning, automatically, without stimuli to beg them to do so, without hesitation, out of the body's predisposition for growing. This is what I mean by "a will to grow." And so we close the class with a truncated experience of authentic movement and announce a schedule of beginning contact improvisation sessions alongside the academic discourse about dance's cultural studies so that we know what our own cellular expectation

5. *Power and politics, writ throughout this description, becomes a dimension in and of itself vis-à-vis postmodernist perspectives on the world. Power/politics flows in modernist definitions in only one direction, while in postmodernist dimensions it flows in multiple directions. The power of postmodern bodily knowledge is precisely the radical political work it can do, and because it is of the body it challenges not only the logophallocentric ideologies but also systems of evaluating representation as if it were "the body." If those in power cannot grasp the (assumed) object (universal) Truth of bodywork; if they cannot locate the essence, interpret the language, and therefore figure out what is true about the world revealed through bodily-kinesthetic studies; if they have not experienced the world through the body, relying on the simulated distance of the intellect instead; if they search for the rational, empiricist temperament of experts rather than some loosely defined and constantly shifting creative/ inventive temperament; then they resist allowing the flow of power to move not to or from the "right person" but through reason/science, language/humanities, and the body/movement.*

of movement is (both alone and in relationship) when we watch the dance patterns of other cultures. They begin to understand "othering" in the de Beauvoir sense: that we are all "others" to things we have not been or done.[10]

By the third class, four teams offer their twenty-minute presentations. There is excitement in the room; these works are entertaining yet eloquent. They illustrate what the students have determined are the traditional boundaries as well as what they think stretches beyond. We begin to talk about midbrain development—when does it feel more appropriate to bring the head into vertical alignment with gravity, and when do we choose to bring it into line with our own spine? They ask why I am talking about this: what does it have to do with research? I ask them what is the nature of gravity? What is the nature of ourselves? How as researchers can we distinguish when it is safer or more reasonable to acknowledge the power of the one and when the other? They ask me if we can ever do one without the other: know ourselves without knowing gravity/know gravity in any way other than through ourselves? They are confused but excited. Their excitement spreads to me; I am confident this will be a wonderful semester.

In the twenty minutes that remain, I present to them one theory about women's intellectual development. We breeze through options: from silence through received knowledge, subjective knowledge, procedural knowledge, and constructed knowledge.[11] While the author's team emphatically states these phases are not linear, that they spiral back and pick up more meaning as we twist and turn through knowledge acquisition, I am reminded of Bonnie's insistence of the same sort of thing in developmental movement. So we close the class with a return to tonic labyrinthine reflexes, check in regarding our groundedness, identify the labyrinthine head-righting reaction, optical-righting reaction, and body righting acting on the head, and I ask them rhetorically where they perceive themselves as researchers of cultural studies, where along the developmental parallels we are journeying. The assignment is for each person to explore what she needs to learn and what she needs to trust so that we can proceed together. They create a chat room online for this exploration and bat it about for forty-eight hours.

By the fourth class, nine class days into the semester, I bring in a syllabus that integrates what they know, what they are interested in, and what is available in the area for us to experience. The two days of preparation for this are grueling for me, in much the way raising my children had bursts of intensity that were forty-eight-hour affairs of the heart. Since they are already online for their own discussion I am able to check in with them hour by hour, getting virtual feedback and criticism, so that by the opening of this class I think we have agreed on the contract through negotiated, multileveled, multidirectional, full-bodied communication. Already we have sampled decentering ourselves as subjects, rejected and reconceived many ideas about what dance's boundaries are, actively created space for bodily-kinesthetic investigations, established a need for and a desire to work toward a shared vocabulary that in turn challenges previously held beliefs about "fact" and "value," and refocused our dominant/subordinate ideologies in the classroom. We are behaving, subtly, as postmodernists in our approach. I call their attention to the fact that *behaving* is a contraction of *being* and *having*.

The third week (classes five and six) begins for us in the forebrain. We are exploring our territory and surroundings with much more personal confidence in the process. Because we can shift our centers of weight (something we have already shown each other we can do in the negotiating of topics and presentation and the semester-long contract), we know two new things: (1) that we can maintain our balance, and (2) that a loss of balance is not so much risky/dangerous as much as it is risky/fun. Over the next four weeks we rely on assignments that encourage the elicitation of equilibrium responses. One assignment asks us to deliver an argument that is counterintuitive, something that does not "fit" with our previously taught notions of cultural expressions in dance. Inviting the students to identify their political beliefs and then requiring an unfamiliar response helps them smile at the loss of internal balance. For example, some students are assigned an exploration of cultural rules of homosexuality from 1890 to 1930, the context in which the "buff" men dancing with Ted Shawn found themselves at Jacob's Pillow. Other students are assigned to reverse their typical methods: to experience a new form of/in movement if they are trained as academic researchers, to use only the library if they are trained as concert performers.

To ask a student who has been successful at writing papers to explore Native American dance by spending the weekend at a pow-wow and then speak from the heart about that experience, or, conversely, to ask the dancer to use two-dimensional library sources to find out about Argentinean/Parisian tango and its transmigration across oceans and class structures removes their external support systems and asks them to sense the ground rules of another arena.

Still others are assigned topics in environments they claim to have no interest or background in, which entails searching out the context as well as the form. The parameters of the assignment (how long, what language, which audience, what method of presentation: spoken/written/performed) are made by drawing choices out of a hat. An assignment of capoeira to the Irish step dance champion in our department pushes her in ways she was not expecting, and she is momentarily mortified to learn that she has to share what she learns with the class through a game of charades. A final group is assigned to make a deliberate connection between their majors and their research in this class—in order to stretch all the way out to, say, the chemistry faculty in exploring the value of Middle Eastern belly dancing in the biologic development of the reproductive process. One student in this group finds herself returning to her advisor, asking the (male) faculty member there to help her create an appropriate research question. He is confused about the links and where to find adequate literature to review, but, in short order, a group of dedicated chemists help her imagine something new. Linking theses arenas is asking the student to bear witness to the politics of any situation, and is drawing her well beyond her experiences in a cultural examination.

The class proceeds for twenty-eight sessions. Over the course of the semester we read like crazy, pull out and examine language, learn to manage the digital equipment, interview artists who come to campus, attend several concerts and openings (formal and informal), assign Judith Butler's term *performativity* to every event, create performance works ourselves, continue to make assignments to each other, and rejoice in the stretching.

Last year we retitled the course "Gender and Performance," organized and sponsored a conference of the same name, successfully sought funding, brought in a videographer to teach us how to document events and how to edit tapes, worked for two weeks with ten improvisers (six dancers, one musician, one lighting designer, and two documentarians), interviewed them and a number of nationally prominent feminist theorists about gender and performance, hosted a conference of 158 participants (professionals, faculty members from various departments, and students from several schools), and then created two fifteen-minute documentaries pulling that information into a "Special Reports" story for an imagined small local television audience using the footage from our tapings. Each of the pieces of these assignments was designed to practice some aspect of the "perceiving" alphabet and integrate it into more and more complex research activity. We moved from simple postural tone through crawling and standing to walking and running by the time the semester was over. No child was left behind.

This story is revealed here to make concrete the statement "I don't teach Body-Mind Centering; it teaches me." I use this material in a comprehensive sense to inform my approach to the courses I create. I believe the body knows how to survive, accommodate, substitute, and grow, and the body's paradigm serves as a model for me. Examining each course design and each request of students within those courses, I ask myself: What does this assignment encourage a student to approach/try/learn/do/experience/embody?

The Study of BMC in the Academy

Richard Grossinger, author of the 1995 two-volume tome *Planet Medicine (Planet Medicine: Origins* and *Planet Medicine: Modalities)*, claims that Bonnie Bainbridge Cohen is "a modernist in the sense that her work defies systemization and crosses traditional boundaries." For example, Grossinger claims, BMC includes dance, performance, voice, and sports while also employing therapy and classical bodywork. To convey this, he continues, Bainbridge Cohen "shifts from ceremonies to treatments, from improv session to classes." He asserts that she is not "systematic in . . . an academic fashion."[12]

I would argue the contrary on both accounts. At first glance, Bainbridge Cohen's work seems to be modernist for historical reasons. *Modernism* implies a period roughly between the mid-nineteenth century and the time when dance and women's studies programs successfully infiltrated colleges and universities. Not coincidentally, the height of the modernist era in academia coincides with the time Bainbridge Cohen first started promoting her unique approach to bodywork (the 1970s). More aptly, the period of modernism was characterized by radical new attitudes toward the past and the present (these attitudes generally reflected the breakdown of traditional sources of financial support: church, state, aristocratic elite) and consequently by the release from a fear of losing or offending financial backers. Modernism arose as an attempt to come to terms with urban, industrial, and secular society. As such, it approached purity and refinement of essential qualities. Inherent in that post-war progress, however, was a built-in obsolescence.[13] These characteristics both supported and encouraged intelligent/creative/intuitive people such as Bainbridge Cohen to innovate. So in that sense BMC can easily be seen to reproduce philosophies held dear during this period. Multifaceted investigations, however, are not particularly "modernist." Instead, they are commonly equated with postmodernism.

As might be expected as well, the working fashion of Body-Mind Centering (as a discourse) is highly academic when one compares it to a liberal arts agenda and specifically to a dance or women's studies program. While professional training institutions such as conservatories and graduate school programs take as their charge making/turning young bodies into élite performers, such is not the agenda for a liberal arts school. We seek, instead, higher-order intellectual and creative competencies to engender certain transferable behaviors: challenging assumptions, creating new ideas, and deriving meaning from these studies. Unlike conservatories or graduate schools, the liberal arts version of "in-depth" is rarely more than a quarter or third of any one student's course offerings, and these studies sit next to just as many general education practices and an equal palette of electives. All of these studies, then, are situated in a residential agenda that promotes civic responsibility and citizenship. In other words, the experiential factor is an important aspect of liberal arts. Comparatively, then, these programs promote breadth rather than depth. Even so, what distinguishes liberal arts environments from arts conservatories and graduate schools should not be misunderstood to be simply "ineffectual depth" but rather completely different missions.

Liberal arts schools actively resist selecting prospective students based on one narrow albeit well-exercised and fine-tuned potential. Instead, they consider arts education as one opportunity among many, any of which is poised to teach independent thinking, to expose students to wide ranges of content and modes of inquiry as well as variations in human culture, and thus to develop increasingly informed understandings of the global world. As a somatic practice, Body-Mind Centering has a similar mission.

Beyond the differences between liberal arts education and conservatory training, the Western academy, beginning with Harvard in 1636, created a tradition of separating into divisions (rhetoric, grammar, and dialogic)[14] in order to construct systematic approaches to knowledge. For the most part, more recent faculty continue to find comfort in containing our discussion and evaluation of theories within the limitations of our own formal training and understandings. It is for this reason that most colleges and universities separate the knowledge they intend to impart into "divisions," "disciplines," and "departments." It is also for this reason that they attempt to make available a reconciliation of life's experience by asking each student to cover a variety of studies through general education requirements. The actual merging of knowledge has usually been left to the conceptual skills of the student.

Currently, however, contemporary faculties have begun to value interdisciplinary studies, areas of overlap, such as black studies, women's studies, environmental studies, and international studies. These collaborative approaches encourage professors to bring many perspectives to bear on the same topic and to see complex layers of influence interacting three-dimensionally. We understand that the disciplinary boundaries help us to isolate and explore fragments in depth, while the interdisciplinary studies help us integrate and interpret complex patterns at work. When we privilege the act of integration as an actual part of the study, the curriculum urges faculty and students to explore many arbitrary approaches side by side.

When I look at BMC, I see a similar philosophy at work. Practitioners and authors analyze the work of BMC in two large and general brushstrokes: the body systems and the developmental work. Collections of essay/interviews such as Bonnie Bainbridge Cohen's *Sensing, Feeling, and Action* support this division in the reading of the contents. Books such as Linda Hartley's *Wisdom of the Body Moving: An Introduction to Body-Mind Centering* organize their offerings in this way. Deep theoretical knowledge of specific issues begins with the more traditional exploration of the systems, whether systemic or regional (e.g., Gerald Tortora's *Principles of Human Anatomy* or Frank Netter's *Atlas of Human Anatomy*). However, applications of the work demonstrate patterns and invite us momentarily to suspend the one while dwelling in the other (e.g., Lenore Grubinger's *Neurodevelopmental Movement Patterns and the Central Nervous System* or Annie Brook's *From Conception to Crawling: Foundations for Developmental Movement*). BMC teachers and authors consistently stress that categorization is for the purpose of, to borrow an earlier statement about postmodernism, "fragment[ing] and localiz[ing] information in order to gather a larger picture."

The work I do at the academy all hangs around/off of/on gender and difference. I am curious about how we are and what we do that identifies us as culturally coherent and distinct and about the membranes that surround that decision making, something that occurs most substantially at a cellular level. This investigation haunts me equally in women's studies as well as in dance. The first I experience as the theoretical exploration of gender and difference, the second as the physical embodiment of that exploration.

Women's studies programs/departments and dance programs/departments in the academy have reason to celebrate their thirty-five-year-deep kinship. To quote feminist theorist Margrit Shildrick, "the body has long been the unspoken abstract theory. [...] Feminism has been deeply concerned with the body—either as something to be rejected in the pursuit of intellectual equality according to a masculinist standard or as something to be reclaimed as the very essence of the female. A third, more recent alternative, largely associated with feminist postmodernism, seeks to emphasize *the importance and inescapability of embodiment as a differential and fluid construct, rather than as a fixed given*"[15] [italics mine]. I spend much of my academic energy working to integrate these ideas or, at the very least, to share these ideas across borders. Both feminist postmodernists and Body-Mind Centering practitioners illustrate in their work that human experience is multifaceted and reveals itself in complicated twists and turns that constantly spiral back to pick up new information. Our gendered performativity is further explained as a postmodernist ideological corporeality. I can't help but wonder: How far can this kinship between the academy and BMC training extend? What could this parallel mean to a somatic curriculum appearing as a foundational investigation anywhere in the academy? At the moment when colleges and universities find themselves risking integrated approaches, is there a timely opening for BMC-based studies, particularly those not intended to train practitioners but rather to inform faculty and students about approaches?

This story of Body-Mind Centering in the academy is a story of extraordinary possibility. It is a story of listening to the gifts of each individual student. It is a story of journeying with each person who agrees to take that journey, of finding a place for the exploration of movement and consciousness in the academy. Good teaching, like Grossinger says about BMC, "does not rely on the programmatic way to attain either postures or functions or even a sustained set of educational etiquette. It is a process of going deeper and deeper into the natural, intrinsic possibilities of movement and somatic expression."[16] The commitment to learn BMC is the work of learning an approach to working in the academy. While one summer's training is hardly adequate for the purpose of becoming a practitioner,

this new approach may open academic faculty to unfamiliar pedagogical possibilities. BMC belongs in the academy because it introduces us to a multifaceted, postmodern approach to teaching and
learning, to reading our students, to playing with overlapping layers
of information, and to accepting our missions as excursions through
mazes that invent and reinvent themselves constantly, spontaneously, and improvisationally.

Learning the Fundamentals: The History of Rhythms and the "Natural" Mind

~ **Kate Tarlow Morgan**, USA (2009)

Now, forget everything that you learned....

—Bonnie Bainbridge Cohen

Making the Connections

In 1987, while studying with Bonnie Bainbridge Cohen at The School for Body-Mind Centering, I realized that I had entered a new world that was using an older language of experiential learning with which I was very familiar. This was very exciting for me, as I felt I had my hands on both the roots (past) and the fruits (present) of a philosophical revolution. This article reviews the process by which two disparate times in history fused under the common theme of "natural move-ment," which became for me one of those rare synthesizing moments. I realized that I was the connecting link between these two very similar systems of thought separated only by time—Ruth Doing's Rhythms (or Rhythmics) Program for children of the 1920s and Bonnie Bainbridge Cohen's Developmental Movement Patterning of the 1970s.

In order to continue, I want to define "natural," a word that will be used throughout this article. When I use this term, I am referring to that which comes naturally and without direct instruction, that is, that which we do not have to remember how to do. Thus I include Bainbridge

Cohen's provocative quote above, which is an invitation to the learner to be guided by that which he/she already knows, "naturally."

While the somatic discoveries that fall between these two innovators have been many, most significantly I think of the work of Arnold Gesell (1934), whose pioneering research on the movement development of the child paved the way for the connection of natural movement and the brain.[1] Gesell inspired several offshoots of physical therapeutic work; to mention a few—the Doman-Delacato work,[2] Jean Ayres' *Sensory Integration*,[3] and the more commercially known "brain gym."[4] The Bobaths' work with cerebral palsy in England[5] (with whom Bainbridge Cohen studied) perhaps also built on Gesell's research. Gesell elevated physical education into the field of academics by documenting the necessity for children to have the time and space to move. Exercise was not just fun, he proved. It also developed the brain and helped children think.

Health benefits derived from movement is obviously not a new idea. It is documented in ancient Greek history and peaked again in the late nineteenth century, as the Physical Culture movement took hold. My grandmother was a product of that time, receiving her training from settlement house camps for immigrants and becoming a professor of Physical Education at Hunter College at the end of World War I. Joining in the Progressive Era's Health Reform Movement, but able to side-step the Temperance Movement, she favored the less rigid alternatives of dancing and enjoying the out-of-doors at Camp Moodna in the Catskills, where she met her marvelous husband. Together they founded Camp Orinsekwa, also in the Catskills, based on many of these progressive principles.

The Progressive Era

The Progressive Era was a time when the body was celebrated, exercised, and cared for. There was an aspect of "keeping control" which in some circles became synonymous for "healthy." In other circles, however, "healthy" stood for "freedom" and this is where our study begins. By the 1920s, a new style of urban architecture became popular by providing good light and good air circulation as the "old law" tenements were replaced by newer, healthier spaces for immigrants. The invention of the "airshaft" was a godsend to families who had lived with windows in only the front and back rooms of their living spaces.

The seeds of Modern Dance were also planted during this time. The front-and-back verticality of Ballet was giving way to the three-dimensionality of a curved spine, as if the body were being allowed more options to move in space, to move more "naturally."

Simultaneously, along with more air for tenements and more room for the body, dress styles were changing. The corset was phasing out while "ready-made" suits for women who were going to work were for sale in new ."department stores."[6] Paralleling the invention of the "full-length mirror" where consumers could reflect their entire physique, the field of psychology was exploring the connection of the body to feelings and the concept that memory could be stored not just in the brain, but also in the body. And so, with the shock of World War I and perhaps the internalization of the full-length mirror, psychologists continued to negotiate the world of symptoms through the lens of physical well-being.[7]

"Rhythms" in That Time

While the psychologists and health reformers dominated the field of mind/body studies in the early twentieth century, it was a New York-based music teacher, Ruth Doing, who came up with the first comprehensive skills-based movement class for children that both nurtured their developing bodies and inspired an individualistic journey toward the creativity of the mind. Her antecedents, Jacques Dalcroze in France and Rudolf Steiner in Germany, also utilized the word "rhythm" to describe their systems. But while Dalcroze's *Eurhythmics* and Steiner's *Eurhythmy* were similar to Doing's work, at the core,

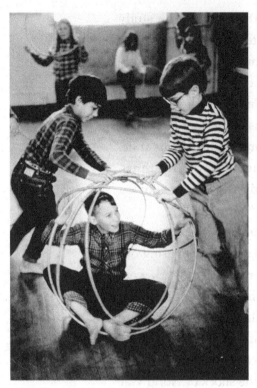

Boy inside hoops, c. 1966–67. This photograph shows Srikant Dutt, Steve Zeichner, and Matthew Cohen, elementary school classmates of the author.

Dalcroze intended to train young musicians, and Steiner used movement to teach the complexities and poetry in language.

In contrast, Doing's *Rhythms* was far more holistic. The student was free to go beyond music and language, and was encouraged to form "his/her own inner rhythm,"[8] thereby formulating an individualized, personal language for movement within the fail-safe template of what came "naturally"—rolling, crawling, creeping, climbing, standing, walking, running, leaping, and jumping.

In 1922, Doing was lucky enough to have The City and Country School in New York City as a laboratory for the development of Rhythms. Consistent with her teaching philosophy, she chose not to patent the name or codify her system. This decision echoed other educators at the time.[9]

Doing's Rhythms work spread through a chain of apprenticeships that produced a small group of educators who taught in schools throughout the twentieth century. Sylvia Miller, now ninety-six, was one of Doing's students. Joan Zuckerman Morgan (my mother) was exposed to Rhythms as a child from 1930 to 1937 directly with Doing and later with Miller. At age forty-one, Morgan became the Rhythms teacher at The City and Country School after Ms. Miller retired. She taught there for thirty-seven years and, overlapping, at Fieldston Lower School for forty years. Miller was also my own childhood Rhythms teacher at The City and Country School, and later I studied with Morgan, my mother. I am the last graduate of such a direct-line apprenticeship.

Recapping Nature: The Fundamentals

Doing's ideas about movement were profoundly influenced by Haeckel's Recapitulation Theory (1866): "Ontogeny recapitulates Phylogeny."[10] This theory describes the development of the human fetus as undergoing an evolutionary journey of all species—from fish to apes. Since its introduction, this theory has been biologically disproven (that is, humans do not share the same genome as fish), but there are definite aspects of our movement development that archive the phylogenetic parade that preceded us. We only have to look at the classic ontogenetic texts to associate the biomechanics of a new infant with that of swimming water life, a seven-month-old with crawling land life, a toddler with a climbing monkey, and possibly some faint recognition of a pair of vestigial wings during those moments when we manage to fly through the air. Modern biology recognizes numerous connections between ontogeny and phylogeny, and explains them using evolutionary theory without recourse to Haeckel's specific views.

Ruth Doing took "recapitulation" as a guide for human movement patterning. She then built an entire movement system upon it, a system she named "The Fundamentals." The Fundamentals was a movement series that included eight Basic Patterns with at least five accompanying variations. These are charted in Table 1.

Doing saw The Fundamentals as solid movement training for child and adult alike. In her time, both scientific and philosophical research pointed to the healthful benefits of being fully engaged in the "building blocks" of one's physical signature—that is, a developmental plan. Around the same time, Irmgard Bartenieff developed her set of Fundamentals consisting of six exercises,[11] and Mabel Todd published *The Thinking Body*,[12] demonstrating the idea that dancer and non-dancer alike could achieve optimum postural health by supporting the natural curves of the spine and the foot. Movement, they both contended, should be *natural*.

RHYTHMS FUNDAMENTALS	NOTES & COMMENTS	DRAWINGS
Rolling (from center of spine or navel)	This pattern is done on the floor in the horizontal plane.	
Shoulder Roll (from prone position)	This pattern is done, belly down, with upper body raised from floor like the cobra position in yoga. The upper torso shifts from side to side by sliding chest across the floor to one side and lifting upper body into a central cobra position and back down again on the opposing side. It remains in the horizontal plane with beginnings of the vertical plane. Sagittal plane is underlying	
Spine Roll or Undulation (on knee)	Body is upright, with kneeling legs under pelvis. Head and tail extend away, as chest leads down to floor. Curling back up, the head and tail condense towards one another. Sagittal plane.	
Spine Roll or Undulation (on hands and knees)	Continue flexion and extension of head and tail but in the vertical plane with sagittal underlying.	
Crawling Bear (travel across floor, body prone, limbs follow spine movement)	The spine is the primary mover for this pattern. During the flexion phase same side arm and leg are drawn along from the spine until extension must occur. The next flexion phase draws on the opposite side of the body. Sagittal plane.	

Table 1: The Fundamentals according to movement educator Ruth Doing.

RHYTHMS FUNDAMENTALS	NOTES & COMMENTS	DRAWINGS
Walking Bear (walking on feet and hands following spine undulation)	Sagittal plane.	
The Frog	This is a very strenuous pattern that requires lifting of the central pelvic area off of the legs into the air. Upon descent opposite leg to arm extends outward to floor (leg) and air (arm). Done as continuous alternating jumping.	
Wings	Wings is done standing, initiated from the spine. The arms move as a reflection of spinal flexion and extension, or undulations. Arms formally move in homologous patterns, but can branch out to all other patterns.	
The Spirals	The Spirals are patterns which can be done in sequence or can be interspersed throughout the basic Fundamentals.	
Leg Spiral (lying on side)	Sitting Spiral II (one knee bent in front, other knee bent to the back)	
Sitting Spiral II (legs straight, sitting in second position)		
Spiral from the Knees		
Standing Body Spiral (standing)		

Arnold Gesell deepened our understanding of the relationship between natural movement and the brain, and Bonnie Bainbridge Cohen incorporated similar ideas and movements in her series, "The Basic Neurological Patterns."[13] Susan Aposhyan, somatic psychologist and long-time student of Bainbridge Cohen, has written, "Natural movement is the manifestation of natural intelligence."[14]

BMC's Basic Neurological Patterns (BNPs)

Bonnie Bainbridge Cohen defines her fundamental work thus:

> The Basic Neurological Patterns (BNPs) are movement templates that first appear in the womb and continue emerging and integrating through infancy. Their emergence in humans parallels the evolutionary development of movement through the animal kingdom (prevertebrate and vertebrate).[15]

The prevertebrate patterns such as vibration, sponging, and navel radiation (a pattern that is clearly visualized as the fetus connects to the umbilical cord, free to move/float in the direction of any limb, head, or tail like a "starfish") establish a flow and suppleness to the body that "underlies the organization of the nervous system" as well as helps to establish a sense of "tone and fluidity."

The vertebrate patterns "move our bodies through space." They fall into four main groups:

a. Spinal Patterns—which integrate the vertical axis of the axial skeleton.
b. Homologous Patterns—which integrate the upper and lower body and establish midline.
c. Homolateral Patterns—which integrate both sides of the body and establish lateral line orientation.
d. Contralateral Patterns—which integrate the diagonals of the body.

These four patterns build on the prevertebrate patterns and work together to enable the human being to move freely through three-dimensional space with "awareness, desire, and motivation."

Progressive Education and Developmental Movement(s)

Doing's pioneering work was given free rein to grow and develop at one of the great progressive schools of the twentieth century, The City and Country School in New York City. But the philosophical underpinnings of Rhythms could not have continued without the ongoing support of Progressive Education ideals, which included the important premise that children were individuals with a voice, and that the best way to educate such individuals was in a democratic community. It was through real experiences that the student realized the need for "skills" (such as reading, writing, and arithmetic), not, as we observe in many contemporary schooling techniques, the other way 'round.

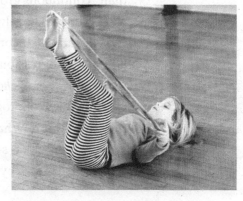

Girl with a hoop explores navel radiation.

John Dewey, one of the progenitors of progressive educational thought, introduced into the Chicago public schools this democratic ideal that *"learning by doing"* could be achieved. Howard Kilpatrick, a colleague of John Dewey, coined the term *"project-based learning"* in 1918.[16] These ideas have reached the majority of U.S. public schools only in the last fifteen years. Dewey and Kilpatrick's mission—to build strong citizens and strong bodies with independent minds—was a moral one, but the groundwork was experiential.

Three-quarters of a century later, Bainbridge Cohen's work builds on Dewey's educational experiment viz. her commitment to gathering knowledge by moving and sensing physical experiences. "Experiential anatomy," a term used frequently by teachers and practitioners of

Bainbridge Cohen's work, is the embodiment of anatomy through the study of the body itself—not as object, but as subject. Experiential anatomy invites the student to don the ethnographer's hat and become an observer/participant in his/her own body.

In addition to anatomical explorations, the embodiment of developmental movement reflects a specific quality or sensibility, often referred to in the Body-Mind Centering community as "mind." Meanwhile, Bainbridge Cohen's brilliance lay in her ability to transmit, either by language or somatic journey, the practice of "project-based learning" in the body. "That was it!" she would say. Like Dewey, Kilpatrick and Doing, Bainbridge Cohen is also a Progressive thinker.

When John Dewey spoke about education as "unfolding" rather than "continuous growing," he understood that development of mind and body does not always occur chronologically or along a linear path.[17] His educational theory clearly resonates with the subtlety of the "overlapping" progression of the Developmental Movement Patterns. This is why, or perhaps *how,* Doing's Fundamentals were easily accepted into the milieu of progressive education: her program sought to release the student into what was natural and basic. At the same time, the approach provided sequencing and skills-building without forfeiting a person's "inner rhythm."[18]

The Delicate Organ

If we say here that our philosophy embodies self-discovery, development of the whole child, learning by doing and the flowering of individual creativity, then Rhythms makes the most of it. All children have an organic urge for rhythmic motor activity. Since each child is born with [his or her] own individual muscular, intellectual, creative rhythm, each Rhythms class aims to reinforce and strengthen these, so that each child may experience harmony of body, mind and spirit. How about that as a challenge!!

—Joan Zuckerman Morgan, 2004[19]

In the Rhythms Room, what starts off as the science of Origins (inspired by the now defunct recapitulation theory) soon becomes a workshop for creative work. This is the core project—to build not only physical skills but also innovative minds. The only way to achieve this is to develop a theory and practice for Creativity—how to mine it, how to extract it, and how to preserve it.

Doing called creativity "the delicate organ of expressive need"[20]—an ornate phrase, which when read over a few times becomes an exciting and provocative idea. Creativity is embodied as an organ, and a delicate one at that, one which must be protected. The purpose of this organ is its expressive need, a need that all humans have to create and express.

In the true Progressive vein, the preservation of the Creative Spirit was also a moral task—as important, if not more so, as Democracy itself. Doing claimed that "all the direct instruction possible cannot match what is achieved when a child knows what he or she is working on in that moment of 'absorption.'"[21] These words speak to what I would offer is the most fundamental tenet of both *Rhythms* and BMC's Developmental Movement Patterning: to create an environment in space, time, relationship, and physicality where this "absorption" can take place. In other circles, this is called *knowing*.

In the last months before my mother died, I sat with her on the side of her bed, seeking the secrets of Rhythms. We had already been dialoguing for twenty-five-plus years on the subject. In January of 2005, my mother said to me, *"Watch them—the ideas come from the children...."* This did not mean that a Rhythms teacher never gives any directives; nor did it mean that one doesn't have a plan. It meant what it meant: "Watch!" I was not surprised to find later that my mother was reiterating an earlier exhortation from Ruth Doing:

"Children's hearing is fresh and unprejudiced. Before they become self-conscious they give out very freely what their real response is. *We must watch them learn.*"[22]

Joan Zuckerman
Morgan, Rhythms
teacher.

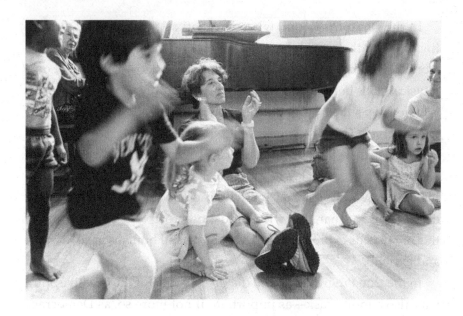

Half a century later, Bonnie Bainbridge Cohen's work adheres to this principle as well. She brings young children into the classroom and labels them our "teachers." Her approach provides the space to experience one's own learning that is unadulterated and uninterrupted. Body-Mind Centering felt familiar to my early experience as a child in Rhythms—the Rhythms that I inherited from Ruth, from Sylvia, and blessedly, from my mother. Bonnie's work reinvests in this kind of teaching and maintains a deep confidence in one's own learning through "absorption." Thus, a fundamental principle of the "natural" mind.

What's Your Next Move?
Consult Your Reflexes

~ **Michele Gay**, USA (2008)

Grandmaster "Soshu" Shigeru S. Oyama said to me after my first knock-down competition, "Beginner fights like baby, always grabbing. He can't help it."

How right he was.

In karate—as in life—reflexes are our most basic natural responses, taking us away from danger and toward our desires. They are our first nervous system reactions to stimulus and are rooted in the spine and lower- and mid-brain, and as such are beyond our conscious control, much like our first fights as white belts.

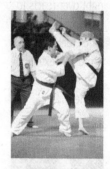

The fighter on the left defends with a lead counter-punch that is supported by crossed extension in the arms and legs.

If, over and over again, you find yourself flinching, ducking, and overreaching when confronted with an aggressive technique, you will appreciate the power of your reflexive reactions. Reflexes, at their worst, are uncontrollable and render you even more vulnerable. At their best, reflexes are quick and effortless, making you feel more stimulated and focused. They are quick because they act below your consciousness and are not inhibited by thought. They are effortless because, as nervous system responses, they travel the muscular-skeletal path of least resistance. They are the hardwiring with which you are born. They provide the roadmap for your basic neurological patterning, the building blocks of all your volitional movement.

A baby's first movements are primitive reflexes that can also be recognized as foundational movements that support good fighting postures and skills. Some of these reflexes and their karate counterparts are:

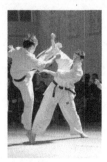

The fighter on the right over-reacts to the attack with a block fueled by protective extension in both arms and legs.

- **Physiological flexion** (fetal position)—fighting stance
- **Moro reflex or startle response** (limbs scattering wide, accompanied by a cry, immediately followed by limbs gathering toward the midline)—attack/defend with kick, return to fighting stance
- **Sucking reflex**—chin tucked in and down
- **Grasp reflex**—fist
- **Babkin** (two fists coming to midline on either side of the mouth)—hands-up fighting stance
- **Babinski**—the side-kick
- **Toe extension reflex**—front snap-kick foot
- **Flexor withdrawal**—chambering punches and kicks, shin-block
- **Extensor thrust**—straight punching and kicking
- **Hand to mouth and asymmetrical tonic neck reflex (ATNR)**—lead punch, reverse punch
- **Abdominal, Galant**—side-bending to facilitate shin-block or elbow-to-hip block
- **Crossed extension** (when one arm extends, the opposite arm flexes; same with legs)—punching with pull back, kicking, shin-block

So here is the challenge: How do you learn to overcome the "thoughtlessness" of the reaction and still use the effortlessness, lightning speed, and intelligence?

First, identify which reflexive reactions are active for you and under which circumstances they are evoked. Once you have this information, you can begin the transition from involuntary reflexive reaction into voluntary conditioned reflexive responses. In other words, you can mold your strong, quick, intuitive reflexive reactions into successful techniques by utilizing what is already present as a foundation and then reshaping it to fit the situation.

Once you understand and recognize your own reflexes, you can also more easily identify and elicit the responses that are outside of your reflexive preferences, giving you more and more options for negotiation in a fight.

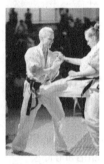

The fighter on the left integrates the freeze response to support grounding and left-side abdominal Galant reflex to further protect the exposed flank.

Fighter Example #1

"I find it hard to take a kick. I always kind of pull back or flinch."

This is flexor withdrawal. What you can do about it: If it is your natural inclination to flinch, go ahead and turn it into a full-blown getaway. Pull the leg all the way back and out of the way. Then immediately follow it up with your favorite attack combination. For some, taking a kick is easy; for others it takes practice.

Fighter Example #2

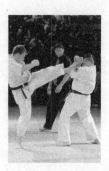

The fighter on the right defends his face and body midline with underlying support from physiological flexion.

"I am a fighter who has a hard time staying in a fighting stance when attacked. My arms tend to fling out from my body. I push my chest out and stand squarely and openly in front of my opponent with my chin out." This is often accompanied by a surprised yelp, sometimes with a quick jump backward.

This reaction is related to the startle reflex, which is a two-part reflex. The first part stops you from doing whatever you were doing and tells you to pay attention, as all four limbs reach out into space. It is a kind of reverse chambering to prepare you for the second part, which flexes your limbs back toward center where you are safer. (I believe that people who hyperventilate are overusing the first half of this reflex.) Picture the baby ape surprised mid-suckle by his mother's need for flight. He stops what he is doing. Eyes wide, he momentarily releases his grip before grabbing again, this time for dear life because momma is swinging through the trees.

What you can do about it: This is a highly mobilizing reflex. You can start by appreciating how your whole body is responsive to your situation. You can begin to rotate the reflex 45 degrees, so that your first response of widening actually makes you a much thinner target. At the same time, you can turn one of those flinging arms into a counter-attack. (I would start with a lead punch.) You can grow that yelp into a blood-curdling *kiai*. And if you notice that you jump back, you could work on shortening your jump so that you can still reach your opponent or be able to take the jump to the side. Whatever you

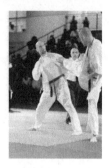

The fighter on the left demonstrates the initial widening and lengthening response of the Moro reflex as he attempts to defend against an oncoming kick.

decide to work on, you must follow it up with a nice deep fighting stance: hands up, elbows close, fists tight, and knees bent.

Fighter Example #3

"I am a fighter who sees a low kick, but I can't move out of the way. I just stand there." This might have to do with the flight, fight, or freeze response, which is very evident in the beginning fighter. It often surfaces in more advanced fighters when confronted with certain techniques or opponents. The freeze response tends to lower your center of gravity and brings your whole body into flexion or a standing fetal position. It is a natural defense position and as such has lots of stabilizing potential.

What you can do about it: Following this pathway, you can increase flexion to cover up and use your body as a bumper to "take it intelligently." Realize that you are only frozen for a moment and that this moment can work in your favor. You can learn to work with it and use it to see the spaces created by your opponent during the attack, to gauge your next response, or to use that low center of gravity to fuel your next attack.

Mastering your reflexive responses is one way that you can master yourself. It is part of the discipline that comes from consistent, intelligent martial arts training. Paying attention to reflexes is a way to listen to your internal workings. If you try to suppress these reactions, you will be frustrated time and time again. If instead you cooperate with them—even welcome them—you are on the road, not only to being a better practitioner, but also to appreciating how much you can do already!

Playing Over the Changes:
Integrating BMC and Music

~ **Michele Feldheim,** USA (1998)

I have always loved being around artists of all types. Art in all forms is the inner expression of our being, and I have been trying to integrate spirituality, the practice of art, and somatic practices in my own life for many years.

When my working situation shifted away from the bodywork practice of car-accident-injured people, I wondered what I was going to do with my Body-Mind Centering (BMC) experience. I sensed that, to some degree, BMC had turned me into a much better teacher in anything I taught or even tried to explain to someone. I felt I had developed an innate sense of when someone was full, when they were overwhelmed, or when they were feeling inadequate and simply needed support. Intuitively, I had also begun to understand learning style and pacing within not only one lesson, but also over the course of a month or a semester.

My BMC education was effortlessly filtering my professional life. I was thrilled. But it wasn't until this semester, teaching for my third year at Amherst College, that I realized how profound this merging was. The following are some examples, insights, and information gleaned from my teaching experiences.

I am a pianist. In the course of my musical explorations, I have developed what I call a "basic piano sound," an even mezzo-forte legato tone on the keyboard from which the pianist can branch off and shift to accompany any other tone or sound. This was something I developed and named on my own, through teaching, as I realized that the student needed a place from which to spring. In retrospect, I know that it was in helping students develop this basic piano sound that I started employing BMC principles in my teaching in a way that was clearly identifiable.

At first I was using the principles of finding weight through the bones, levering through the bones of the fingers into the ribs, and finding the rebound in the hand at the bottom of the keyboard. Trying to have students get these basic principles of the skeletal system is actually enough material for a whole semester. However, I couldn't spend all the lesson time with this kind of content, as the students had varying levels of interest and desire for this. In their minds, my primary role was as a "piano teacher," and this work fell outside their expectations. Increasingly, the students became receptive, and soon I started bringing in six-inch soft balls, then three-pound weights, and eventually a physio-ball to explore these concepts. Finding weight through the bones proved to be a major ally. When the students found this, even to a small degree, they started to know how to release into sound.

I have also found that people's learning abilities and disabilities show in a lesson of this type, a situation in which they are making themselves vulnerable to a teacher who is inviting them to expose their deep yearning for creativity in their lives. This is especially true at a place like Amherst College, where students are under tremendous pressure to find themselves in a high-paying career track within the four years. Time to explore, express, ponder, and wait—which is what is necessary for any artistic or contemplative practice to develop—is not a given. In fact, I believe that when students are confronted with a teacher like me—someone who gives them space and support without too much pressure and has an honest interest in their creativity—they must confront their creativity in a way that brings up its tone, sometimes for the first time in their lives.

Unfortunately, at this point, most academic settings do not include the somatic process as a viable and important aspect of the learning process. From my perspective, however, it is clear that BMC can augment a variety of learning experiences, both creative and academic. To be more specific, I will explain how I used BMC principles in teaching classical piano.

We all know intuitively that different composers evoke different styles of sound, as well as technique and performance principles, in their works. I discovered that if I could identify the system(s) the composer was primarily working within when creating a given piece, then I could teach this with a student. For example, take Frédéric Chopin. To my perceptions, Chopin often wrote in a compact-bone type of sound, with cerebrospinal fluid as a support for phrasing; for clarity, I believe his work needs some ligamentous touch. On the other hand, Ludwig van Beethoven, known for his passionate, robust, and dramatic piano writing, would never be satisfied with this sound. His work demands a lot of muscle, blood, bone for density, and nervous system intensity.

When I tried employing this kind of thinking to get what I wanted out of my students, I found that when I could get the message across—that is, the "how" to do it—students could understand it for themselves. The challenge is getting the material across without going into depth with the BMC vocabulary.

I'm learning to trust my instincts in finding such translations. For example, for any beginning piano student, the practice of looking at the sheet music for two-handed piano while playing with both hands seems to be difficult for everyone, even if they are already proficient at another instrument. During a lesson this semester, I began feeling really frustrated and thought, "I've got to come up with some way for my students to deal with this!" I couldn't go on imagining that each year I would just have to sit there and practice with students trying to master this rudimentary skill, one that is second nature for me. Suddenly I thought, "Oh, crossing over the brain—right hand to left brain, left hand to right brain!" and I started experimenting. I asked the students to focus on the part of the brain where the tracts cross over, and not focus so much with the eyes glued to the written music. I even put my hands on their foreheads and had them imagine this, telling them to relax into this part of their brain, imagining the tracts crossing easily over from eyes to brain to hand. For the students who were willing to work with this on their own, this method worked miraculously.

One of my jazz piano students had a tremendous breakthrough this semester. It was another indicator of how profound this type of integration can be. I was working with a male piano student from Hampshire College who has been studying with me for more than two years. He had been making slow, steady progress, but his melodic improvisational-skills work was frustrating both of us. A few weeks before the end of the semester, he was practicing improvising during the lesson, feeling depressed, as was I, about his ability to integrate all the practicing skills he was doing on his own during the semester. All of a sudden I yelled out, "Play over the changes! Assume you know the changes. Move higher in your brain and play without thinking!" I went on like this for a bit when, suddenly, he had a tremendous breakthrough and starting playing like a mature jazz pianist, beautifully integrating melodic ideas that synthesized the material we had worked hard on all semester. It was really an incredible thing to see and hear. He played in this new paradigm for ten minutes and then we stopped and tried to identify what it was, exactly, that he had done within his bodymind. At the next lesson we tried to recreate this shift. We were able to get about half the way to the same place but, still, we both felt very successful in what had transpired. Finding this place of integration once was enough to feel the *inspiration* to find it again.

In this process of exploring the integration of somatics and piano teaching, I am realizing that not only is BMC very helpful in teaching technique, it is also great for developing a teaching style; for working with learning differences and disabilities, both cognitive and musical; and for working with injuries having to do with the instrument. To codify all of this would take writing a book, and at this point I am still learning, editing, and in need of more experience. However, I am ready to stretch other people's definitions of a "music instrumental teacher." I postulate that the piano lesson can be used as a diagnostic tool to discover a lot about both the strengths and weaknesses of a person's learning style and where a challenge is in the case of a learning disability. A lesson of this type could also show motor-skill difficulties and strengths and one's ability to modulate between motor/sensory and parasympathetic/sympathetic systems. This is true because in learning to play, one needs to listen as well, and there are delicate shifts that need to happen in order to improvise. Students need to have their motor skills going and, at the same time, be able to soften into their sensory and parasympathetic systems in order to *hear* a melody in their minds *and play* it. In this sense, in any kind of lesson where one's physical, mental, and creative desires are combined, the same diagnostic principles would hold by changing the ear apparatus as part of the motor-system loop to the eye, the whole body, and so forth, depending on the art form.

In closing, I would like to say that I am now interested in working with artists who want support of this kind. I can offer guidance in solving technique problems and support in finding depth of creativity and expression. I can also counsel on injury prevention and I hope, over time, to be able to address learning problems relating to someone's individual art form, using Body-Mind Centering as a base. We all struggle with these issues in our own forms of expression in work and life. The struggle is one that requires a patient sense of compassion to hang in there with this kind of learning. I have not found this type of support in the educational system anywhere so far, but it definitely is in us from our BMC training; it is something we have to offer.

I recently got some feedback from Myra Avedon, a BMC-certified teacher, as I was sharing my experiences with her. The feedback was helpful in terms of interpreting BMC language into a movement, and then giving an example of a famous musician who clearly does this movement in his body while performing. Stevie Wonder, as Myra pointed out, moves his head back and forth in the horizontal plane, with an organ-like rhythm. Perhaps his movement integrates his right and left sides and helps him stay in his organs and out of an intense nervous-system flood. The possibilities of this approach are well worth investigating. Body-Mind Centering offers us an incredible resource at hand, a huge blossoming of wisdom, if we can only be patient enough within ourselves to find it.

Mentoring from a Distance

〜 **Gill Wright Miller,** USA (2009)

The impact of mentoring is not what people learn, but rather how it changes people.

Somatics is something we tune in to through experience in our own bodies in the present moment. The concept of "distance mentoring" seems oxymoronic in relation to a somatic learning journey. Is there a way for professionals in the field to bring their expertise to college classrooms in rural locations? Can distanced learning adequately mentor students who are new to the idea of a somatic process? Can an on-site teacher guide a multi-directional learning process? My recent experiment in "distance somatic mentoring" shows that the college classroom can become a laboratory for translating practitioner/client ideas; certified mentors can articulate expectations of their experiences in lay terms; students can explain something they just learned to a third party; and the classroom teacher can serve as guide, interpreter, and supporter of the learning process rather than as an ultimate evaluator of student performance.

This essay explores a pilot study in which technology facilitated the mentoring of college students new to the practice of somatics, specifically the practices of Body-Mind Centering. A six-week-long academic project rotated the leadership role among teams of primary players (field professionals, students, and a faculty member), promoting deeper and more meaningful teaching/learning events and encouraging group activities through which explanation, exploration, and experience were shared among the participants.

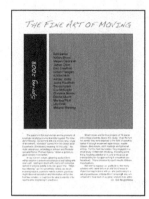

The students in Dr. Miller's experiential anatomy/ kinesiology class did individual research projects and then published them in a text called "The Fine Art of Moving."

This is a story about thirty-three people of various ages bumping into each other for a few short weeks to experience and exchange information about a somatics exploration. It is a story about identifying expertise and acknowledging support at the edges of our intellectual capacity. It is a story about the wonder of discovery in a process that is, initially, intentionally confusing. It is a story about exposure: "meeting" the risks of learning and "allowing" the challenge of teaching.

"The Fine Art of Moving," an Honors seminar in Experiential Anatomy, was offered in Spring 2008 at Denison University (Granville, Ohio), a small liberal arts college of twenty-one hundred students where I have been teaching dance and women's studies for nearly thirty years. While I've taught anatomy since the beginning of my tenure at Denison, in the early 1990s this course transformed from one that focused on learning to identify the interactive skeletal and muscular systems to one that incorporated all the somatic work I felt qualified to introduce. The course added a new dimension, distance mentoring, in the Honors curriculum in Spring 2008. Sixteen students enrolled—fourteen females, two males; four seniors, five juniors, four sophomores, three first-years. The students' majors were heavily concentrated in the sciences and, to a lesser degree, the arts. Nine were natural science majors, three social science majors, three humanities students, and one undeclared. Three had second majors in dance; two claimed minors in dance. The course met for two hours twice a week for fourteen weeks. Additionally, there was a final exam period of two hours in Week 15.

The first eight weeks of the semester served as preparation for a final class project. During that time, the students read Don Hanlon Johnson's *Bones, Breath & Gesture* for general context, Linda Hartley's *Wisdom of the Body Moving* for an explanation and summary of Body-Mind Centering concepts and approaches, and several essays from Bonnie Bainbridge Cohen's *Sensing, Feeling, and Action* for focused attention on reflexes and developmental movement. This academic work was accompanied by field experiences in water play, juggling, sledding, wall climbing, and ice skating—each movement experience selected to expose the students to reflexes and developmental movement in "less familiar" movement contexts.[1] Students were then invited to identify a movement exploration of their own design, one in which they could more closely examine a personal movement experience in the context of reflexes and developmental movement.

The final project was designed to extend through the last six weeks of the semester. In the first two weeks of the project (Weeks 9–10 of the course), each of the sixteen students named their *Intention* and *Attention*. (What did they want to consider, and how did they want to attend to it?) I then posted the list of sixteen projects on an Internet list serve, asking Body-Mind Centering (BMC) practitioners if they would volunteer to be "temporary mentors" by selecting a project that resonated with them and making a two-week commitment to the student. By the end of the third week of the project (Week 11 of the course), each student had been matched with a certified practitioner in the field of Body-Mind Centering.

The profiles of the professional volunteer mentors paralleled that of the students comfortably. Fourteen identify as female; two as male. They represented the field's "spread" of most experienced to least experienced (with certification having been granted more than twenty-five years ago for one; just under one year ago for another). They each identified movement explorations of their own design that they had developed into a professional focus or practice.

The students were novices to the field of somatics. None of them had studied this work previously, but each was genuinely curious about movement in some form or another. Their movement explorations varied greatly, looking at the activities of golf swings, sprint mechanics, bench pressing, playing the violin, competitive swimming "starts," horseback riding, learning to cartwheel and to ride a bike. Several students looked at more internal quests: yielding weight in a *plié*, the secrets of performing *fouetté* or *pirouette* turns, or the tendency to walk only on the ball of the foot rather than the whole foot. Three sought an understanding of "core support"; one addressed a previously encountered knee injury.

Like the students, the volunteer mentors represented a wide range of interests in the professional field. One had been in private practice since 1975 and was certified in BMC as long ago as 1982. At the time of this study, she offered workshops and specialty classes in breathing, vocalization, and movement applications for voice.

About half of the practitioners were certified in the 1990s. Their post-graduate work took them in different directions: one taught BMC at the University of Minnesota and maintained a private practice working with adults and children. Another pioneered contemporary dance in Ireland in the '70s and '80s and had consistently experimented with collaborative art as a professional artist and therapist. Claiming a deep connection to nature, her current work was based on the practice of Authentic Movement along with Body-Mind Centering. A third had a private practice in bodywork and movement therapy, newly renamed "Bodylearning," where she focused on children with cerebral palsy.

A fourth mentor worked as a Movement Therapist, Craniosacral Therapist, musician and writer/producer in western Massachusetts, New York City, and Seattle. A fifth, who had extensive training in dance, Reiki/energy medicine, yoga, herbology, nutrition, and counseling, had maintained a private practice in BMC for more than a decade. A sixth had created his own program, The Center for BodyMindMovement, co-directed the Embodied Performing Arts Program in London with a colleague, and taught regularly in Mexico through the Center for Choreographic Investigation and the Instituto de Psicología Profunda en México, and in Brazil and Ireland.

The remainder of the mentors were much more recent graduates of the BMC certification program but often had worked in tangential somatic fields for years: one was a Reiki practitioner, teaching experiential anatomy, meditation, and dance; two spent much of their time teaching embodied yoga classes and workshops in various places on both U.S.

coasts; a third was in the beginning stages of building a BMC private practice, along with teaching and assisting in certification programs.

The partners—one student and one mentor—spent Weeks 4 and 5 of the project (Weeks 12 and 13 of the course) communicating through email correspondence. As the faculty member, I created a linked address to an individual video and/or uploaded material to YouTube so that this correspondence could be supplemented with video exchanges. The mentor helped the student consider *Assimilation* and *Retention*. (What experiences from early developmental neurological practices could support accomplishing a specific movement goal, and how would that newly-practiced pattern be retained in the current adult state?) In Week 6 of the project (Week 14 of the course), the students wrote up their experiences of both movement and mentoring with a required statement of *Extension* (how will this work be carried out into the future?) and presented the results to each other.[2]

Once these individual mini-research projects were completed, I collated them, dumped them into an iWork/Pages file, copyedited each one of them, and sent them back and forth to the students for re-reading, revising, and re-integrating. This process, while paralleling an expedited professional publications process, was designed to accomplish several "post-project" aspects of learning as well. Students were able to see their work with some distance, having been away from it for a week. They were asked to answer minute questions of clarity, since a new reader was trying to make sense of their writing. As they checked each other's work for errors, they were exposed to each other's writing and needed to make sense of their own in the context of their classmates'. Finally, as in any writing project, the very act of working with the written word over several drafts helped to clarify and deepen the drafts.

In our final-exam time slot, we created a sort of "fair," with stations where a third of the students at a time presented their projects as active studies, demonstrating what they had learned, leading their classmates through an exploration of at least one physical exercise, illustrating the relationship between theory and practice. In this way, each student experienced the teaching of his/her own material and was a student for several other classmates' material. This form of a final exam gave the students an opportunity to expand the concept of a "poster program" (familiar in the sciences, the home discipline of many of the students) by combining the illustrated explanation of their exploration with physical activity.

"Somatics" comes from the Greek word Σωματικός (Somatikòs) meaning "of the body." Somatic awareness, according to scholar and Feldenkrais practitioner Thomas Hanna, "allows a person to glean wisdom from within." In our quick-paced, rather impatient U.S. culture, gleaning wisdom from within requires an uncustomary sitting with one's self. Getting in touch with one's self unfolds quietly in its own good time. "Attentive listening" can be a somewhat evasive practice; a person new to somatic practices might discover sensation and information within the first few minutes, or might not be able to identify it for months after practicing the discipline of it.

While the pedagogy of somatics lends itself easily to a traditional college curriculum, the content of somatics does not. First, any and all students are invited to enroll, regardless of background. Some come to a new course with a high level of technical skill in a movement field. (In this Honors class, one student was a superb baseball player, another a highly competitive swimmer; one was a graceful and skilled wall climber, while six were beautifully trained dancers.) Others in the class enrolled less due to their commitment to specific movement practices and more due to their intelligence and curiosity as individuals with accomplished academic records. (In our Honors program, students are given a short list of courses from which to choose.) Some had been exposed to bits and pieces of somatic practices; others had never heard the word before. This variation in preparation, while challenging, is typical in a liberal arts setting. But it means that traveling through the syllabus as a group may be problematic.

Second, a specific timetable is imposed on the learning process. All events related to the teaching must begin at the start of the semester and be completed by the end of the semester, a fifteen-week window. Each class meets two or three times a week, but must start and stop at a specified time. Each student is engaged not only by this study but by three other courses or more, so long periods of concentrated commitment are unavailable and unreasonable.

Finally, the very concept of "grading" in its traditional understanding seems antithetical to the kind of support a somatics exploration might warrant. On what will the students be "measured"? How can the observer (in this case the teacher) know when and whether an authentic experience will "pay off" within the semester? If a student is coming to class prepared every day (having read the assignments, having studied the pictures, having spent quiet time with himself or herself, having written a journal entry), there is still no guarantee she or he will have an "ah-ha!" moment within the soma. And so, teaching Experiential Anatomy with a heavy dose of somatics invited a tension between exploring and expanding, with an acceptance of whatever discoveries were made within a given and limited framework of time, and evaluating concrete and quantifiable progress toward "an understanding of oneself from the inside out," rather than mapping that progress as work of A (excellent), B (good), or C (average) quality.

Adding to this inherent dilemma for any liberal arts class was the assumption that Honors students are more skilled at the academic game than the average student, and therefore are expecting to receive better grades. The Honors Document, which guides the structure and implementation of Honors courses, implores faculty to realize that Honors seminars should place a premium on students who are highly motivated. Faculty expect high quality in all student work while using texts/materials that are especially challenging. Honors students expect to be unequivocally successful at tackling/conquering/embodying new information. They are asked and want to reach beyond the average agenda. For some students, this means making the scaffolding of the academic game so crystal-clear that they are sure to win it. Ironically, some students find it difficult to accept taking what they assess as "un-do" risks, not knowing where the journey will lead, as a feasible part of the bargain.

And yet, Denison's Honors Program has other goals and characteristics [see table] that include a significant research component, promotion of student initiative, and cultivation of a profound sense of intellectual intimacy. The program encourages courses on more experimental topics, or conventional topics with more experimental course designs, and asks that faculty address the topic(s) of the seminar in ways that may seem unorthodox or outside the box. These goals and characteristics encouraged me simultaneously to risk submitting my students to the professional somatic community and the professional somatic community to my students. I believed the students were prepared for a more challenging conversation in Body-Mind Centering than I could provide for each one of them, and I believed the BMC mentor/practitioners would be generous enough to find wonder and awe in successful students who were curious about a journey of gleaning wisdom from within.

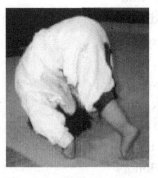

The student researcher sorted through her own family pictures to find evidence of her early relationship to "yielding" and "groundedness." Pictured here, she experiments with somersaulting.

Student Explorations

BB (students are identified only through a set of initials) was exploring her sense of groundedness, the connection of her lower torso to the earth. Ultimately, she named this "a desire to yield [her] weight into gravity." Her work showed that she understood the continuity from her own youth-through-adult activities, took on precise challenges, and kept her sights on her specific inquiry in several situations. Through a range of actions, from *pliés* to downhill skiing, she applied what she was learning about her homologous push with the lower limbs.

KB was curious about a new sport (golf) that she was just beginning to explore. Her more experienced friends often told

Goals and Characteristics of Honors Seminars at Denison

- Each semester, there should be diverse course offerings, across divisions, and across all undergraduate classes.
- We encourage Honors seminars on special topics, as well as special sections of regular courses.
- Ideally, seminars are limited to 15 students. (We recognize that individual faculty and departments may wish on occasion to expand these limits.)
- Ideally, seminars are limited to Honors students. (We recognize that faculty may wish on occasion to admit other students. We encourage faculty to look especially to students with strong academic records, special expertise, and/or with exceptional motivation in the area.)
- Honors seminars should place a premium on students who are highly motivated and intellectually engaged in creative and scholarly work.
- Seminars ought to include a significant research component and/or artistic endeavor. They should promote student initiative and disciplined practice.
- Faculty should be able to expect high quality in all student work.
- Faculty should be able to use texts/materials that are especially challenging.
- We encourage courses on more experimental topics, or conventional topics with more experimental course designs.
- We especially encourage courses that feature multiple intellectual and/or disciplinary perspectives. How can we address the topic(s) of the seminar in a variety of ways, that may seem unorthodox or outside the box?
- We encourage courses that are team-taught (rather than with separate modules taught by different instructors) and/or "linked courses" on related topics (where students register for two courses simultaneously).
- A major goal of Seminars is to achieve a profound sense of intellectual intimacy and a shared delight in exploring a topic in usual depth. We encourage the use of venues—whether for special events or regular class meetings—that foster conversation in a relaxed setting and/or acquaint students with specialized resources or technology.

Denison University's Honors Program has created guidelines
that steer the creation of any course being offered.

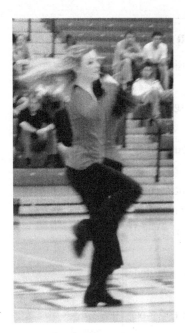

The student in this illustration is twirling in a dance routine. She noticed the pull from the upper body in several named movements from dance class.

her that she needed to keep her head down while swinging. She focused her project on reflexes that supported connecting her upper limbs with her core. Her work started with floor exercises and gradually spiraled to standing.

A highly accomplished ballet dancer, MC noticed that she "pulled from the upper to initiate a push from the lower" during *fouetté* turns. She had been trained to rely on a visual check in the mirrors. In this exploration, she realized she had organs. "Focusing [on] my body's postural tone led me to realize that organ tone is directly underneath this postural tone. My body's inner 'soma' feels the organs touching my skin from the inside...."

Her close friend and classmate, CM, is also a highly accomplished ballet dancer. She sought perfection of her *pirouette* turn. Earlier, using the third-person perspective so typical in ballet training, she determined she would "shift back into the soma" to work with the undesirable "falling off vertical alignment" before she completed multiple turns. Unfortunately for this accomplished dancer, she injured herself during the semester and had to wait to test out her theories. Nevertheless, somatic methods allowed her to work on several aspects of this exploration, even without accumulating them toward her own goal. She continued working, just on a different level. As is often the case with a forced shift in plans, this opportunity allowed her to investigate far more thoroughly some underlying reflexes: tonic lumbar reflex, and lumbar reach reflex in particular.

The college's most decorated baseball player, JC, decided to investigate his physical training regime in the 30-yard dash. Previously training on a microcosmic level (looking at sprint mechanics, dorsiflexion at the ankle, and Achilles stretch reflex), he was encouraged to consider larger movement patterns and to integrate his efforts at a whole-body rather than brain level. Although his results were a bit disappointing, he began to understand that over time he might well be able to shave off fractions of seconds in his sprint by running "with his whole body" instead of just using his lower limbs.

DC was a bench presser who found himself "left stuck, repetitively performing the movement yet lacking the ability to progress to higher weights." He hadn't considered approaching his work from any system other than muscle. Opening to this new possibility led him to more fully integrated reach-pull patterns involving the pinkie-scapula relationships, and to "numb areas" of his sensory awareness, thus passing his 200-pound threshold.

During this particular semester at Denison, our Vail Series (which brings world-class musicians to perform at Denison) brought to campus the cellist Yo-Yo Ma. One of our students had played violin as a child but had let go of that interest years ago. Reinspired by Mr. Ma's performance, she decided to investigate how certain principles in BMC could help her begin to play again. She reports:

"When we practiced homolateral movement through the 'lizard' movement in class, I had trouble connecting my neck and head to my arm and leg. My six limbs (arms, legs, head/tail) lacked any type of fluid coordination together. Homolateral patterns are important to playing a musical instrument because they are associated with the hindbrain, namely the cerebellum and pons. This brain region is involved in the control of muscular movement patterns and coordination, and thus it was imperative that I make improvements in this area. I began on a more simplistic or 'primitive' reflex known as asymmetrical tonic neck reflex (ATNR). I practiced regaining this reflex until it felt comfortable to me. I then moved on to more complex movement patterns by practicing the 'lizard' pattern of homolateral movement." Parenthetically, this exploration also helped her understand her hesitations about the communal ice-skating attempt, an experience in which she had politely refused to participate because it seemed too dangerous.

KH was an exquisite and accomplished speed swimmer, a student scholar/athlete of much renown. Her work here was to shave milliseconds off the start of her race, presumably by not going as deep into the

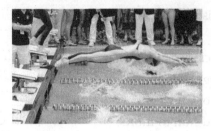

The student pictured in this competition is one of Denison's top student swimmers. Her research project worked toward shaving milliseconds off her entrance to improve her overall time.

water. By the end of her exploration, she was talking about "mouthing patterns" and "spinal reach and pull." The class got to watch videotapes of her head pulling her spine/tail through space in a smooth and connected arc, something she was virtually incapable of doing earlier in the semester. But equally compelling was a switch in her mental imagery. Instead of entering the water through a single and small hole, her mentor suggested that she imagine taking flight and skimming the surface. About this shift, the student remarked: "When I thought of this during my practice sessions, I found I was in fact diving less deeply. I don't know whether this is from my change in thoughts or a result of my other explorations and work."

These narratives illustrate some of the explorations this class undertook. Each one demanded a different set of theories and practical advice from mentors and the classroom teacher alike. As the students began to get information in their bodies, they also started coaching each other. The relationship with mentors (akin to private tutorials) gave each student the sense that he/she had "privileged knowledge." As a group, they enjoyed sharing with classmates the secrets divulged from mentor to student, clues to unlocking movement understandings that weren't necessarily described in the textbooks. The excitement of having been exposed to something no one else in the class had heard before increased the curiosity and motivation for work on their own projects while providing a sense of community.

Intellectual Growth as a Developmental Process or Bilateral Learning: A Two-Phasic Process

The individual stories represent a wide range of interests and modes of learning very typical in a liberal arts classroom. The collective process, discovery, and benefit of having a professional mentor who was new to these students' processes is significant, as is the way in which those individual relationships might have influenced the results of the students' investigations.

Over the course of the four months, these students shifted gears several times. The most consistently used process, named in eleven of the sixteen projects, involved a principle called "matching." Elizabeth Behnke defines "matching" in her 1988 essay, included in Don Hanlon Johnson's *Bones, Breath & Gesture*, as (1) an awareness of something in one's own body, (2) an inner act of matching or aligning oneself with this, and (3) allowing something to change. Behnke summarizes the process thus:

> ... I must be genuinely focused each time on simply matching what is there; trying for a specific outcome only gets in the way. Thus I have to allow myself time to feel whatever presents itself and to match it just as it is, rather than immediately trying to "fix" it or getting caught up in comparisons between the way things are and the way I think they should be.[3]

The students found this principle a good starting point for understanding their somatic experiences, regardless of the techniques, reflexes, or Basic Neurological Patterns they selected to process what they discovered.

Twelve of the sixteen students also discovered the BMC concept of "mind," evidenced in the way they described their results. That they could "place" their understanding and perspective in any location/system of their bodies, and that they could perceive the world through this location/system was a completely new concept, met at first with skepticism. Near the middle of a class on grounding, I asked a student if her feet were on the floor or whether the floor was under her feet. "Whoa! Wait a minute," she asked. "Are those different? Because they feel really different." Half the class was experiencing a shift in perspective; the other half was confused. More typical, however, was the shift that occurs when many in the room are in the same mind. For example, when we worked from a particular bony layer, the room's countenance would shift, and those who were struggling to understand were carried along. A week later, perceiving from the mind of the muscle, different students were carried along. This form of co-teaching made all of us smile.

In the fifth week of the course, we had two guests visit, Pat Ethridge and Kate Tarlow Morgan, both longtime BMC practitioners. The students attended a weekend workshop where Ethridge and Morgan introduced thumb-chest connections, middle finger-inferior angle connections, and pinkie-scapula connections. I began to see the students connecting Behnke's "matching" with Bainbridge Cohen's "mind." To quote one student, "After sensing this high tension and stiffness [in my shoulders], I entered the mind of the shoulders and joined in with the tension. I did not try to physically change the placement of my shoulders or restructure anything; instead I let the tension happen. As I explored the tension through heightened awareness, my shoulders were able to experience a movement and placement change of their own."

A lovely dialectic began to develop between the students' identifying more fully with their bodies ("embodiment") and their re-appropriation of the traditional Western separation of mind and body. Comments like "This observation displays the significance of the interplay between a (conscious) mind and an (integrated) body" were sprinkled throughout their reports as they worked to integrate these two seeming contradictions.

The mentors, too, shared their experiences of this process. Choosing to participate was a personal decision for some, a professional experience for others. One participant reflected sensitively on her own past:

> I remember my own experience in the Laban program and how esoteric all the material felt until we had a guest who came in and talked about how she actually used the work ... it was so hugely practical, and useful, and not nearly as heady as I had thought.... I do love the heady stuff, and learning for the sake of learning. But also having the material grounded in practical experience is intoxicating in its

own way. . . . So when there was the opportunity to help someone ground their learning in experience (what a great assignment in the first place!), I wanted to be a part of it. . . . I also have a huge amount of respect for teachers who make other points of view available to their students—I think it shows a lot of respect for the students' potential ability to navigate apparently conflicting information.

Another shared the kind of excitement this collaboration generated:

The level of excitement I felt about the project really was an eye-opener for me. I've never considered working with college-age people before, mainly because I never wanted to teach college-level art. But to work with movement as the subject (which actually was what I, myself, was studying in college more than art) seems wide open and very interesting. You really awakened a new sense of possibility for me personally, for which I'm very grateful!

A third corroborated:

An opportunity to contribute to a student's curiosity is always a learning process for me. They tend to think of things I would probably not by myself. And help me organize what I may have forgotten. Then there are the surprises. Since I know and respect [this faculty member's] work, I even expected surprises.

I asked the mentors to identify and describe one of the most positive aspects of this mentoring relationship. By far the most common response illustrated that participation deepened one's own relationship to the material and to a teaching/learning cycle. Comments ranged among the following: "I loved watching myself notice the pre-motor focus, pre-conceived ideas and expectations my student/mentee had. I smiled in recognition; I know that place. I go there often." And: "Even without knowing much of her process ahead of time, I was touched by the way C found her own value in principles I am passionate about. I thought her writing was excellently done and described revelations in learning.

I feel the satisfaction of knowing that learning happened." This final response summarized the experience of many: "I was so thrilled to do it, thoroughly enjoyed engaging with the student's questions, spent much longer on generating suggestions than I really should have, given my schedule—but I just couldn't resist! It's such rich territory." These remarks, then, illustrate that the teaching/learning process was shared among students, faculty, and mentors, to everyone's benefit.

College teaching is about sharing knowledge, imparting it and receiving it, with a constant kind of "flow" among all participants. In the undergraduate classroom, however, there needs to be a designated "convener," i.e., the professor, someone whose responsibility it is to monitor the experiences of all concerned, notice and name the activities, evaluate progress, determine if the journey is too slow, too fast, or just right, and gather up those who seem to be falling off the edges. In this educational setting, students often agree only to be active passengers along the journey, for they do not know the terrain well enough to be guides. They expect the learning to begin at a certain time and end on a certain date, whether or not they have reached the destination. Finally, they expect the directions and the expectations to be concise and within their reach. College teachers and college students have a contract (called a "syllabus") that serves as a roadmap for this journey. The challenge for the professor is to serve as creator of the course while also serving as guide, imparter of knowledge, convener, mentor, evaluator, disciplinarian, and timekeeper. Drawing on the resources of a distance mentor supports and extends these roles, increasing the probability of meeting each student where he or she is along the journey.

For the students, working with mentors makes the work of professionals in the field not only accessible but also applicable, and students' names and field interests become known to the field at large. The small liberal arts college traditionally promises that students will come to know faculty members intimately and that faculty members will shepherd their move from the institution into the professional world. But it is equally empowering to realize that professionals actively working in the field might take seriously the questions posed by college students. In fact, exposing mentor/practitioners to the questions that educated college students ask also benefits the professional somatic arena, since these students are the future of the field itself.

There are deep and meaningful benefits for the individual practitioners as well. One of the traditions of BMC and other somatic fields is the offering of "private sessions." A temporary one-on-one relationship is *de rigueur*. However, there is a difference in the roles of "practitioner" and "client" in the private session and the roles of "teacher" and "student" in teaching workshops. In the former, the "client" is expecting some sort of personal result—perhaps we could call it "healing." In the latter, the "student" is expecting an experience of the practice—perhaps we could call it "learning." The mentor/student relationship sets up a third possibility, in which students offer themselves as willing participants available to "receive," "experience," and then "question" the presentation. Because these students were relatively naïve in the material but highly experienced as active learners, they served as wonderful resources of critical feedback for the mentor/practitioners. In this relationship, the mentor/practitioners also had the opportunity to present new findings (whether in content or pedagogy) to these informed student/clients for the benefit of both parties. Perhaps we could call this "exchange," ideal in the arena of teaching/learning and in the somatic study of Body-Mind Centering.

Over time, the benefits gained through the mentor/student relationship are exponential. They are experienced not only by the students but also by the practitioners. At the heart of this experiment in mentoring is a philosophy basic to Body-Mind Centering—that sharing responsibilities and offering one's own gifts are part of what the work is about. I hope that as a community, we will continue to explore distance mentoring as a process that offers benefits for all parties involved.

Two Great Lights: The Spiritual Potency of the Teacher-Student Relationship (excerpt)

~ **Diane Elliot**, USA (2006)

For the past five years, in addition to teaching Body-Mind Centering both independently and as part of the faculty of The School for Body-Mind Centering and maintaining a private somatic therapy practice in San Diego and Los Angeles, I have been matriculated in the rabbinical program at the Academy for Jewish Religion. Rabbinical studies, culminating in ordination as a rabbi (a two-thousand-year-old "job description" available to women only since 1971), are largely framed within an academic context. They encompass ancient and not-so-ancient texts (*Torah, Talmud, Midrash* or "commentary," and *Halakhah* or "Codes of Law," studied in the original Hebrew and Aramaic), philosophy, history, liturgy, poetry—a vast compendium of information that must be, if not mastered, at least dipped into. More recently feminist studies (focusing on women's relationship to cultural norms as well as tracing the Divine Feminine in canonical literature), creative life-cycle ritual, and spiritual counseling have also become part of the curriculum.

The *rav-talmid* (master-disciple) relationship, that powerful dynamic called into play when one person agrees to guide and mentor another's journey, serves in many spiritual traditions as one path toward Truth. (The path of the mystic—receiver of unmediated, direct transmission—is another.) What happens when two people, or one person and a group of people, commit to this intense and risky process of together entering the unknown?

As we know so well within the Body-Mind Centering framework, no participant in the intimate dance of teacher and learner is left unchanged. In one story from the sacred literature, a student's ultimate rebellion, after many years of engagement with his honored *rav*, causes the teacher to sicken and die. The level of emotional closeness and even, at times, physical closeness between student and teacher may approach that of married partners. Yet it is the agreement on the part of both master and disciple to a power differential, with the *rav* being asked to expand to what often seems super-human dimensions, while the student agrees to temporarily dim his or her own light to make space for the teacher's wisdom, that renders this complex and potent relationship a training ground for the human-divine interaction.

I offer for your consideration and contemplation an exploration of the nature of the *rav-talmid* relationship focusing on two of my most important teachers. Many of the quotations with which the sections begin are from texts that my class at the Academy studied together. This essay represents, in effect, an effort to weave these teachings into an understanding of my own life experience. I have revised a bit and translated terms and quotes as necessary to make certain passages more comprehensible for a general readership. But I've tried to keep the original spirit of the piece intact.

Clearly, this view of master and disciple grows from within a particular religious and cultural context; yet I feel it illumines dynamics that are universal in nature. We in the Body-Mind Centering world are grappling with the effects of learning with a charismatic teacher. Many of us have found in Bonnie Cohen a *rav muvhak*, an extraordinary teacher. How we allow this privileged and powerful relationship to transform speaks to the future of the work, to the forms it will take, and to the way it will be transmitted.

i

Regarding the measurements of aron ha-kodesh [the Ark that contained the tablets of the covenant], all of them are something-and-a-half. Why? So that the talmid khakham [wise, gifted student/teacher] will know that he is not complete and always lacks his other half. The teacher lacks a student, and the student lacks a teacher. The Talmud teaches: "There is no before or after in the Torah." Therefore neither the teacher nor the student has precedence or preference over the other, since the student receives from the teacher and the teacher is sharpened by the student.

—attributed to Olalot Efraim in *Itturei Torah*, vol. III, p. 212

We begin with *"aseh l'kha rav v'kaneh l'kha khaver"* ("Make for yourself a master and acquire for yourself a friend," *Avot* 1:6). We begin (and end) by *making* for ourselves a teacher, a different process, the sages of *Pirke Avot* tell us, than that of *acquiring* a friend. The energy of the friend exists, perhaps, outside ourselves in the world, a familiar face waiting to be recognized, to be drawn into our sphere, to engage with us in the give-and-take of human companionship. The *rav*, the *rebbe*, is an ever-elusive being, a screen upon which I project my deepest spiritual yearnings. S/he rises to my occasion from the space of myth and dream, of desire, joy, and loss. We make for ourselves a teacher and perhaps, if we are fortunate, we find—many years later, sooner sometimes—that we (and s/he) have been able to penetrate the opacity of our own projections; that we each have, after all, acquired a *khaver*— a friend, a companion, or a mate.

The *rav-talmid* "process," as it has developed over time, serves as crucible and anchor for a depth and urgency of spiritual yearning that, if not contained and disciplined, witnessed, and guided, could drive an aspiring student—or teacher—mad.

ii

You can't live without a rav.
Make for yourself a rav, "v'yitkayem talmud'kha b'yadekha," for
then your study will be sustained by your hand.

—Rabbi Moses Maimonides' commentary to *Avot* 1:6.

By *your* hand....

For so many years I was searching for the *one,* the *ones,* the *One* whom I needed. I vaguely sensed that it was *my own hand* that must first reach out if I wanted to be truly sustained, to truly progress. As a young person I loved the teachers, the ones in grade school and high school, who saw and held me. I strove fiercely to make contact and to serve with a force that I would only many years later be able to name as *yirat shamayim* (literally, "fear of heaven"). During my first semester in college, my English teacher told me that the ferocity of my efforts scared her. "You give too much," she said. At the time I couldn't articulate, even to myself, that though I had left my hometown Jewish community behind, I was on a spiritual quest, even when not practicing religion. Straining toward unseen support, I threw myself into the void with hopes of meeting the resistive push of a spiritual mentor whose pressure on me would give "me" back to myself and, ultimately, back to God.

But I wasn't fully met, partly because I so feared the meeting and partly because that wasn't the way our Western, secularized culture worked in the latter half of the twentieth century. We were to be "cool." So I grew wary, and I held back, and the buffer zone around me grew deeper, lonelier.

iii

I've been dancing since I was three and teaching dance since I was eighteen. For many years, while also a performer, I taught technique, movement improvisation, and choreography. Though these disciplines were my "excuse" to teach, my classes became a forum for sharing the richness of my perceptions, the depth of my curiosity about life, love, the body, mind, and spirit. When, pretty early on, my ego latched onto the role of teacher, innocent enthusiasm began to be soured by judgment born of fear. As a young dance teacher I spent many hours planning each class. I didn't teach students, I taught "material." The harshness with which I judged myself as an artist and a person was applied to those I taught; I pushed, I challenged, I was smart and tough, I cut to the bone. I saw my students with sharp eyes.

My students loved me for my talent, intelligence, and presence, but I didn't know how to love them back. Not wanting to be held "responsible" for the people who studied with me—who invited me year after year for teaching residencies in Indiana and North Carolina and France and Canada—I never allowed myself to fully feel the poignancy of their struggles or to truly *kvell* (to rejoice, with a tinge of personal pride) at their successes. I traveled the country—the world—teaching, performing, staying in touch with friends and students by letter or phone, avoiding spending too much continuous time with any one group of people, fleeing intimacy with my students—and myself. Maybe my students from those days would say that they really did feel seen and nourished and cared for. After all, I was a young teacher doing the best I could. But *I* knew how uncomfortable I was in my skin, and I sensed that there were many further levels to be traversed. I didn't yet know that I couldn't traverse them alone.

iv

Obligations of the rav:
- *Commitment*
- *Devotion*
- *Seeing*
- *Holding*
- *Bringing the students close*

You can't be a rav if you've never been a talmid.

My first *rav muvhak* (special teacher who agrees to take you on as a student, sees aspects of you that you can't see in yourself) was Bonnie Bainbridge Cohen. In the summer of 1983 I began my studies with her, which continue to this day, with a two-week summer course at Naropa Institute. The work she created is called Body-Mind Centering, and it involves a detailed experiential study of the quality of "mind" inherent in each of the body's anatomical structures and physiological functions, with the aim of becoming more fully and joyfully "embodied." In class after class, over years of study, we practiced moving from our bones, our organs, our fluids, our nerves. We chanted and sang from our endocrine glands. We re-tracked the developmental pathways from conception through the reflexive movements of birth, from the first lift of the head and the first rolling over to belly crawling, creeping on hands and knees, and rising to vertical with new legs beneath us. We learned to perceive the subtlest internal movements and to touch others in ways that could evoke healing and enlightening experiences of body-mind connection within them.

This work is brilliant and profound, but what really drew me into it was the way Bonnie saw and held her students, the great spaciousness in the room for us each to be who we were. She knew everyone's *name,* and not just the ones we had been given. Somehow, even in a roomful of one hundred people, you knew she was speaking directly to you, to the particular question, perhaps unasked, that you were holding in your heart. She seemed to sense when a word or a touch might open a whole new world for a particular student. Many times a few minutes with her would shift my whole perspective, precipitate a healing in my body-mind, realign my sense of self and purpose. I remember things she said to me years ago and tell the stories of my encounters with her over and over.

When I first began to teach and practice Body-Mind Centering, and for many years afterward, I would hear Bonnie's voice speaking in my head, encouraging me to stay present, coaching me how to handle scary, unknown situations with my students or somatic therapy clients. Even now, touching a client, I can sometimes sense the soft intelligence of her hand in my hand. I still hear myself saying, "Bonnie says ..." or "Bonnie would say ..." much as the *khakhamim* (wise men) of the *Talmud* speak *b'shem ha-rav* ("in the name of the Master"). Not until meeting her and engaging with the amazing group of students from all over the world that gathered around her had I seen modeled the vulnerability required of both *rav* and *talmid*. Here, among this somatic community, I began to understand the role of the true *talmid*—the requisite humility, the willingness to trust, to serve, to question, to expose oneself, to go beyond the limits of what feels safe or even possible. Because in large part she herself was so seemingly transparent, I sensed a space safe enough to strip away layers of disguise I didn't even know I had taken on.

V

Amar rav khisda: "kol ha-kholek al rabo k'kholek al ha-shekhinah"
... Amar rabi khama b'rabi khanina: "kol ha-oseh merivah im rabo,
k'oseh im shekhinah...."

Said Rav Khisda: "Anyone who challenges his rav, it's as if he challenges the Shekhinah [indwelling, Feminine Presence of God]"
... Said Rabbi Khama in the name of Rabbi Khanina: "Anyone who picks a fight with his rav, it's as if he picks a fight with the Shekhinah...."

—Babylonian *Talmud*, Sanhedrin, 110a

I believe these interpretations intend not to teach that we are *not* to challenge or fight with our teachers (for as we learn in *Bava Metzia* [a tractate of the *Talmud*], "you shall surely rebuke...."), but rather to make clear that *when* we do, it is as *if* we are wrestling with Holy Presence herSelf.

There may be no more Abrahams in this world to welcome the divine visitor at the tent flap (see Genesis 18:1–3), nor Jacobs to engage the divine messenger in hand-to-hand combat in the open field (see Genesis 32:25–30). How telling that the sages of Sanhedrin invoke not "*ha-Shem, Y-H-V-H*," or another of the divine names, but "*shekhinah*," the indwelling Presence, god's most intimate manifestation: "*v'asu li mikdash v'shokhanti b'tocham*" ("make Me a holy Temple and I will dwell in their midst," literally "within them," Exodus 25:8). In the absence of *avot* (ancestors), of *n'vi'im* (prophets), of a *mikdash* (temple) of stone and wood with its altars, layers, curtains, and Holy Ark, what could serve as the "container," the lightning rod for drawing holiness into this world?

The space between *rav* and *talmid* becomes as the space between the *keruvim* (the cherubim facing each other over the Ark of the Covenant in the inner sanctum of the Jerusalem Temple) once was—a lacuna, a sacred emptiness that, resting upon the covenant, invites ongoing relationship with the Transcendent.

vi

It was a number of years before I found another *rav muvhak*. It was the day after Yom Kippur, 1996, and I was in the midst of a spiritual "crisis," unable to see my way clearly. After practicing *vipassana* meditation for many years while continuing to learn and to teach Body-Mind Centering, I had spent the past year and a half birthing a theater piece that threw me back into the European Jewish milieu that my grandparents and great-grandparents had fled nearly a century before. Eight Jewish artists—dancers, playwrights, actors, singers, composers—unearthed and retold, through poetry, movement, song, and dialogue, stories of our ancestors that reflected our own journeys as artists and Jews.

In the course of working on this project I'd become quite ill. It was as if these figures from my past had taken up residence in my body and were feeding on my life force. I postponed a residency in Hungary and canceled another in Berkeley in order to regain my health and inner balance. After having spent *Rosh Ha-Shanah* (the first of the Jewish high holy days in autumn) at a friend's synagogue in Oakland, I impulsively drove up to Seattle to spend the fast day of *Yom Kippur* with Rabbi David Wolfe-Blank, a teacher whose work had touched me. I felt the same vulnerability, spaciousness, and heightened vibration with him that I always felt with Bonnie.

Reb David's writings, a mix of Hasidic lore, Lurianaic *kabbalah*, Zen wisdom, psychology, and blazing flashes of intuitive insight, were way over my head. But during that Yom Kippur, his first in Seattle, Reb David managed to embody the energetic trajectory of the day in a way that carried me to a depth beyond any I'd ever experienced in a Jewish prayer setting. We finished well after sundown, and though a tempting break-the-fast potluck awaited in the next room, no one rushed to the food. Instead Reb David suggested we go outside to bless the moon, and everyone poured out onto the lawn, ecstatic, dancing and singing, drunk on prayer and night air. I had never experienced a holy day so infused with spiritual energy.

At the end of the evening, when David came over to say good-bye, I found myself reaching out of the car window to hug him. Not wanting to let go, I blurted out, "Do you think you could see me tomorrow?" I didn't know what had possessed me; normally I would have been too shy to ask for time with a rabbi I hardly knew, and on the day after Yom Kippur yet, when he must be exhausted. But I was scheduled to leave the day after, so he agreed to meet with me after dinner at the home of the friend with whom I was staying, a member of his congregation.

Rav David, a brilliant student and chess prodigy, trained in *Yiddishkeit* (Jewish learning) with *Chabad* (an American orthodox movement stemming from a European Hasidic lineage) and was a favorite of the late Lubavitcher Rebber (last charismatic leader of the Chabad movement). Ultimately finding the world of orthodoxy too confining, he had left Chabad to study Zen for five years, then trekked across the country, where he participated in the early days of the Aquarian Minyan (one of the earliest Jewish Renewal groups) in Berkeley. During that time he earned a master's degree in somatic psychology, writing his thesis on Feldenkrais (a modality of somatic work sharing some aspects with Body-Mind Centering) and spirituality.

The night after that amazing Yom Kippur, I poured out my heart to Rav David, trying to describe the confused impasse at which I found myself. He offered to guide me in an interactive visualization, and from somewhere deep inside me surfaced a powerful image from the ocean of the collective Jewish unconscious. I saw myself imprisoned within a kind of grotesque giant beneath whose scaly skin my own tender-skinned, vulnerable self was hidden. "It's a *golem*!" I exclaimed, not even sure what that was or how I knew that word. (Later I discovered that *golem* referred to a man-made creature brought to life through shamanistic magic. A famous *golem* was the powerful giant supposed to have been created by the seventeenth-century rabbi, Judah Loew ben Bezalel, to protect the Jews of Prague.)

"What needs to happen?" David asked.

"I need to kill it, to scratch this ugly skin off of me!" I exclaimed.

"What will you do with it?" he asked.

"Bury it!" I answered.

"But won't it just come back to life if you try to kill it?" he prodded gently. I saw that he was right; I couldn't do violence to this monster who had only grown up around me to try to protect me. In a flash I knew that the "*golem* skin" needed to shrink, while my true, vulnerable skin must reach out to meet it. If the two skins could merge, then I could enter the world feeling at ease with myself—*bien dans ma peau*, "well inside my skin," as the French say. As I told my insight to David, I could feel its rightness. The next day, when I left to return to Minnesota, I developed a red, itchy skin rash that lasted a month!

Never before had I encountered a rabbi who could work intimately with me in this way. In the middle American Reform Jewish world in which I grew up, there were no *ravs* or *rebbes*. While I respected and feared and sought to please the charismatic rabbi of my teenage years, the one who confirmed me and whose eye I always tried to catch when he stood high up and distant on the *bima* in his perfectly tailored suit, white shirt, and tie, he was not a teacher with whom I could feel personally engaged in a deep commitment to mutual learning and growth. He gave me much—intellectual challenge and a great feel for the spiritual possibilities of the Jewish path—but the relationship was too formal, too one-sided.

Blown away as I was by this encounter with David Wolfe-Blank, it took a couple of months to realize that I wanted to study with him, and a few more months for him to rediscover my letter at the bottom of a pile on his desk. By the following August I was driving cross-country again, this time to spend two months as a *talmid*, a *hasid* (disciple) of Reb David.

vii

d'hineh h-shem yitbarakh bara m'khitzot-
m'khitzot, v'kol malakh she'nikhnas lif nim
m'khitzoto nisraf, shehishtalshlut ha-olamot. . . .

And behold, the Blessed One created container after container, and
any angel that goes beyond its container burns, in traversing the
worlds. . . .

—R. Levi Yitzkhak, *Kedushat Levi*

Rabbi David was killed in a freak automobile accident as he and his wife and son returned from vacation. For no apparent reason the car spun out of control and rolled over twice on a dry, straight road in broad daylight. David was driving with his young son Uri beside him, belted into the passenger seat, while his wife, Elaine, lay unbelted, taking a nap in the backseat. Uri and Elaine survived the crash with fairly minor injuries, but David sustained massive head wounds and internal injuries. Paramedics jump-started his heart and airlifted him to a hospital in Seattle. There he was declared brain dead, and after Elaine made the decision to take him off life support, he died within a day. It was hard not to wonder why he was taken. Had he overreached in some way? Was he needed elsewhere?

My *rav*'s death is perhaps his greatest teaching, and it is still unfolding. Never have I felt such a wrenching sense of loss. The night he hovered between life and death with his congregants keeping vigil at the hospital, I tossed and turned in San Diego, feeling a sickening pull in my chest. As morning approached I sensed that he was gone. Anger surged through me. How could he leave? How could he leave me? And what was I to do now? Only in his absence did I begin to feel how much I had given over to him, how much I was depending on him to shape my Jewish spiritual path. I would not have to learn to read all these arcane texts—the *Torah*, the *Talmud*, *Midrash*, and *Zohar*—because he would do that part. I could stick to what I was good at—singing, dancing, healing ritual—and absorb bits of the tradition as needed.

A year after David's death I helped a new *rav* conduct high holy day services in San Diego. Eight months after that, having never become bat mitzvah (literally, "a daughter of the covenant"), I chanted *Torah* for the first time—from my birth *parashah*, Metzorah. (The portion of the *Torah* being read during the week a child is born is the one from which he or she will chant when becoming bar or bat mitzvah.)

viii

> *... yesh malakh m'muneh sham gam ken*
> *d'gafif v'nashik lah, u' ma-lah otah l'olam*
> *v'heykhal ha-elyon....*

> *... There is an angel responsible there, similarly, to hug and kiss it*
> *(the prayer) and raise it to the next higher world and palace....*
> —Reb Schneur Zalman of Liady, *Siddur ha-Admir ha-Zaken*

I had never fully understood before the intimacy, the eroticism of the *rav-talmid* commitment. I feared it. I longed for it. On the afternoon of Kol Nidre, in the year that I had helped Reb David conduct high holy day services, I had a meltdown. Nervous about dancing Kol Nidre, rattled because we were still planning the evening service at 1 p.m. and because I didn't know where I'd eat dinner before the service or how I'd get through the twenty-six hours of dancing and singing without food or water, I began to sob. David hugged me and held my head in his arms as I cried. He told me, "The *rebbes* teach that if you don't cry during the Yamim Nora'im (Days of Awe), something's wrong. I don't know why I haven't cried this year."

As a therapist I knew very well about the "hugging" job of the *rav*, the creating of container, of witness. I had often been the ear that elicits the story, the eye that unleashes the dance. But "kissing" was new to me—the meeting of souls, mouth to mouth, that could carry the "prayers" and insights of a person's being to a higher or deeper level. David taught me more about how *rav* and *talmid* synergistically augment each other's soul offerings. Among my most treasured legacies are the practice tapes I made of him teaching me Shabbat and high holy day liturgy, especially the haunting melodies of S'likhot. I had to set them aside for a while, but now, when I need to reconnect to the pure *kavannah* of those prayers, I listen to the tapes. These songs, in his voice, are like kisses, the prayers infused with love. When I sing them I try to empty myself so that the same *ruakh ha-kodesh* (holy spirit) may move through me.

ix

am'rah y'reyakh lif nei ha'kadosh barukh hu,
"ribono shel olam, ef shar l'shnei malakhim
she'yishtamshu b'keter ekhad?" amar lah,
"l'khi u-ma-atai et atzmakh."

Said the moon, before the Holy One of Blessing, "Master of the
Universe, is it possible that two monarchs should make use of the
same crown?" He said to her, "Go and shrink yourself."

—*Babylonian Talmud*, Kholin, 60b

We wear many different hats during one lifetime. The agreement to
step back, to do *tzim tzum* (the kabbalistic concept of contracting the
self) so that someone else's gifts may be amplified and fully received,
is essential to the *rav-talmid* relationship. In order to become the *talmid*
I must both reach out and "become all ears," as it were. Even in my
speaking I am listening, holding the space for my *rav*'s wisdom to blos-
som. And as a *rav*, the skill of knowing when to hold back, when to
invite students to come forward in the freshness of their perceptions,
the excitement of their learning, is a great art. It is of deep comfort and
benefit to know that my masters have masters. And that even as I sit
at the feet of a *rav*, my students are benefiting. A chain of loving purpose
is thus created, a chain with many *nekavim*, many spaces, into and
through which waves Shekhinah/Kadosh-Barukh-Hu, the Wholly One
of Blessing.

How gifted I have been with so many exquisite teachers! When I
can give back even a small portion of what has been given to me in the
way it has been given, I feel blessed. When students appear who wish,
in love and compassion, to draw out the best I have to offer—what joy!
Just as the chain of teacher-student-teacher is so essential to the Jewish
spiritual path, with teachings always attributed to the specific masters
who spoke them, I have noticed that Bonnie Bainbridge Cohen always
takes great pains to credit and to thank her teachers, the somatic and

movement therapy pioneers, the yoga and Aikido masters, whose work fed into hers.

We make for ourselves a teacher, investing a man or a woman with the power to hold our inner wisdom in trust for us as we expand the boundaries of self, becoming more than we ever dreamed we could be. And then, in the ever-shifting dance of student and teacher, the balance may change, the agreement shift. A teacher becomes ill or dies or breaches our trust and is no longer there in the same way to hold the larger vision of our selves.

We are left floundering, it seems. Suddenly, we notice someone approaching. We notice that someone has been sitting for three days on our doorstep, waiting for an appointment. We notice that someone needs our guidance. And the *rav* who I thought had left me, the teacher whom I was sure I had left behind forever, is speaking gently to me, through me, hovering just above my left shoulder or standing right in front of me, smiling and smiling. And I am flooded with gratitude and relief.

BMC and Yoga:
Breathing into Form

～ **Doug MacKenzie**, USA (1998)

From early fall 1996 to late fall 1997 the author had an inspiring opportunity to meet regularly with Bonnie Bainbridge Cohen, Michael Ridge, and Margaret Guay to explore and respond to sundry vital needs. Each of the four had different strengths and weaknesses—yet they met each other where they were. From the differences arose many creative modalities for finding balance and ease within the systems of the body, and there emerged a shared form that served to contain and further their activity. They called it yoga, a practice that focuses on the integration of mind through the initiation of breath and sequencing of movement.

In this practice, though we study and incorporate our understanding of the work of many others (most essentially the resplendent heritage of Sri T. Krishnamacharya as described by his son T.K.V. Desikachar, and student A.G. Mohan[1]), we discover yogic principles in our own language through Body-Mind Centering (BMC). We begin by approaching a state of awareness of respiration, both *lung* or *external* respiration and *cellular* or *internal* respiration. Here we feel life force; breathing and moving are two partners in one inner dance. From this general flowing state, which shows us where we are and generates countless possibilities—"a labyrinth of ramifications"—we practice mindful sequencing into intentional movement, toward *specific* goals that address our needs.

While the emphasis in BMC is exploring the possibilities, the emphasis of yoga is harnessing the mind.[2] Engaging both simultaneously, we develop the capacity to approach each chosen moment with an attention and clarity that is based upon the comfort of balanced physiological tone. Dormant sensitivities awaken. I find the integration of activity and effortlessness, a new keenness of perception, and the motivation I need to bring my internal vision to the external world.

We can experience how beautifully the classical yoga asanas emerge from a developmental matrix and how both the *developmental series* and yoga serve as containers to hold all of the BMC principles. That is: in the first year of life our strengths and perceptions grow in movement patterns, much like asanas, that integrate all of our body's systems, and we learn how to learn. These patterns cohere in a continuum that echoes the evolutionary progression of the animal kingdom as it guides and supports our orientation to this world. Playing with these patterns of our earliest movement, as the first yogis may have done intuitively, we find more coordination, ease, and choice in the way we move. Because any problems in early movement will present themselves as obstacles to the fulfillment of our potential—imbalances in skeletal alignment and the body systems, and problems in perception, sequencing, organization, memory, and creativity—we can practice either the developmental series of BMC or yoga to address such problems at a basic level.

As we practice, we explore principles rather than collect techniques. Our intention as practitioners is to meet each fresh situation with mindfulness. When a situation arises that asks for attention, we invoke such maxims as "support precedes initiation," "even and consistent joint space," "fluid/membrane balance," or "systems in shadow versus systems in expression." We then harvest what we can learn from the situation and about the principle.

I am inspired by the potential to apply or modify this practice to support anyone who is attempting something—*anything*! Please let me know what you find in your practice and what you add or change. How do you balance inner and outer activity, find your cells, and sequence toward your goals?

Cellular Breathing

At a cellular level, breathing and moving are intertwined. An elementary look at the physiology of movement will reveal that cellular breathing, with the support of nutrients and other processes, forms the metabolic basis for the production of energy and movement. Perhaps surprisingly, we can feel it. Our experience—what we are aware of in daily living—can reflect this and other cellular phenomena in various degrees of resolution. For most of us it makes sense that when our tissues' cells are fueled and breathing well (say, for example, when eating, sleeping, exercising, and enjoying ourselves), we feel vital. Body-Mind Centering demonstrates another emphasis and point of entry: when we *feel* the breath and vitality of our cells, our tissues can find support, homeostasis, and balance—and dynamic new options in wellness and expression are possible.

The explorations in this essay begin from the foundation of cellular breathing. If you have not experienced cellular breathing and would like to, I suggest you consult with a BMC practitioner.[3] What follows of these explorations is an introduction, but it is a condensed version. Take all of the time you need with each step! You will reap what you sow. I will introduce many of the breathing principles, describe how breathing integrates with moving, and then present the movement principles. After this, I will guide you through the specific movement sequences. I encourage you to try each principle as you read, and to integrate all the preceding principles in practice as you progress through the movement sequences.

Rhythm of External Breathing

Remove potential distractions before you start. Begin by sitting comfortably or lying on your back in a place you have dedicated for practice.

- As you breathe and notice your lungs breathing, feel also your blood pulse rhythm. Notice how many times your heart beats per inhale, and how many times per exhale. Take your time with this phase of just noticing; listen and feel for your own organic rhythms, shifts, and cadences.

- Begin to suspend your breath after each inhale and after each exhale. Do not hold your breath by closing off your epiglottis, but rather, keep it open—suspend.

  – Inhale . . . suspend . . . exhale . . . suspend . . . inhale . . .

  – Let the duration of your suspension be equal to half of the number of pulses of your active breathing, so that if you inhale/exhale, say, on six pulses, then suspend for three. (This work with breath rhythm comes from the Krishnamacharya lineage. See T.K.V. Desikachar, *Heart of Yoga*.)

- Gradually extend the breath to 8-4-8-4, or to a ratio that you find is close to your cerebrospinal fluid (CSF) rhythm.

  The fluid in your spine, cerebrospinal fluid or CSF, ebbs and flows in a subtle but measurable, palpable rhythm, like a wave. This rhythm (named the Primary Respiratory Mechanism by William Sutherland, DO, in 1939) has particular qualities in the spine and head, and an effect throughout the body that can indicate many essentials of homeostasis, including the relative state of balance of the nervous system. In BMC we influence the quality of this rhythm not only through gentle touch, as you may experience in cranial osteopathy or craniosacral therapy, but also through direct internal exploration. Again, contact a BMC practitioner if you want to experience this approach to embodiment.[4]

  Begin to be aware of the coordination of your respiratory, circulatory, and CSF rhythms.

- Generally coordinate all fluid rhythms as you breathe.

Sequential Breathing

As in Desikachar's yoga style, we begin filling sequentially on the inhale from the upper body to the lower, and emptying sequentially on the exhale from the lower body to the upper. We layer in BMC principles, originating breath within and sequencing breath through various physiological systems.

Perhaps the most colorful and vast of BMC explorations is the experience of each system's particular qualities. We breathe into, feel, and follow the inherent movement of the various tissues (like the kidneys, the thyroid, the suprachiasmatic nucleus, and so forth). The movement we find reflects that tissue's quality, or consciousness, which can be accessed not only in the quest for homeostasis and health, but also in the pursuit of expression in art, music, dance, athletics, and daily living. This comparative enquiry into the systems refines our sensitivities, clarifies our strengths and weaknesses, and widens our palette of choice in everything we do.

Here are some suggestions:

Organs

Inhale: from thoracic organs to pelvic organs
Exhale: from pelvic organs to thoracic organs

Skeleton-Muscles-Ligaments-Fasciae

Inhale: from head to tail (breathe down and/or along the spine)
Exhale: from tail to head (breathe up and/or along the spine)

Nervous System

Inhale: from brain down the spinal cord to tail (through cauda equina)
Exhale: from tail up the spinal cord to the brain
Inhale: from reticular system to the spinal neuropil
Exhale: from spinal neuropil to the reticular system

Glands

Inhale: from pineal gland to the coccygeal body
Exhale: from coccygeal body to the pineal gland

Fluids

As you practice, continually encourage your fluids (CSF; blood pulse and venous return; external and internal breathing; lymph and interstitial) to move throughout your whole body. Be aware of the movement of one fluid, and then combine fluids to see how this affects your attention/intention and abilities to sense, feel, and act. Notice the subtleties of each fluid rhythm as you coordinate it with others. Integrated fluid rhythms provide an inner symphony of ease and attention that supports all other exploration.

Explore this sequencing *developmentally* by reaching through the head on inhale, and reaching through the tail on exhale. Notice the counter-support of this movement. As you inhale the breath energy moves down your spine and your head moves up; as you exhale the breath energy moves up your spine and your tail moves down. Do you find a gentle ease and lengthening of your whole spine? Do you find more space for your intervertebral disks?

Throughout these explorations, maintain and channel breathing energy within the body. Do not disperse it out of the body.

Sequential Internal Breathing into Movement

While external lung breathing is through the medium of air, internal cellular breathing is through a fluid medium very close in composition to seawater. As you breathe in your lungs, feel the wind on the water; as you breathe in your cells, feel the waves and tides and currents of the sea. How do these rhythms interact with each other? And what else happens when they do? Let yourself be carried by the ocean while you feel the wind within you.

Allow the nutrients and nourishment that you want to pass through your membranes into your cells to support your creativity; release the goods of your creativity from your cells to manifest their further purposes. Take in and release what is appropriate for you and as you need to, but do not limit yourself only to that which is familiar. You do not need to take in what is not appropriate.

Gradually allow your awareness of cellular breathing to focus on one skeletal joint (your hip, for example).

- As you breathe in that joint, allow the joint to release into movement through space.
- As that joint moves allow cellular movement to sequence throughout your body, carry you wherever it will, and come to settle on a new joint.
- Begin again, continually breathing and releasing into movement.

Some important aspects of breathing are:

1. The rhythm of external lung breathing (inhaling and exhaling rhythm);
2. Internal cellular breathing at the focal point of the movement; and
3. Sequential internal cellular breath traveling through the whole body.

Coordinating these aspects in practice leads into effortless automatic movement and sense of well-being. It encourages other positive phenomena as well. When these aspects come together,

Rhythm of external lung breathing

Mitochondria
ATP & water
"Nectar of well-being"

Internal cellular breathing at the focal   Sequential internal cellular breathing
point of the movement   traveling through the whole body

I feel flow and sustained vitality which spreads through my whole body like nectar. Bonnie has called this the "nectar of well-being." It has the quality of kindness and grace. I feel the same grace when, exploring subcellular processes through BMC, I feel mitochondria producing ATP and water (power and flow), rather than free radicals (stress and toxicity). I imagine this is something like the movement of chi, as it beings to feel like tai chi chu'an.

As we channel this flow into intentional movement sequences, we are able to encourage strength, address imbalances, and pattern integration and coherence with ease, choice, and specificity.

Breathing and Moving

The movement sequences that follow developed in coordination with breathing. Breathing is the initiation of the movement. The breathing rhythm is the duration of the movement. The quality of breathing is the indicator of the quality of the movement.

The sequence of breathing in each phase is circular:

1. From cellular breathing at the place where we initiate the movement,
2. To external lung respiration (and sequential cellular breathing traveling through the body) as we sequence movement through skeletal joints,
3. To suspension of external breathing (continuation of cellular breathing) as we suspend the movement.

In each movement there is an expansive, opening phase involving extension (generally, but not always, an inhale) and a condensing, closing phase involving flexion (generally, but not always, an exhale).

Our practice of expanding/extending/opening on the inhale and condensing/flexing/closing on the exhale encourages the movement of arterial and venous blood flow. Together both phases also support the CSF rhythm and generally help blood and CSF to come into balance with one another. One can also switch to condensing/flexing/closing on the inhale and expanding/extending/opening on the exhale. This emphasizes different fluid rhythms. Condensing on the inhale brings up interstitial pressure, and expanding on the exhale directs the interstitial into lymph.

The breathing supports the movement.

The movement supports the breathing.

The movement sequencing principles we use are:

Knitting together: As we move, whether peripherally or centrally, we maintain a sense of connection from center to periphery and periphery to center and in all dimensions throughout the whole body. This connection is facilitated by the knitting together (modulation between the sliding and binding factor) of the transverse abdominus in breathing. As we knit together we are modulating between two BMC principles, the *sliding factor* and the *binding factor* of muscle dynamics, which are based on experience and congruent with a molecular model of muscle contraction. The spirallic action and myosin molecules within muscle fibers alternate between sliding past each other and binding to one another for leverage. We can emphasize either aspect or mix them to the appropriate degree. Muscle contraction (or lengthening) is more subtle, specific, and efficient when we initiate within muscle fibers rather than engaging the entire muscle mass as a unit. The attitude is of *connecting,* not holding. The belly remains soft to allow full organ expression in breathing.

Balancing eccentric and concentric contracting within movements: To maintain even and consistent joint space and integrity within joints, we focus on balancing the side of the joint that is lengthening with the side of the joint that is shortening.

Distal initiation of limbs with proximal support of spine and torso: As we move our limbs through space, the initiation sequences from the most distal joint to the most proximal. As we move our body against the floor and gravity, the sequence is the opposite: from proximal to distal. Moving in this way can enable a shift in attitude and attention. Lengthening occurs easily and loosens both physical and psychological holding patterns. It is easy to do, but the attitude takes practice.

Balance and alternate each movement with its opposite: If a movement we do is a flexion movement, we alternate with an extension movement in the same area of the body. We are always seeking to balance one side of the body with the other—as well as front with back, and upper with lower. We look and feel for the integration of the body as a whole, and for the coordination of all systems and all three spatial dimensions.

Building and progressing: We progress from simple to more complex movement patterns. We build long sequences from shorter ones. We telescope inside of the sequences as well, to find balance within the short segments that make up longer sequences.

The Movement Sequences

The foundation of integrated breathing that supports all of the movement sequences is as follows:

- Begin by either lying supine or sitting. Take some time to rest and breathe as you are.
- Gradually bring your focus to your breathing, and if you can, notice the number of heart pulses per breath. If you cannot feel your heart pulse, approximate it by counting slowly to yourself as you breathe.
- On the inhale, begin to fill from the upper cavities of your body to the lower (head, chest, abdomen, pelvis). On the exhale, empty from the lower to the upper (pelvis, abdomen, chest, head). Retain the energy of your breath; do not disperse it into your surroundings.
- As you inhale and the breath moves down your spine, gently and fluidly reach with your head away from your tail. As you exhale and the breath moves up your spine, gently and fluidly reach your tail away from your head. You can feel your spine lengthen in both directions, and an easy agreeable counter-support between your spinal structure and the direction of your breathing.

- Gradually expand or rarefy your inhale and exhale until you are breathing in your optimal range—for example, 8 pulses inhale and 8 pulses exhale, or 6 pulses inhale and 6 pulses exhale, or the number of pulses that feels appropriate for you. *Do not force your breath!*
- Introduce a suspension of breath between inhale and exhale that is equal to half the duration of the breath itself. Your ratio might be 8-4-8-4, or 6-3-6-3.

Keeping aware of all of these aspects of breathing, progress to the movement sequences. You will find that these specific breathing principles form an integrated foundation that supports and informs the movement in surprising and wonderful ways.

Sequence 1: Bellows

Begin lying supine with arms at your sides, palms down (Figure 1). Knit together within your abdomen by allowing the fibers of your transverse abdominus to slide and engage rather than hold. Find a comfortable cohesiveness and allow your breathing to support this knitting.

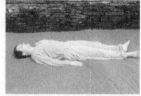

Figure 1

Feel your fingertips, and when you are ready, inhale and then initiate from your fingers as you raise your arms above your head (Figure 2). Take the full 8 pulses (or number of pulses that is right for you) to move through your range. Acknowledge the range of your movement with respect to your fasciae, and go only as far as your fasciae remain integral—if there is even slight tugging within your arms then pause there; do not push through it. Suspend both your movement and breath for 4 pulses.

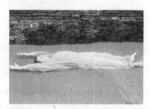

Figure 2

Initiate again from your fingers, exhaling on 8 pulses as you return your hands to your sides (Figure 3). Suspend for 4 pulses. Begin the sequence again.

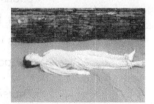

Figure 3

Repeat six times, and deepen your awareness as you go.

Transition: As you suspend your breath after your last exhale in Sequence 1, bring your knees to your chest. (See Figure 4.)

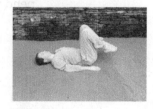

Figure 4

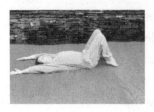

Figure 5

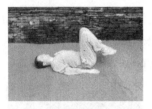

Figure 6

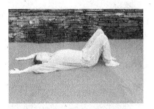

Figure 7

Sequence 2: Clamshell

Prepare and initiate as in Sequence 1. This time, while raising your arms overhead on the inhale, *current* your psoas minor upward and your psoas major downward, and lower your legs until your toes touch the floor (Figure 5). Suspend, and return on the exhale (Figure 6). Repeat six times.

Currenting is a BMC way to direct the internal energy of muscles. Imagine and feel two jets of a fountain, one rising from the right outer edge of your pubic bone, and one rising from the left. Each jet splashes into your spine at the level of your bottom ribs and the water falls down, over your pelvis, to the inside of your thigh. The jet rising from your pubic bones to spine corresponds to the psoas minor. The water flowing down and along your spine to the inside of your thigh corresponds to the deeper and larger psoas major. Do you feel more support? Is your psoas complex in a better state of readiness for activity?

Because the psoas minor originates at T12/L1 and inserts on the pubic bone, you can use it to stabilize your pelvis. Do not allow your pelvis to tilt anteriorly! If your pelvis begins to tip, back off: pause and suspend right there—there is no need to go all the way to the floor. As your psoas minor stabilizes your pelvis, free your psoas major to elongate downward and control the extension of your hips. Keep your abdominals knit together but soft and breathing freely. This is a way to release the abdominals and to lengthen and tone the deeper psoas muscles.

Transition: On the last inhale of the last repetition of Sequence 2, lower your legs to the floor and raise your arms overhead. (See Figure 7.) Suspend your breath and then begin Sequence 3.

Sequence 3: Jackknife

As you exhale, lower your arms to your sides and simultaneously move your leg as follows: Initiating movement in your right toes, slide your foot along the floor until your leg is fully extended, and then raise it up in the air in one continuous movement (Figure 8). Free your hip and sequence from the distal joints to the proximal joints of your right leg: foot, ankle, knee, hip, pelvic half, then tail. While you suspend, your tail lifts and reaches up. Your left leg can ground with the ball of the foot or, if you prefer, the whole foot including the heel can remain on the floor.

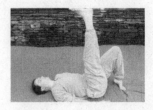

Figure 8

As you return on the inhale, initiate again from the foot, sequencing through the joints. Bend your knee and then your hip to return your foot to the floor as you raise your arms (Figure 9). Repeat with the left leg.

Alternate right and left three times.

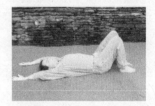

Figure 9

Transition: On the last inhale of Sequence 3, only lower your leg. Do not raise your arms. Knees are bent, hands are by your sides. (See Figure 10.)

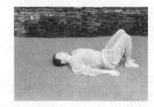

Figure 10

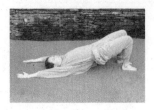

Figure 11

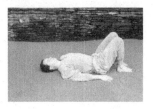

Figure 12

Sequence 4: Pelvic Lift #1

As you inhale, begin by filling your chest and let your breath initiate the lifting of your arms. Simultaneously, sequence the breathing energy through your torso to your tail, lift your tail and, vertebra by vertebra, lift your spine into the air (Figure 11). Breathing in your chest lifts your chest and shifts your whole spine toward your head. Do not work the muscles of your buttocks—keep them released. Suspend.

As you return on the exhale, initiate with breathing in your tail and shift your tail toward your feet. Drop your tail toward the floor and, vertebra by vertebra, gently return your spine to the floor (Figure 12).

Repeat six times.

Sequence 5: Helpless Insect

On the inhale, as one leg extends, sequencing from distal to proximal joints, open your arms to the side (Figure 13). Free your hip. Suspend.

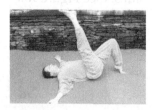

Figure 13

Exhale and return to the original position (Figure 14).

Repeat with the same leg two more times, then with the opposite leg three more times.

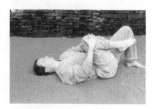

Figure 14

Sequence 6: Sit-up: Preparation for the Plough

With knees bent and your mid-back supported by a 9–15-inch ball, focus on maintaining equal length between the front and back of your body (Figure 15). Focus also on knitting together, and especially on *widening* through, the transverse abdominus by allowing your muscle fibers to slide eccentrically. Flatten your navel to your spine as you breathe.

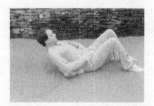

Figure 15

Initiate a sit-up keeping your spine long and integrated. Do not round your shoulders forward to come up; instead, reach your head upward (Figure 16). Feel the weight and shape of the bottom of your liver and allow the fullness of your liver to support the sit-up.

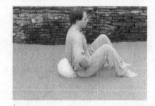

Figure 16

There are two sit-up variations:

1. Place your hands on your belly with elbows wide in the vertical plane, and sit up straight in the sagittal plane (as in Figures 15 and 16).

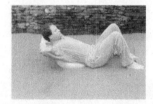

Figure 17

2. Place your hands behind your head and sit up straight in the sagittal plane (Figure 17) and then turn from your obliques in the horizontal plane so that your elbow touches the opposite knee (elbows stay in the vertical plane relative to your head) (Figure 18). Be careful not to use your elbows to pull yourself forward.

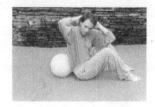

Figure 18

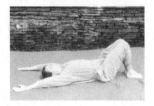

Figure 19

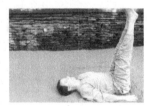

Figure 20

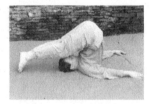

Figure 21

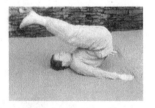

Figure 22

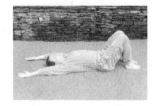

Figure 23

Sequence 7: Plough

Begin lying on your back with arms overhead and knees bent (Figure 19).

Lower your arms on the exhale and simultaneously let your toes lead your legs into the air as your heel follows an under-curve (Figure 20). During the first four counts of the exhale your palms reach the floor, your legs straighten, and your hip joints come to 90 degrees. During the last four counts of the exhale your spine flexes, lifting your pelvis and carrying your feet toward your head and beyond (Figure 21).

Suspend for four counts. On the inhale, lower your spine on the first four counts (Figure 22), and lower your legs and raise your arms on the last four counts (Figure 23). (So for the duration that your spine is away from the floor, your hands will be on the floor.)

Throughout the movement, but especially as you flex your spine, *flatten:* keep knit and wide through your abdomen. Only go as far as you can with ease and regular breathing. Effort means you have gone too far. If you cannot easily lift your pelvis, begin with the support of a ball under the pelvis. Swing your legs over it while you flatten your belly.

Repeat six times, gradually and easily progressing further.

Sequence 8: Uncurl and Reach of the Sitz Bones

Lift your legs and flex your spine similarly to Sequence 7, coming into the plough (Figures 24, 25, and 26). Pause and allow your breathing to assume a comfortable, easy rhythm. This does not need to be according to pulses.

Reach with your sitz bones toward the ceiling to lengthen your spine, and reach with your feet toward the ceiling to straighten your legs into a shoulder stand (Figure 27).

Continue to reach with your sitz bones and lengthen your inverted spine toward the ceiling while you flex your hips and reach your feet away above your head toward the floor (Figure 28). When you have reached your end range, grab your toes with your hands (Figure 29). Releasing your psoas and reaching with your sitz bones, fold your hips and uncurl your spine one vertebra at a time (Figure 30). Should you have a blockage in an area you can rock slowly back and forth, alternately flexing and extending through that vertebra (while breathing) to release it. Keep your shoulders wide and your front and back of equal (long) length.

When your tail reaches the floor, gently lower your legs to the floor and rest (Figures 31 and 32).

Do not strain. Strain will only defeat the purpose and be contrary to this practice of effortlessness, flexibility, strength, and coordination. Good practice both depends upon and develops self-awareness and self-responsibility. It is up to you to keep these elements in your practice. Do not set unrealistic or imagined goals. Work up to it!

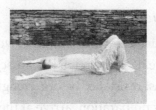

Figure 24

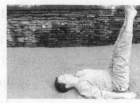

Figure 25

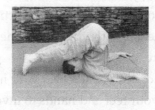

Figure 26

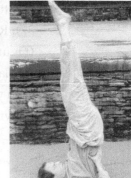

Figure 27

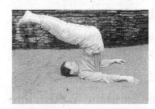

Figure 28

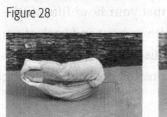

Figure 29

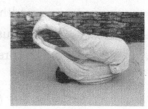

Figure 30

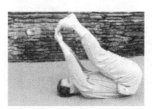

Figure 31

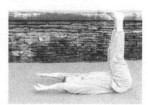

Figure 32

Sequence 9: Backbend

Practice the backbend after you can do the plough effortlessly, not before. If you stretch the muscles on the front of the body and spine against resistance before strengthening them, you may injure yourself.

As preparation, arrive at the shoulder stand as in Sequence 8, supporting your low back with your hands (Figures 33–36). From the position of your thighs in vertical, bend your knees forward (Figure 37). Reach with your sitz bones and drop your feet flat on the floor (Figure 38).

Place your hands over your head, palms down (Figure 39), and push with your feet and hands to invert into the backbend. At first leave the crown of your head on the floor while you connect your:

> head to tail
> feet to head
> hands to tail
> feet to hands

Then continue to push into extension through your hands and feet so that your head lifts off the floor (Figure 40). Maintain length and width in front and back of your body. Keep knitted in the front.

Suspend.

Breathe easily and return gently to the floor (Figure 41).

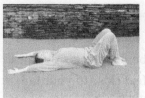

Figure 33

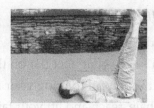

Figure 34

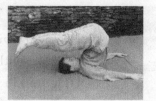

Figure 35

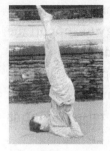

Figure 36

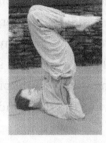

Figure 37

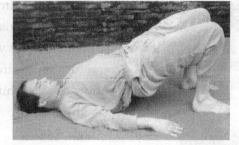

Figure 38

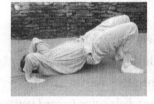

Figure 39

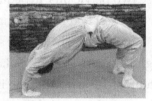

Figure 40

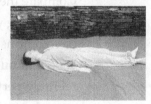

Figure 41

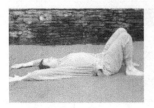

Figure 42

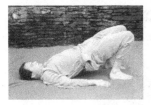

Figure 43

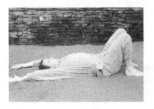

Figure 44

Sequence 10: Pelvic Lift #2

Compare with Sequence 4.

Start with knees bent, feet flat on the floor, arms overhead (Figure 42). It is helpful to bring your feet close to your tail.

As you exhale, reach and lift your tail toward your feet, shifting your spine toward your tail, and lifting your spine from the floor one vertebra at a time (Figure 43). Connect your tail to your hands and allow this sequence of energy to support the lowering of your arms to your sides. Suspend.

As you return on the inhale, lower your spine through the breath—allow the breathing down your spine to soften each vertebra as you lower toward the floor and raise your arms overhead (Figure 44).

Compare these two pelvic lifts: in Sequence 4, as you *inhale* you begin filling your chest and letting your breath initiate the lifting of your arms. Simultaneously you are sequencing the breathing energy through your torso to your tail, lifting your tail and, vertebra by vertebra, lifting your spine into the air. Breathing in your chest lifts your chest and *shifts your whole spine toward your head*. In Sequence 10, as you *exhale* you are reaching and lifting your tail toward your feet, *shifting your spine toward your tail*, and lifting your spine from the floor one vertebra at a time.

Try both patterns and explore how your breathing supports the movement of your spine differently in each.

Sequence 11: Preparation for Spinal Rotation

Begin lying on your back, knees bent with feet on the floor, arms out horizontally to the side with palms up (Figure 45).

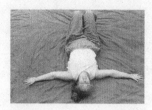

Figure 45

Initiating from the feet, ankles, and forelegs, exhale and lever your femurs to one side, releasing your knees and lengthening eccentrically through the psoas major (Figure 46). Pause as you suspend your breath. Return to center on the inhale (Figure 47).

While your ankles remain stable, initiate by rolling inside and outside the foot and deepening in the hip joint rather than initiating by lowering/lifting the knees. Maintain the length of the front and back of the body. Do not arch or press your back into the floor! Maintain the kidney/adrenal/bladder triangular balance. Let your head remain in the midline and your spine remain calm. Stay grounded in your sacrum/bladder.

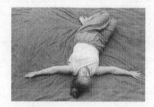

Figure 46

It is not heavy knees that pull the pelvis: lower your knees only as far as you can maintain stability of the pelvis and integrity of the spine. Keep your weight in the inside of your legs and inside your hip joint—not outside or in the greater trochanter. Practice articulating each leg individually and then combine them in tandem. Control each leg independently.

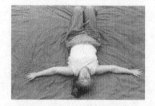

Figure 47

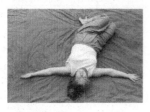

Figure 48

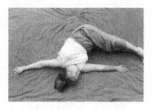

Figure 49

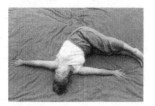

Figure 50

Sequence 12: Spinal Rotation through the Legs and Arms

Begin as in the preparation (Sequence 11): exhale and lever your legs to the floor on the right side (Figure 48). As you meet the end of your range, slide your feet along the floor and straighten your knees, which will rotate your pelvis and lumbar spine. At the same time, turn your head to the right and rotate your right arm by reaching with your hand so that your palm faces down (Figure 49).

Inhale and rotate your left arm by reaching with your hand so that your palm faces down. At the same time, turn your head to the left side (Figure 50).

Suspend.

Exhale and move your left arm along the floor over your head to meet your right hand. Turn your right palm up to meet your left palm. Rotate your head to the right (Figure 51). Your spine straightens.

Suspend.

Inhale and return your left hand to the left side and rotate your left arm by reaching with your hand so that your palm faces down. At the same time turn your head to the left side (Figure 52).

Suspend.

Exhale and rotate your right arm by reaching with your hand so that your palm faces down. At the same time, turn your head to the right side (Figure 53).

Suspend.

Inhale and, initiating in the feet and tail, return your legs to the starting position: knees bent with feet flat on the floor (Figure 54). As you suspend your breath, return your arms to the starting position by rotating your palms up (Figure 55).

Repeat this sequence to the left side.

In practicing this spinal rotation, find maximum counter-rotation between ribs and pelvis (maximum rotation of lumbar vertebrae) as you maintain your ribs and thoracic spine in restful/breathing stability. The rotation of the waist facilitates strengthening of the kidney/adrenal/bladder complex. Maintain the length of the front and back of the spine and the integrity of the spinal axis as you rotate your waist. While the dome of your diaphragm expands eccentrically to maintain maximum stability, your crura will rotate to keep your pelvis connected to this support.

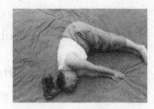

Figure 51

During the movements that combine reaching and rotating the arm with turning the head, initiate distally: let your head turn your neck and your hand turn your arm. Both the head and arm meet at the heart/breathing center, and both are supported by and initiated from breath. Find rotation of the cervical vertebrae as you maintain your ribs and thoracic spine in restful/breathing stability.

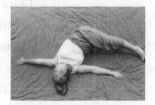

Figure 52

Leave your feet on the floor for the entire exercise. It is very important to keep extending through the feet and tail, and to feel and move from the anchor provided by their counter-supports. Throughout the exercise keep your tail active in initiating countermovement toward the feet. The reaching of your feet and tail provide a constant anchor. Keep the weight and energy in the inside of your legs.

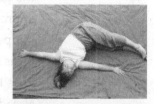

Figure 53

The arm and hand that remain stable in this movement also provide essential counter-support. The counter-support will change from hand to hand depending on which side you initiate from. Use the counter-support of the stabilizing arm/hand to widen through your back and anchor your reach through the moving arm/hand.

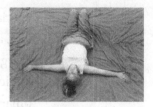

Figure 54

As you rotate your moving hand from palm up to palm down and palm down to palm up, maintain awareness of the

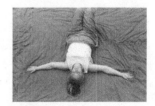

Figure 55

back of your palm on the floor. Initiate the supination/pronation from the ulna, brushing your little finger along the floor in an undercurve.

Conclusion

Few subjects are more potentially vast and at the same time more potentially simple than Body-Mind Centering and yoga. What both Bonnie Bainbridge Cohen and Desikachar emphasize primarily is fitting a practice to the individual, rather than the individual to the practice. There is room within each tradition for anyone to find a practice that suits him or her. However, a practice that works must be continually distilled from an infinity of possibilities.

One big piece of learning for me has been witnessing and sharing the benefit of Bonnie's mastery in finding and choosing simple but appropriate pursuits in response to what is needed. As we share how our perspectives can shed light on each other, my hope is that practical ideas will become more accessible to all. What do you practice? How does that work for you? What do you add or change? What do you already do?

Special thanks to my yoga teachers Edwina Ranganathan, David Schonfeld, and Sri T.K.V. Desikachar. And, of course, to Bonnie, Michael, and Margaret for their brilliance, strength, patience, and wit. This essay is dedicated to Bonnie and Len Cohen with gratitude for their extraordinary vision, dedication, and generosity.

Yielding Toward Presence: Dynamic Relationships in Dance Performance

~ **Darcy McGehee,** Canada (2003)

Growing up in the ballet studio world, I accepted living in a high-adrenal state. Controlling the flight/flight/freeze response in order to please was also part of the package. In that world, life became a performative act; my relationships with need and with real desire were often put on the back burner. Cultural and aesthetic images of lightness and flight and constant, elusive movement fired my very active imagination.

Three-year-old aspirations.

My cortical motor systems were highly connected to my high-brain smarts. Independence, drive, and discipline were applauded early on, from walking at nine months to pushing the limits of exhaustion through my teen years. I was the high-extensor-tone kid who found physical containment in hypertonic power muscles and lightness in anorexia. I did not perceive my health as something that I had anything to do with. Illness and injury were the result of invasion by forces beyond my control.

I loved dancing. Flying, defying gravity, and the feeling of transcendence gave me great joy, but the truth was that I had no way to land or to come back home again. Trust issues emerged—I either completely threw myself into the influence of others or backed off entirely into my own world. I would either attempt to control myself and

349

everything around me or escape to fantasies that allowed me to disconnect from the real world. Fantasy can motivate, but it does not support a more fundamental corporeal awareness of moving into support to reach and grow.

Thirty years ago, I temporarily left behind the verticality of ballet to revel in the modernist trajectories of suspension and fall, but I never quite moved past being a gaze-receiving object. Then, as a faithful postmodernist, I twirled the kaleidoscope of my bodymind view of performance and did my best to extricate myself from feeling good as the tragic heroine. Disconnection and a lack of metaphor only added to my brave suffering.

The second half of my dancing life was about perpetual inversion. I was engaged in the myth of falling, desperately trying to find ground through high-brain intention. I began to realize an acute urge to be horizontal and to pause. The trouble was, I did not know how to do this.

Research into somatics and neurodevelopmental theory has taught me that I was doing a lot of unsupported motoring then. I was out in the world without a way to transition back into rest, comfort, and desire. Through these musings, it began to occur to me that performance is, in fact, a social relationship that has to do with communication at very subtle as well as very obvious levels.

Somatic experience told me what fifteen years of looking at anatomical representations of the body had somehow failed to reveal—my cortical, imaginative brain had to make connection with my locomoting body through my brainstem, my low brain, and my mid brain. Without the integration of sub-cortical brain systems, my action was lacking in the subtleties of genuine communication. I was not fully present; I was lacking relationships in the performing moment.

The reflexes that underlie movement depend on the proprioception of gravity, providing a basis for relationship to self. Relationship to self gives one person the basis for relating to another. I needed to rediscover gravity.

My journey of learning and research through Martha Eddy's Somatic Movement Therapy Training program, Bonnie Bainbridge Cohen's School for Body-Mind Centering, and somatic practice—particularly observing babies and children—has led me to understand a primary concept of moving into support. This affords me the pleasure of modulating movement and focus between inside and outside in body systems and developmental movement patterns, and it affords me a subjective voice in a performance relationship. The simple and powerful concept of yielding into a relationship with gravity and exploring the astonishing ability of the body to be in dynamic reciprocity with self and other now forms a basis of my teaching and practice.

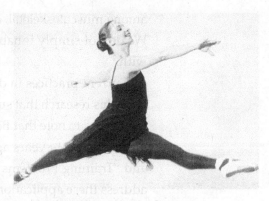

Looking for a place to land.

I am intrigued by the similarities between movement markers for diagnosing developmental delays and historical representations of the dancing body. I recall the aesthetic dancing body of my youth: little spinal rotation, thoracic hyperextension, toe walking, frontal-plane weight shifting, arms held up, no midline crossing, defending through the senses, restricted gaze shift. I also recall my own difficulties with connecting vocally to communicate. Perhaps being engaged in the myth of falling was a "stim," a stereotypical activity for me, much like the repetitive actions that autistics engage in. These behaviors often signal a stuck attempt to stimulate neural support.

Research in neurology is redefining motor learning and beginning to situate expression and aesthetic in embodiment.

Indeed, there are no externally fixed representations of the external world in the "motor systems"; rather, it is under the guidance of both internal and external factors with important linkages to frontal, parietal, cerebellar, basal ganglionic, and cingulated gyrus areas that subserve cognitive and motivational activities. The motor system, including related structures, is a self-organizing dynamic system contextualized among musculoskeletal, environmental (*e.g.*, gravity), and social forces. We do not simply inhabit our bodies; we literally use them to think with.[1]

Current practices in dance pedagogy and performance can benefit from this research that supports developmental movement theory. It is interesting to note that Bonnie Bainbridge Cohen addressed these connections twenty years ago in her manuals "The Dancer's Warm-up" and "Training Problems of the Dancer," two treatises that eloquently address these applications of Body-Mind Centering.[2]

The population I teach currently is comprised of eighteen- to twenty-something-year-old university students. I endeavor that our work together helps them to become aware of the need to explore concepts of centering, grounding, and the subjective voice in movement and performance. I teach them that a dancer's warm-up can consist of many Body-Mind Centering principles of developmental movement, all of which support efficient artistic practice. Cellular breathing, yielding various body surfaces and tissues to gravity in tonic lab, and balancing the autonomic nervous system through the opening and closing patterns of simultaneous condensing and expanding yield gently awaken primary connections to support action.

All of these are necessary precursors to dynamic balance and the development of mature righting reactions and equilibrium responses necessary in dance performance. Mouthing, nosing, and gentle scanning begin to connect the senses and perceptions to gut-brain impulses and are foundational to spatial intent. Yielding to push establishes weight shift from a supported, connected place, providing proprioceptive support for eccentric muscle contractions in movement initiations toward gravity and in transitions to reaching in space. This fine-tuning of basic patterns allows well-integrated reflexes to support complex, creative sequences of movement.

Classes for children can incorporate more experiential learning based on developmental movement principles. Many studio dance classes for children, whether in contemporary or ballet forms, consist of imitation or mirroring, which is often relationally one-sided and draws a child's attention away from sensing and honoring her or his immediate experience. The child attempts to meet the teacher, not vice versa. The improvisational component of dance class, while it connects gesture and movement to imagination, may not establish relationship with corporeal sensation or with the environment. The imagination is often developed in isolation, and its development is unrelated to the kinesthetic, emotional, and social development of the performative dancing body. Playfulness may not be embodied and movement becomes mimetic or symbolically representational, without a sense of metaphor that connects it to a sensing and feeling present moment.

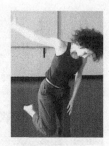

"Inside reaching out."

Most children can enjoy the awareness of dynamically shifting internal sensations and movement in the body. For those challenged to do so, the opportunity to play with this shift is critical to their development. These experiences allow children to begin to modulate attention, intention, and action in time, space, and quality of movement. They can learn to bridge inside and outside relationship and understand how to "get back home" again by acknowledging a changing self in relationship to a changing world.

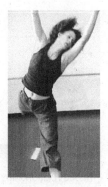

"Outside reaching in."

An infant discovers a supported relationship to gravity through being held, being moved, and shaping and molding to a caregiver. A baby learning to travel measures time and space from this initial support as well as from his or her own center of gravity. A child moving in space begins to establish a more independent relationship to gravity, to self-nurturing, and to self-care. This is an important transition that we continue to re-examine as we mature. Exploring moving into active relationship with gravity and connecting feeling, sensing, and doing should be an integral part of any movement class for any age.

Science now explores what a typically playful child innately knows: movement is critical in organizing us in time and space and supports the emergence of social, emotional, and cognitive function. Yielding opens up dynamic, interdependent patterns of possibility. As I learn to yield to gravity, I learn to bond and defend based on a respect for

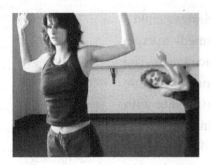

"Searching for the transition between inside and outside."

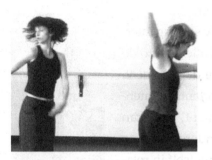

"Missed relationships."

my experiences and the experiences of others. I am capable of the pause of presence and relationship.

In theatre, the concept of "The Play" is integral to performance. My current experience of weaving dance and theatre through movement and text is informed by my somatic practice. I try to balance a sensing awareness of inside and outside (self and other) with action that is mediated through feeling.

Exploring this option in a recent piece with two dancers and an actor revealed to me a new kind of virtuosity that was simultaneously very vulnerable and very powerful. The resulting piece, "Shift," frames the question of how to honor a sense of both self and other in a dynamically shifting landscape of interaction. In this piece, performers embody a representation of the ethereal, disconnected bodymind searching for connection.

The process of choreography and performance brought up developmental issues of feeling unsupported in transitions, highlighting the courage needed to trust self and other and the intricate connections between perceptual and motor development. It distinguished the global focus of awareness and the more specific focus of embodied attention.

We explored ways of debriefing from the character bodies we were assuming in this process. A web of simple rhythms emerged in our explorations that mirror the basic physiological and developmental processes explored in Body-Mind Centering: moving in to go out as I condense to expand, moving out to go in as I expand to condense, and moving down to go up and up to go down as I explore the cycle of yield to push to reach to pull to yield again.

This exquisite dance of opposites has its basis in a seemingly simple, but sometimes elusive, relationship to gravity. This experience gives me insights into the possibilities of a more conversational relationship with an audience in performance.

BMC and Dance

~ **Mark Taylor,** USA (2005)

As a choreographer and Body-Mind Centering practitioner, I was recently challenged to think in a different way regarding my assumptions and values about dance. My habit had been to discount work that didn't conform to my value structure—my *worldview*, as BMC practitioner Jan Cook would say—and I'm thinking about the ways in which what I considered to be my aesthetic values were perhaps really a limitation in my vision. The interesting challenge came in seeing Alonzo King's *Lines* ballet company a second time, and it has given me the opportunity to rethink my BMC-infused values about dance and performance.

Lines is a company that I saw four years ago in a festival context, in Dusseldorf, Germany. At that time I disliked them and pretty much everything they represented. Their performance epitomized a set of values about dance and performance that I felt I had rejected; I saw it merely as beautiful bodies pumping out a spectacle of virtuosic but meaningless movement with no sense of engagement with the audience or themselves. A short and somewhat exaggerated statement of these values might include the following ideas:

- There is an ideal physical conformation of the body that a dancer should train to achieve, emphasizing verticality and the musculoskeletal system.
- The bodies and movement should appear uniform at the expense of individuality.
- Choreography is based on a codified movement vocabulary (ballet, jazz, modern, "release," and so forth).

- Dancers have the active role in performance, and the audience is passive.
- Dance technique serves to entertain and dazzle the audience.
- A performer displays or pretends to be in relationship with a partner rather than fully living in relationship in the moment.
- Performance requires constant teasing, manipulation, and overpowering of the audience's emotions.
- The artist is the choreographer; dancers are tools for the communication of his or her artistic impulse.

It was a surprise to me that in a recent performance of the same company I saw something totally different. In spite of the fact that Alonzo King's choreography remains grounded in these traditional values and forms—a combination of ballet and early postmodern movement manipulation techniques—and entirely lacks content and meaning other than the display of movement, nonetheless the performance communicated something essential about the resilience of the human spirit. I was deeply moved, and I felt the audience respond as well. In our kinesthetic identification with these demi-gods doing these amazing things, we were able to feel the potential of fullness and ease within ourselves.

The dancers embodied the display and virtuosic technique stemming from rigorous ballet training, yet the best of them also had release, articulation, weight, and a relationship to the heavens and earth that was profoundly satisfying to watch and communicated something like a state of grace. I saw the individuality in the performers' approaches to the material. I saw some experimentation and risk-taking, pushing the boundaries of the ballet vocabulary. I felt the dancers' generosity and commitment. So there I sat, appreciating what I thought I didn't value at all.

The experience led me to several questions. Had the company really changed that much in three years? Were new and better performers finally doing what King had intended all along? Or was the change in me—a new willingness to suspend my preconceived notions and really take in aspects of the work I hadn't opened to before? (Was it the Perceptual Action-Response Cycle at work?![1])

What do I do with this change in perception? I have been involved in choreographing and training dancers for many years. The values that evolved over those years for me might be summarized as:

- Each conscious movement of my body is dance and can be valued.
- Experimentation and innovation within a form is more important than the form itself.
- Dance is for everyone; it is not just the province of professional dancers.
- Movement is an expression of the whole person; the more deeply individuated I am as a mover, the more I have to share.
- As a teacher, I facilitate my students' process of self-definition and self-discovery rather than make choices for them about movement.
- Rather than learning or teaching movement from motoric objectives, we can train from sensory experience.
- The moment of performance occurs somewhere in the dynamic field between performer and audience, rendering the audience more active and the performers more reactive.
- Choreographers and dancers can have a partnering relationship that empowers and satisfies both parties, thereby strengthening the choreographic work and allowing the performers to deepen their relationship to material.

As a choreographer in New York, before I began to explore my work within a BMC context, I was interested in maintaining some traditions of Western theatrical dance. Yet I was also drawn to celebrate the individuality of dancers, to work with an expanded notion of movement possibilities, and to create a more integrated relational field between performer and audience.

In Pittsburgh, and under the influence of Bonnie Bainbridge Cohen and the BMC approach, I began working with non-traditional casts, incorporating untrained performers and specific populations in my work. I entered into a series of deep collaborations with dancers and artists from other cultures (Hawaii, India, the Caribbean) in order to understand other performance options than the one I had inherited. I anchored my work in the experience of specific communities. I worked to empower my collaborating dancers in themselves as movers, performers, and humans. Then, two years ago, I chose to leave the Pittsburgh company in order to develop my work in BMC as practitioner and teacher, while retaining loose ties to the dance community as an occasional choreographer and teacher.

Recently I've begun to work more in dance again, choreographing some small works and teaching in university settings. The day before the Lines company performance, I had the opportunity to teach three classes at a university dance department where the curriculum is fairly traditional. Afterward, I felt that in loading my classes toward the improvisational and experiential I didn't meet the students' need for self-identification as dancers. It disoriented them not to have the safe container of their *pliés* and *tendus.* Then I saw many of these students at the Lines performance and witnessed their self-identification with the angelic technical performers, and their desire to morph into similar beings. Since I am capable of meeting their expectations of a traditional "technique" class, I'm now questioning why I should try to impose my values, when I can see value in what they're hoping to achieve.

I guess what I need to learn is something about context and shades of gray, where I had been seeing the issues in black and white. I had pretty much limited myself to thinking that if I am true to my value system of utilizing dance as a tool for personal growth, then I need to reject proscenium-based theatrical spectacle as an option I can support and enjoy. Now I'm thinking that maybe I can embrace those values again in some way that doesn't deny the inherent worth of either approach. The softening and blurring of value systems feels good to me, and it's helping me look forward to reentering dance more deeply again.

This experience led me to these questions: How do we negotiate the integration of movement from a BMC perspective with older, inherited traditions? How do we acknowledge, accept, enrich, and appreciate older forms we've worked in, as our perceptions and souls shift in the process of embodiment?

Unfracturing: An Interview with RoseAnne Spradlin

~ **Gill Wright Miller,** USA (2004)

I wanted to make myself and others feel better
about accepting the transient nature of life.[1]

Body-Mind Centering certified practitioner and teacher RoseAnne Spradlin won a Bessie Award in Fall 2003, making her only the second Body-Mind Centering artist to do so. (Gale Turner won a Bessie in 1990 for her performing with Meredith Monk.) Spradlin and Turner sit in esteemed company. Since the award's inception in 1985, Bessies, which honor outstanding innovative achievements in dance and related performance, have signaled exceptional artistic achievements and bring attention to the issues and challenges that face artistic communities in New York and nationally. Bessie Awards have been given to such revered dance artists as Trisha Brown, Donald Byrd, Ann Carlson, Ping Chong, Chuck Davis, Garth Fagan, Molissa Fenley, William Forsythe, Guillermo Gomez-Pena, David Gordon, Bill Irwin, Bill T. Jones, Anne Teresa de Keersmaeker, Meredith Monk, Mark Morris, Steve Paxton, Gus Solomons, Jr., and Robert Wilson, a list of presenters that is a veritable Who's Who among the "downtown dance" scene in New York. Spradlin's choreography has been produced at Danspace Project, The Kitchen, Dance Theater Workshop, Joyce SoHo, Dixon Place, and The Club at La Mama. Her work has also been produced in Atlanta, San Francisco, and London, and she has been invited to teach at the American Dance Festival (Durham, North Carolina) and Dance in August Festival (Berlin) and in both England and Greece. Born and raised in

Oklahoma City as she was, I can't help but ask how Spradlin made her way through a training maze that included undergraduate and graduate school in Ohio, the Laban Movement Analysis program in New York, and finally the Body-Mind Centering program in Massachusetts, all in unanticipated preparation for the "downtown" New York dance scene and this coveted award.

A Journey

In December 2003 I was fortunate to interview RoseAnne about her journey. "After finishing a visual arts undergraduate degree at the University of Oklahoma, I went to graduate school at Ohio University. I had been dancing all through undergraduate school, but in Athens I saw a lot of modern student choreography, so I enrolled in another undergraduate program in dance." The program was chaired by long-time Alwin Nikolais dancer Gladys Bailin. "I already had an idea of what I wanted to do, and it wasn't making dances like Nikolais did," RoseAnne shared. "Besides, I was older and was restless to get out of the undergraduate position." Still, she says, she got solid training and a great deal of support from the OU program. "I started coming to New York, and in 1982–83 did the Laban Intensive (two summers and the January in between). While doing that program, I stumbled onto Bonnie's work." Certified Movement Analyst Ellen Goldman, who was one of her teachers at LIMS, had studied with Bonnie Bainbridge Cohen. Bainbridge Cohen and Sandy Jamrog, and eventually Martha Eddy, had made guest appearances in the New York program. Spradlin says at that time she followed up her interest by checking out the "Organ Manual" and the "Skeletal Manual" from the LIMS library, but she thought studying with Bainbridge Cohen would never happen.

Then, one weekend, Bainbridge Cohen arrived in New York to teach a workshop on the spine. "By Friday night I wanted to do the whole program. I was thirty-two or thirty-three at the time. That was the average age of the students enrolled in her program." For well over a decade, Spradlin spent every summer in Amherst ... that is, until recently, when she started a four-year degree program in Chinese medicine at Pacific College of Oriental Medicine.

Draw a Bigger Circle

"When I started studying BMC I had no intention of becoming a 'healthcare practitioner.' I really considered myself a choreographer and dancer. I was trying to understand myself and my movement. So many questions I had, and nobody had answers. I went into the BMC program for my own self as a dancer. I did also feel this pull toward healing work, but I didn't feel like I could do it. That happened along the way."

There is a pause in our interview, as RoseAnne revisits another era, embodies another voice, draws a new breath initiation. "**'Draw a bigger circle.'** Did you ever hear Bonnie say, 'Draw a bigger circle'?" Spradlin asked me. "Everything I am doing and everything I am studying fits if I just draw a bigger circle. It's all about movement." The confirmation of being awarded the Bessie seeped back into her consciousness then. "The way this fall has gone, I didn't feel the conflict anymore."

To Athena Malloy, one of her dancers, Spradlin's complex journey seemed logical enough. "For someone like RoseAnne, who's really steady in her conviction about her work, it makes sense that this is the way her career would happen."[2]

Artful Somatics: Frames for Her Work

Cutting-edge dance artists are often involved in several different forms of movement exploration. They tend to explore anything that transports them closer to the inside, closer to an understanding of how and why they work the way they do. So it makes sense that theories about bodywork are integral to Spradlin's choreographic method. I asked her if she talked to her dancers about Body-Mind Centering.

"I didn't at first," she admitted, "but I do now. I make comments like 'Access your notochord here; nucleolus there. You know, the connection into the earth, gravity, and magnetism; lightness and wholeness. Get the experience of some of these things.'" She made a conscious decision to allow the three dancers she now works with, Bessie winners in their own right for their performances in Spradlin's work, to communicate how much they wanted to know. Walter Dundervill, Athena Malloy, and Tasha Taylor each had different technical skills when they came to Spradlin. "He came toward me the most," she said, "and I feel like I've given the most to him." Athena and Tasha were familiar with other theories, work like Zero Balancing, Klein Technique, and Feldenkrais. "They probably wouldn't be working with me if they weren't interested . . . well, if they were just interested in the steps," Spradlin reflected.

Various critics described her 2002 work, "under/world." Each critic hones in on the raw tenderness of human existence. About the dancers, Susan Reiter said, "They let the audience in on edgy, intensely private, at times animalistic encounters that in no way felt refined or smoothed over with a performance veneer."[3] Reiter continues by describing a section of this work. "In one extremely intimate encounter that remained with me long after, Taylor (wearing just panties and a garter belt) and Dundervill (who had donned a black dance belt and dark hooded sweatshirt) alternate rolls and grapples on the floor, with him tickling her mercilessly, and then suddenly stop short with him cradled in her arms, suckling on her breast. They continue between playful, sensual tickling and the mother-and-child image, for a while, before it was time to move on to the next task." Critic Chris Dohse makes these summary remarks: "From [the duet described above] to sections that delight in the naked body's authentically awkward tangle with gravity, 'under/world' never condescends to suburban mockery of fringe sexuality, but rather groans with its urgency, its sweetness, its legitimacy."[4]

Spradlin believes that she is engaged by a process of revealing the dancers with whom she is working, drawing movement out of their

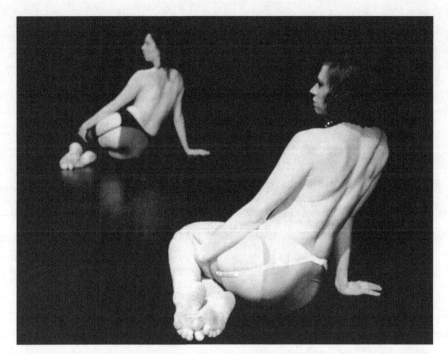

Athena Malloy
and Tasha Taylor
in RoseAnne
Spradlin's *under/
world*, presented
by the Kitchen
in New York City
in 2003.

bodies. "If the audience can see a real person on stage, it's a treat. For
the dancers, well, it's about 'letting themselves be seen,' as Deborah
Hay used to say." Spradlin claims her role is "to figure out how to
support them in letting people see them. I watch them and give them
feedback to get over their own neuroses from dance training—and
just living."

Many a critic has commented on the audience's reception of
Spradlin's methods. Certain words, like "rawness," come up over and
over again. The process is like taking off layers, exposing, getting to
the core, unzipping the coverings and shedding them layer by layer.
"It comes from my background," Spradlin said. "I have a visual arts
background, and the aesthetic [at the time I was studying it] was in
the use of found objects. There is certain 'organicity' there. The goal
was to let the material have its own quality. Don't cover it up."

In 1999, Deborah Jowitt said about Spradlin's work: "I feel the
dancer's turmoil and I can't take my eyes away." To this Spradlin says,

Tasha Taylor on the screen and Paige Martin on the stage in RoseAnne Spradlin's *Survive Cycle,* a mixed-media work presented by Dance Theater Workshop in New York City in 2006.

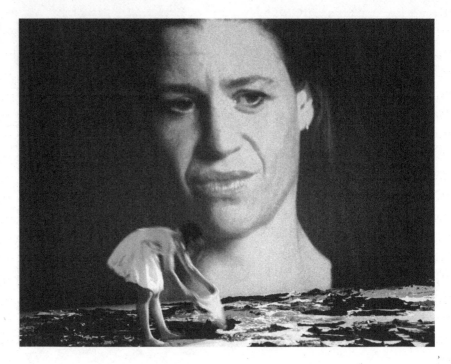

"I'm not trying to make an emotional-type story. I'm more interested in revealing the progress of raw emotions. When this happens successfully, the emotional response is raw as well. It resonates in the tissues, blood, and organs." Because of this Spradlin claims her work does not appeal as much to the cerebral type, those who want to understand the piece as it is unfolding. She recalled one bad review. "The critic claimed there was nothing there. She couldn't write what her own participation was with it."

On the contrary, Spradlin has been working intimately with her own participation. "When I went back to (Oriental Medicine) school in 2001, I thought I was giving up choreography. It wasn't fun anymore. I thought I was done."

So, how is it she just won the most coveted art-dance award in the United States? "There was just some unfinished business," she admits. "I had already applied for an important grant, and then I heard I got it. A door opened. I hadn't let my thinking go that far before." And she wondered, "Could I have an impact on the way other people see things?" Indeed she has.

Shifting on the Membrane

Body-Mind Centering teaches us about community. It is a lesson Spradlin takes to heart. "I need the support of the community. I need to have other people produce my work. I need the bigger structure to hold the choreography rather than have the choreography hold itself." Successful grants have allowed for that, but she admits she isn't comfortable asking for money. "I think it's a good idea to be able to put some money into your projects yourself." By asking for money, she claims, "You make yourself so vulnerable—or you become responsible for paybacks. The whole grant thing is not structured around healthy business practices." For example, when her work was produced at the Kitchen, they profited four times as much as she did, "even though I had to take out a big personal loan to do the work."

In the end, winning the Bessie has challenged her "outsider" status and shifted her location. "I am on the membrane," she said. But that location has brought her more closely to herself. "If you don't know yourself, you don't have a chance," she said. "I *am* an outsider in a way. I'm from Oklahoma—another universe, another planet. And I started dancing late. Well, at least I never felt like I was losing my technique," she mused. "I never really *had* technique."

One of the difficulties with downtown choreography is the vanishing target that artists reach for. "There is no center in the contemporary dance scene." Still, she admits, "Certainly I feel slightly different [due to the award]. The work's the same as it was the day before, the day after. In that respect, nothing really changed." Her voice becomes easy and indirect, more remote. "It was nice to get it."

"One of the things about me when I started BMC: I was very confused inside, temporally, going back to school at my age, trying to get into dance so late. Something about BMC has helped me get caught up with myself." She pauses. "When I was younger, I was together. BMC really helped me put myself *back* together—emotionally, cellularly. It is an integrating moment. The person who managed to get a Bessie was not fractured," she asserted. "That's kind of what it's all about."

Reflecting on the direct relationship between her BMC training and her dancing, Spradlin concluded, "Body-Mind Centering is a jewel. It has come in through the people rather than through the concepts." Cellular indeed.

Section Four

Embodying Body-Mind Centering: Being and Doing

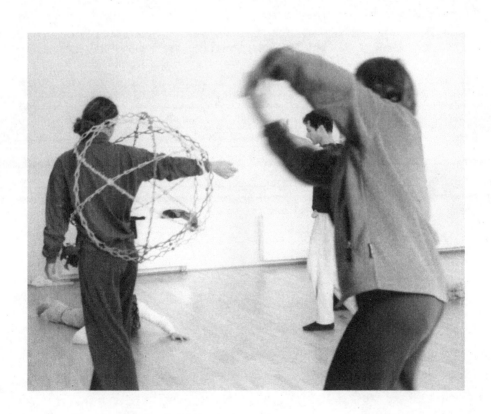

Section Four

Embodying body-Mind Context:
Being and Doing

Body-Mind Centering, Mindfulness, and the Body Politic

~ **Maggie McGuire,** USA (2006)

Awakening to BMC

My first experience of Bonnie Bainbridge Cohen (and Body-Mind Centering) was watching a videotape of her working with an eight-year-old boy who, at the age of four, experienced a drowning accident that left him severely brain injured, with no voluntary movement except for his eyes on occasion. Bonnie worked in unfolding layers, first by simply listening to whatever the boy's mother had to share about her son, and then by being particularly curious about the boy's life before the accident. What did he enjoy doing? Did he have a favorite nursery rhyme? It seemed to me that Bonnie was respectfully entering the dyadic world of mother and child, attuning herself to their energy rhythms, feeling where they could meet her, and she them.

She then moved to the boy's head, which she held in her hands, sitting in quiet stillness for a very long time. Only later, after years of study with Bonnie and BMC, did I fully understand what she was doing: penetrating deeply the layers of tissue, letting her attentive mind be guided by the feel of sensations and movements within herself and within the boy, making contact with parts of the brain that were caught in a reactive pattern, and awakening the mind of the tissue so that it could be freed from its unconscious state and shift into a new movement pattern. Once the connection was made, Bonnie began lightly stroking the boy's cheek, stimulating the rooting reflex. The boy slowly began to turn his head in the direction of Bonnie's hand, while she sang his favorite nursery rhyme.

Deeply moved, tears flowing, I silently said, "I want to learn how to do that." I recognized something I already knew and felt within my own experience of working with others but had not yet been able to articulate. I began studying with Bonnie in 1984, about the same time that I began to study Buddhism and Native American healing practices. I was already immersed in the field of body-based approaches in education and psychotherapy, having been an early childhood/special education teacher who had switched into experiential, body-centered psychotherapy and family systems work.

Body-Mind Centering and Buddhism are both grounded in an understanding of mind as the capacity for being awake to our experience in the present moment. Both cultivate the practice of mindfulness, of being present to our direct experience. A key teaching of both is to accept nothing on faith and instead to investigate for ourselves whether or not these teachings accurately reflect our experience. They each recognize our most fundamental nature to be awake and aware.

As Bonnie worked with the young boy, she demonstrated three qualities of this basic nature: openness, clarity, and compassion. Openness is the indestructible spaciousness in the mind. All experiences—sensations, emotions, thoughts, images—arise in the open space of mind. It is the sense of slowing down and simply being present with what is happening. Bonnie simply established herself in this openness of mind through which she connected with the boy and his mother.

Bonnie's years of study and practice in embodied anatomy and developmental movement allowed her to be present to what *is* in a very precise way. Clarity is the ability to be precisely mindful and aware of direct experience, an unmediated experience not overlaid with thoughts and preferences. Bonnie's focused and receptive attention was guided by acceptance and curiosity. Her intention to discover the primary tissues involved in the injury and to support the mind's capacity to consciously experience itself directly at the tissue level and to self-organize was based on a mutually shared perception, albeit unconscious on the client's part.

Compassion, to feel another's pain and wish to relieve unnecessary suffering, is an inherent part of our fundamental nature. It adds a quality of tenderness that establishes the mind in the heart, allowing us to remain open and connected to experience. The task of the healer is to help others recognize and reconnect to their own brilliant nature.

The Mind in Body-Mind Centering

One of my favorite classes in my training was Mind class. During the first half of the hour we would sit in quiet stillness, practicing steadying our attention to the present moment through resting awareness in the breath or in the subtle shifts in sensation and movement within various tissues of the body or within the cells. During the second half of the hour we would explore the impulse to move, an intimate dialogue of awareness and action, balancing the smallest activity within the body at the cellular level with the largest expression of external movement through space. We were "becoming aware of the relationship that exists throughout our body/mind and acting from that awareness. This alignment creates a state of knowing."[1]

The mind and body in BMC are both the explorer and the subject of exploration. BMC is an experiential journey that guides us in our understanding of how the mind is expressed through the body in movement. As Bonnie describes it,

> There is something in nature that forms patterns. We, as part of
> nature, also form patterns. The mind is like the wind and the body
> is like the sand; if you want to know how the wind is blowing, you
> can look at the sand.
>
> Our body moves as our mind moves. The qualities of any move-
> ment are a manifestation of how the mind is expressed through the
> body at that moment. Changes in movement qualities indicate that
> the mind has shifted focus in the body. Conversely, when we direct
> the mind or attention to different parts of the body and initiate

movement from those areas, we change the quality of our movement. So we find that movement can be a way to observe the expression of mind through the body and it can also be a way to effect changes in the body-mind relationship.[2]

In BMC, using the maps of Western medicine and science—anatomy, physiology, and kinesiology—we identify, articulate, differentiate, and integrate various tissues within the body, lending new meaning to these concepts though our own embodied experience of them. As we bring our awareness to specific layers of the body through touch, somatization, movement, and internal tracking, we get a feel for how each tissue and body system organizes, responds, and expresses itself. When we talk about a nerve or muscle, for example, we are not just talking about a substance but also about a state of consciousness and processes inherent within them. We relate our experience to these maps, but the map is not the experience.

The Foundations of Mindfulness

In Buddhism, mindfulness is key to being present. Without it we stay lost in the wanderings of our mind. Mindfulness keeps us connected to what is happening in the present and, when used skillfully, enables us to realize our deepest desire to be awake, happy, and peaceful. When we are mindful in the present, compassion becomes the natural response to suffering. As we open to suffering, there is a simple and spontaneous movement of the heart to help in whatever way we can. Cultivating compassion as a practice, we strengthen our intuitive response. Through mindful attention to the moment, we see the impermanent nature of phenomena and understand the happiness of non-grasping. Through non-grasping, we experience for ourselves the innate wakefulness of the wisdom mind. Mindfulness, compassion, and wisdom are the essential strands of the path of practice. Non-grasping is the essential unifying experience of freedom.[3]

Guided by a variety of methods and practices, we employ whatever is truly useful in helping someone become free of self-limiting patterns of mind and body that lead to unnecessary suffering. Suffering is an inherent reality in every being's life. Birth, illness, aging, and death are experiences no one can escape. The problem is not in the pain *per se*, but in our relationship to the pain. Most of us have a tendency to hang on to what is pleasurable and to deny, push away, or withdraw from whatever is painful, frightening, or threatening to the status quo in our lives. We struggle to distance ourselves from how things are and how we are in the moment, especially feelings of uncertainty and vulnerability. We seek security in mindless activities. This aversion or grasping is a kind of self-aggression that perpetuates suffering. A sense of ourselves as fundamentally flawed, fed by stories of basic unworthiness, perpetuates our attempts to escape. Each time we do so, we plant the seeds for this suffering to reenact itself.

When we are able to experience the pain or anxiety directly, without judgment placed on top of it, we have a chance to be free from suffering and our endless reactivity. We have a chance to establish a mind that is tranquil and alert, able to bear witness to experience without being consumed or identified by the experience. We are able to appreciate the constancy of change, trust the flow of energy, and become confident in our ability to experience life in the present, openly and directly, with ease. As we learn how to relax the struggle and make friends with the truth of our experiences, we can feel the openness, warmth, and tenderness that arise naturally.

Mindfulness means being aware, in the present moment, with acceptance. It holds within it the qualities of tranquility and alertness: being present, relaxed, at ease with, concentrated, non-aversive, and aware. The foundations of mindfulness refer to the placement of mind, or where we rest our attention. The four foundations, or places of awareness, are body, feelings, thoughts, and mind. Relaxing the body and softening the mind allows us to experience directly the sensations and movements of the body, the feelings of like and dislike, the impulse to move *toward* and *away* from experience, and the perceptions, thoughts, and beliefs we've constructed *about* experience. Most importantly, our mind is aware of itself being aware. It helps us sort out the other three states, threading them into a whole that supports our understanding of how things are and supports our being with what is. In Western societies, where one's sense of connection within oneself and to other human beings and the larger world is generally fragile and fragmented, human connection is vital to spirituality as a means of groundedness and expression. Such connection requires individuation, independence, and openness. Mindfulness is like a spiritual balm that soothes us, helping us guard against loss of self in relationship while softening the overly hard boundaries that construct oppositional posturing of self and other. Both of these elements—self-protection and satisfying connection—are crucial to cultivating strength, independence, and connection.[4]

Mindfulness in BMC

In BMC, we are especially attuned to mindfulness of body, while simultaneously appreciating the changing texture of emotions and shifts in habits of perception and thoughts. We make use of mindfulness in a relational context, through the process of exchange. As we establish a mutual resonance with our clients, we are able to experience within ourselves what is happening in them and are able to support them in connecting to their experience and releasing ineffective patterns.

Movement habits, gestures, and body tensions are commonly exhibited when one is emotionally charged. They signal the engagement of unconscious movement patterns of aversion and desire formed throughout our lives as we move away from perceived danger and harm and move toward perceived comfort and safety. Whenever movement is held back, energy/life flow is impeded and we become sick. When movement is rushed, energy/life flow is distorted and we become sick. Over time, these movement patterns can manifest as aches and pains, chronic health conditions and/or mental distress. These physical and psychological habits become comfortable and familiar, maintaining a sense of self-identify and an illusion of safety and stability. Each time we withdraw our awareness from our body and perform habitual behaviors under stress, we flee from experience in the present moment. We miss the opportunity to access these unconscious movements that hold the unexpressed and fragmented parts of ourselves.

As we cultivate awareness of body in the body, we bring our confused attention to rest in the experience of sensation, including the sense of movement and non-movement. Being fully present with a heartfelt mind allows us to make contact directly with the tissue through which the energy is flowing or held. As we make conscious contact, we support the tissue in being awake to its own nature and its ability to self-organize. Instead of trying to stop the pattern, we join the client in making contact with it, sometimes consciously, sometimes unconsciously, allowing the gesture or internal movement to develop in whatever way it wants to go, until it has completed its movement sequencing. We enable the tissue to move in ways that make sense to it or to be held in ways that reassure its sense of support. We are able to witness the body's incredible power to self-regulate, a process simultaneously expressed in our thoughts and emotions. We are able to awaken and engage our capacity to reprocess, complete, and release traumatic stress patterns, relearn how to feel excitement and pleasure, and engage in activities that nourish.

Coming to Our Senses

Jon Kabat-Zinn, in his book *Coming to Our Senses: Healing Ourselves and the World through Mindfulness,* enlarges our understanding of mindfulness as a political act. He invites us to consider the vital importance of body awareness at all levels of the body, from the microcosms within our body, to our private world of personal and relational body, to the communal body of citizens, governments, and corporations. He addresses in a fresh way principles inherent in BMC and Buddhism.

As humans, we always have a choice. We can either be passively carried along by forces and habits that remain stubbornly unexamined and which imprison us in distorting dreams and potential nightmares, or we can engage in our lives by waking up to them and participating fully in their unfolding, whether we like what is happening in any moment or not. It is only when we wake up that our lives become real and have even a chance of becoming liberated from our individual and collective delusions, diseases, and suffering.[5]

The inner world of our personal aspirations and the outer world of our relationships with others are comprised of the same dream. We all share a common desire to live in peace; follow our creative impulses and private yearnings; to fit in, be valued, belong, and contribute in some meaningful way to the larger good; "flourish as individuals and as families, and as societies of purpose and mutual regard, to live in individual dynamic balance, which is health, and in collective dynamic balance, which used to be called the commonweal, which honors our differences and optimizes our mutual creativity and the possibility of a future free from wanton harm and from that which threatens what is most vital to our well-being and our very being."[6]

The work of healing our planet must always begin with a personal commitment to developing a foundation of mindfulness, through which we are willing to be present to a suffering world and able to find the courage to act purposely and creatively, with clarity and compassion, in all situations, personal and communal.

Boundaries, Defense, and War:
What Can We Learn
from Embodiment Practices?

~ **Linda Hartley**, England (2006)

Just days after finishing this article, I was travelling to London, where I work every Thursday. It was the morning of July 7. As the journey began, fragments of message were filtering through—a fire at the station my train was headed for, an accident, a power surge, then finally, several bomb attacks on the London underground network. Halfway along the route we had to leave the train, as all transport in and out of London was being closed down. Two weeks later, I was again caught up in the transport chaos, evacuated from one of the London underground stations following the second series of attacks. As we had been expecting, the war had come to London.

It was shocking for people here in the UK to learn that the first group of suicide bombers were born and brought up in this country. Is this something like a political autoimmune disorder—the cells attacking their own kind?

A lot of soul-searching has been going on since these attacks as to why young British Muslim men would do this, and what can be done to address the problems and the politics of these disaffected young men. An autoimmune attack is the result of an overzealous immune system, stimulated by sympathetic arousal; the B-cells may not be adequately modulated by suppressor T-cells, and the attack turns upon self-structures, the body's own cells, wrongly identifying them as foreign enemies. As I follow the concerned debate about what these young

Muslims need in order to integrate into British society, I also wonder if we can learn from this what our struggling immunity is in need of. Essentially, they are saying they want a different kind of world, one based on (their own) spiritual values. I can sympathize with the essence of this desire, though not, of course, with their methods or dogmatism. The health of the body also thrives in the presence of what we call spiritual energies—love, kindness, respect, harmony, peace, and joy.

The Interface

As a practitioner and teacher of Body-Mind Centering and a psychotherapist, I have long been interested in the subject of boundaries. In psychology, the skin is often referred to as the primary boundary, that which differentiates self from other at the most fundamental of levels, the edges of the physical organism that I call "me." From the Body-Mind Centering perspective, the cellular membrane can also be included as a primary boundary, being the first membrane of containment and definition as we source back to the earliest origins of embryonic selfhood. Other, secondary boundaries evolve as the membranes of distinct tissues and organ systems develop.

Physiologically, these boundaries are semi-permeable and responsive membranes, places of meeting, communication, and transformation. Psychologically, we are talking about boundary not as something solid and impenetrable but boundary as *awareness*—awareness of what is self, what is other, and the quality of relationship between them. I prefer the term *interface* for this subtly shifting experience of containment, differentiation, and contact. At the interface, two worlds meet and interact. Consciousness arises as awareness is brought to the interface.

I am always amazed at the precision of information that is often revealed when a person focuses her or his awareness within the layers of skin and cellular membranes. Embodying these membranes can reveal the condition of psychological boundaries in intimate detail; through bringing awareness here, subtle but important psychological changes sometimes occur as cells and tissues respond to the attention and intention focused toward them.

Protection

I have also had a long-time interest in the lymphatic system, initially because of my own health problems in this area. As the essential system of the immune response, it is the lymphatic system's task to protect the body in order to maintain the integrity of the organism. Embodying lymph can also engender an experience of being psychologically boundaried, contained, of filling one's personal space in a way that protects from outside "attacks."

It is a deep concern that at this point in time, humanity is collectively suffering a weakened immune system. Many drugs and surgical methods have been developed that protect us from diseases that would once have killed many of us in our early years, and in this we are very fortunate. But some believe that our natural immunity can be weakened by overuse of the "knives, guns, and chemical warfare" of modern medicine. Seeking the unnatural but powerful and effective methods of attack, we may lose some of our innate ability to protect ourselves. This might be a contributing factor in the proliferation of diseases specifically related to immune system dysfunction or failure, such as untreatable cancers, AIDS, multiple sclerosis, chronic fatigue syndrome, allergies, and autoimmune disorders.

Particular stresses of modern life can also weaken the immune system. Mental, emotional, nutritional, environmental, and trauma-related stress all put the body into the resistance phase of the stress cycle, which entails a heightened activation of the sympathetic nervous system at the expense of the recuperative processes of the parasympathetic. As Alfred Hässig's research has shown, excessive and prolonged sympathetic stimulation increases production of the immune system's B-cells, those that "attack the enemy without" through the production of antibodies (antibody-mediated immunity). At the same time, the presence of T-cells is reduced; they are responsible for the "housekeeping," the management of the internal environment, clearing up and removing damaged and infected "self-structures" (cellular immunity).[1] Helper and suppressor T-cells also regulate both B-cell and T-cell activity.

At the psychological level, sympathetic stimulation reflects and enhances a frame of mind in which the problem is seen as coming from outside us. The solution is to attack and get rid of it. Parasympathetic stimulation, which encourages the activity of the T-cells, is that process of attending to the internal ecology of the body-mind—the processing and digestion of difficult experiences and emotions, taking responsibility for our own shadow rather than projecting it out and attacking it in the form of the "other."

The Collective Body and Planetary Body

When I look at what happens in the cell, then see its structures and life processes reflected in the organism as a whole, my attention widens to the macrocosm of the planetary body and I see how this, too, reflects the internal processes, the deep ecology, of cell and organism. And as I reflect on the psychology of embodied skin, cellular membranes, and lymphatic system, and all the problems that we as individuals experience in protecting and maintaining healthy psychological boundaries, I wonder about the collective body and what we can learn from our individual experiences that might have relevance to the overwhelming problems of our world today.[2]

I think of Earth's ozone layer as a kind of energetic outer membrane that is comparable to the energetic sense of boundary around us, the membrane of the aura that we each develop. Our energetic skin can be damaged, weakened, rigidified, and at times lost altogether as a result of physical and psychological imbalance, excess, trauma, and toxicity, reflecting the condition of our primary skin and cellular boundaries. In the macrocosm of the planetary body the ozone layer is also being damaged—we are not quite sure of this—by the excess and toxicity being created here, on Earth, by us humans. As a result, the ecology of the planet is beginning to suffer, the integrity of its structure starting to change. The planetary body may, like the collective human body, be on the verge of a breakdown of its immune system; its own processes for maintaining its integrity in the form that we know it are threatened by our excesses and pollution.

Psychologically, we can see how the process of "attacking the enemy without," instead of owning our own shadow and attending to the internal ecology of our own psyches, is magnified in our relationships and our social groups and between nations on the political world stage. And as in medicine, so too in warfare: as more and more powerful weapons of mass destruction—unnatural methods of defense—are developed to defeat the enemy without, our innate capacity to protect ourselves and resolve conflicts through humanistic approaches seems to be diminished. Individually and collectively, our capacity to maintain healthy psychological boundaries and attend creatively to the internal ecology of our mind is undermined by the dehumanizing of conflict-resolution processes.

Boundaries, Structure, Defense, and War

These interests came together in the spring of 2002, when I made plans to teach a course in London called "Boundaries, Structure, and Defense." It was to run from September 2002 to May 2003. I had no idea that this would be exactly the time period during which the debate about going to war in Iraq, and then the war itself, would be taking place. We have since heard from various sources that U.S. leaders had been intending to attack Iraq for some time, and that the tragedy of September 11 was the "excuse" they were looking for to implement their plan. The debate was already in the air before it was in the public domain.

The course I taught ran for six weekends (roughly once a month excluding holidays) from September through May. On the Saturdays, we studied the body systems that most specifically embodied the themes of boundaries, structure, and defense, using the Body-Mind Centering approach, and we explored the psychological themes and personal meanings expressed through the body systems: how the skin, cellular membranes, fat, muscles, lymph, and nervous system may be used to give us different senses of boundary, containment, and defense; and how bones and connective tissues provide inner structure and form, the solid-fluid architecture of the body.

The Sundays were devoted to the practice of Authentic Movement; this was a time to deepen and integrate the work of the day before, as well as an opportunity to learn the art of clear and compassionate witnessing as taught within this discipline.

Because of the events that were unfolding during this time, I could not help but reflect on how the themes we were addressing at a personal level might also relate to the drama of the debate about war in Iraq. I would like to offer some of my personal reflections. I have no answers, and this is just one perspective, but I hope it might stimulate you in your own thinking, feeling, and embodiment.

WEEKEND 1

Primary Boundaries: Skin and Cellular Membranes

The focus this first weekend was on embodying the different layers of the skin and the cellular membranes through touch and movement and on becoming conscious of where our awareness is when making contact with another. We discussed the nature of primary boundaries and explored personal experiences of this. When the surface membrane is not intact—when it is too rigid, too permeable, unclear or absent to awareness—then an essential layer of protection and a place of healthy interaction with the world are compromised. We must seek deeper within our tissue layers for a sense of boundary and interface.

At a personal level, the woundings of invasive or neglectful care or trauma and an emotionally unsupportive environment *in utero*, infancy, and childhood can damage the experience of primary boundary. As a result, the sense of containment, differentiation, and integrity and the ability to make healthy contact are damaged. Multiplied within cultures, these effects create groups and nations who lack a sense of basic integrity and security, who will need to develop other means of defense to protect their boundaries. Primary woundings are readily reactivated with subsequent trauma or invasion. The tragedy of 9/11 seemed to constellate such a retraumatization for the people of the U.S., in particular, and for the world at large, and a defensive response was perhaps inevitable.

Around the time we met for this first seminar, September 2002, discussions about going to war in Iraq were hitting the news.

WEEKEND 2

Protective Layers: Fat and Muscle

As our explorations took us deeper into the body tissues, we came to experience different qualities of boundary and interface as we embodied subcutaneous fat and skeletal muscles. For some for whom the fat is present, it might be experienced as a soft, nurturing cushion; it might evoke a sense of sinking into a warm, maternal, holding environment. Warmth, energy, and an insulating padding that protects and creates a fluid sense of boundary might be experienced here, when the fat is embraced and embodied.

When skin and fat are not embodied and embraced within our awareness, we may descend directly into the muscle layers, where a different quality of boundary is created. We all use our muscles to some degree, and in different areas of the body, to create defensive boundaries. Wilhelm Reich and his followers based their therapy on the way we somatize character in defensive patterns of muscular armoring.[3] We need this to some degree, but when it is excessive, muscular tension (hypertone) creates a too-rigid interface, which interferes with healthy interaction and contact. Too little muscular tension (hypotone) will leave us feeling unboundaried, and we will have to seek even deeper for protection or we will be left feeling too vulnerable and undefended.

When a person is in a tense, contracted state, the nervous stimulation to the muscles is set too high; then the body's reflexes are easily triggered by a small addition of stress. The expression of this is what is commonly called a "knee-jerk reaction." The events of 9/11 split the whole world in a way that no event in our current times has done; after the initial shock, it opened the hearts of many, who focused love and compassion toward the grieving community. For others, it stimulated a knee-jerk reaction—a sort of "he hit me so I'll hit him back" response. An organism—an individual or a group—already on a state of high alert is usually not able to take the space needed to reflect and reach for other courses of action, but will instead be compelled to react in this way.

WEEKEND 3

Lymphatic System and the Immune Response

It was December 2002 and we came together to study the lymphatic system and immune response. Embodying the lymphatic system through touch and movement, boundaries could be experienced with greater clarity and spaciousness, free from conflict. This practice reminds me of the master of martial arts who does not get into fights because he or she is so clearly embodying healthy boundaries, so integrated and self-contained, that conflict is not invited.

We explored how stress affects the immune system. As mentioned earlier, the body switches to the sympathetic fight-or-flight mode when under stress; this supports B-cell antibody-immunity—the attack on the enemy without. The internal processes of digestion, repair, and recuperation are supported by a parasympathetic state, which also supports T-cell activity. When in the sympathetic mode of attack, T-cell activity is diminished; it is the T-cells that initiate, maintain, and control an *appropriate* immune response. They maintain the internal ecology through rooting out damaged and infected "self-structures" (cells), attending to the balance of internal ecology. The balance, or lack of it, within the autonomic and immune systems can be felt to relate to psychological patterns of protection and defense, physiological and psychological patternings each influencing the other.

During this time, talks were intensifying. Blair was trying to persuade Bush to follow the United Nations procedures; the weapons inspection process needed more time. Bush and his colleagues had their own agenda and did not want to take more time.

I began to wonder about the United Nations' role as the immune system of our collective body. The immunological surveillance cells that patrol the body's tissues, seeking out harmful pathogens and initiating the process of their containment and destruction, clearly reflect the attempts of the weapons inspectors to seek out weapons of mass destruction. The UN tried to work through strategies of negotiation, diplomacy, restrictions, and sanctions—in short, to contain and render harmless the "pathogen" of Saddam Hussein's regime. In the end, they failed. The guns and bombs were brought in before the surveillance team could complete its work, and so it was rendered ineffective and redundant (just as the immune system might be after chemotherapy or radiation treatment, for example). The credibility of the UN itself may have been damaged through this process.

And what about those miracles of the immune system, the memory B- and T-cells? It seems to me they were not given enough of a chance in this situation. I longed to have the elders, those who had negotiated through intractable conflicts in the past, brought in. Could someone like Nelson Mandela have provided a wise and impartial voice, borne out of his own experience, to oversee the discussions? Or the Dalai Lama, maybe? Or could the learnings from peace talks in Northern Ireland, largely successful, have more fully informed the process? These voices were not invited in, not even considered, I imagine. The memory B- and T-cells, those elders who carry knowledge of the battles that went before, were incapacitated by the reflexive stance that had already been taken.

What did not happen at all in the discussions among the Western leaders was a moment of reflection on what our part in the conflict may be. All evil was projected out onto the enemy—first to Osama Bin Laden, then Saddam Hussein. God was assumed to be on our side, and no one dared to look at whether, within all of the atrocities committed, there was a message that needed to be heard. There was no inner reflection, digestion, and integration of the shadow—only the imperative to destroy it by destroying the enemy who carries the projected evil. As we know, this is not unfamiliar within our Judeo-Christian history; it is as if a part of the collective regressed to a more primitive stage of consciousness that had dominated our culture some centuries ago. The mentality of the Inquisition had returned.

This can be seen as an expression of an immune system out of balance through prolonged activation of the sympathetic nervous system, no longer able to attend to the "housekeeping" functions of maintaining the internal milieu in healthy balance and so resorting to primitive fight-or-flight, reflexive behavior. It reflects a psychology of splitting and projection.

WEEKEND 4

Bones as Inner Ground and Structure

It was early February 2003 and a relief to settle into the grounding presence of the bones with the inevitability of war looming, and anger and distress escalating around the world as political splits deepened. Bones as a core of support, strength, and containment—it is good to remember this in times of stress and trauma.

We fear this war will fracture the structure of our world as we know it.

WEEKEND 5

Nervous System: Sensory-Motor Processing

We met again on March 15 and 16, 2003, just days before the war began. We met to study how the nervous system mediates cycles of receptivity, activity, and recuperation; inner and outer; and the balancing of the autonomic nervous system. We explored sensing (taking in) and expressing (moving out) and disruptions to the sensory-motor loop that often occur in our formative years. We looked at shock and nervous system reversals and some primitive reflexes that support the basic instincts to bond and defend.

When our outer membranes do not adequately contain and protect us, we may seek to defend through the nervous system, through a hypervigilance that is born out of fear and the expectation that we will be attacked or invaded, or that there will not be enough, so we must fight for every mouthful. Muscle tone is on high alert and we are ready to be fired off at the slightest provocation. Startle and defense reflexes dominate; the ability to bond is weakened and we may come to feel isolated and at war with the world. As if caught in an incomplete Moro reflex, we have startled and opened but are unable to close, embrace, and find protection and comfort. We can do nothing but attack in order to defend from this vulnerable position.

Just days before the war was to begin, the sky was clear blue and a brilliant sun shone down upon us. There was a full moon at night, piercingly bright. So much light! And so much darkness amassing over Iraq and in our hearts. On Sunday we gathered to practice Authentic Movement together. After Saturday's work, people were full. They named their rage, their fear, their despair, the grief they already felt for the deaths to come, as we gathered once more in the circle. They began to move. Again and again, I saw someone entering the circle full of rage, or fear, or despair. Again and again, I saw them move their pain and fear, and I saw rage transformed into burning passion, I saw grief transformed into overwhelming love, I saw despair transformed into power, and fear into joy and delight. I felt so deeply privileged in all that I witnessed that day, as we came together at the end in joy and awe and deep respect for a process we may never fully understand. I felt so grateful for this opportunity to go with so much light and consciousness into this dark passage. We may never fully know the meaning of what happened at that time, but I felt the darkness so strongly balanced by light that I was given hope.

20 03 2003 (this is how we write the date in the UK)—the day war began. What is the significance of this number? It seems so balanced and complete within itself that I wonder what might be its mystical significance. Reflecting on this and on the intense coincidence of so much light and so much darkness that weekend, I wonder about paradox and a greater source that can contain duality, the opposites so often in conflict. I am reminded of holding a circle of women during one of the SBMC[4] summers where there was great discord and we could not find a meeting place. Then one member of the group asked everyone to name their birth sign. It turned out that we were sitting in a perfect mandala of zodiac signs, balanced in an extraordinary way around the circle. We dissolved into uncontrollable laughter as the mysterious form revealed itself, and the conflict dispersed. When we met the following week, we sat down in the circle and immediately dissolved into laughter again. No more conflict!

Perhaps, in a few hundred years or so, history will look back on this time and locate these events within a greater order, recognize a pattern it was part of, and forgiveness may flow. But for now, the conflict prevails.

WEEKEND 6

Connective Tissue and Integration

We came to our final theme with a body system that could help us move toward integration. Connective tissue, in its many gel and fluid states, connects every part, each cell and membrane and tissue of the body, into a unified whole. Wrapping and flowing around each part, it both differentiates—clarifying boundaries and defining the uniqueness of each—as well as integrates them into one whole. This system embodies the inseparability of the one and the many. As we were nearing the end of the series of workshops, a feeling of warmth was evident within the group, but also a sense of people readying themselves to separate, to part. Embodying the connective tissue helped each one to reconnect to a sense of containment and inner integrity in preparation for leaving.

With so much violence and fracture in the world, we deeply needed this. It was May and we were also nearing the end of the shocking war, at least the "official" part of the war. As I sat on the train on my way to London for our last meeting, I reflected on what it was that could hold me through these terrible events. Immediately my heart came into awareness. I saw-felt its redness, moistness, the strong and vibrant movement of muscle. I felt its deep pulse within me. This is my key, my resource, my savior, that which I must remember and nurture and trust. Then my bones became present—their firm, reliable, ever-present ground, the earth within, my earth-body. Gratitude. On this I can depend.

Concluding Words

The story continues and there is still death and fear and grieving. I feel this war was morally, ethically, legally, politically, and economically wrong; I believe there were other ways to pursue the problems. Yet my own experience of these events also suggests to me a greater and mysterious source that somehow holds it all, both the light and the dark. There is terrible suffering and horrendous cruelty, and yet there is also love and light—they arise simultaneously; they coexist. The best and the worst in humanity have been evoked through terrible events and seem to hang in precarious balance.

Suffering can be transformed—we know this through the work we do. And the shadow can be integrated, but only when there is the will to do so. Scapegoating and projection is easier, more familiar; facing our inner demons, embodying those shadowy, unembodied parts of ourselves that may hold intolerable feelings is a challenge not everyone wants to take. Faced with such magnitude of suffering and conflict in the world, it is sometimes hard to believe that seeking to take responsibility for our own little piece of it—embodying and integrating our own shadow, transforming our personal sorrows into compassion and joy—will help. Yet this is what we must keep on trying to do—it is sometimes all we can do in the face of forces so much greater than ourselves.

Postscript

It is hard to bring this discussion to a close, as these issues are clearly deep, complex, and widespread. The war is now on my own doorstep too, so I am compelled to reflect on the issues. Yet I must acknowledge that there cannot be real closure on these questions right now, as we are still very much in the midst of the unfolding of events that will no doubt shape the future of our world.

The Role of the Arts and Embodiment in Post-Trauma Community Building

~ **Martha Hart Eddy,** USA (2010)

The material in this essay was rewritten from a keynote speech given at the statewide convention of art educators at The Ohio State University in Columbus on September 15, 2001. With permission of the author, coeditors Gill Wright Miller and Pat Ethridge excerpted and reconfigured this talk for inclusion in this anthology.

The Reality of Metaphor

The work of Body-Mind Centering offers the artist/community worker a sophisticated entry into embodiment through its comprehensive understanding of the body in the context of human development.[1] BMC teaches us to note specific areas of trauma and give them voice, allowing a "motoring out" with consciousness of these negative experiences. Physical expression helps the human emotional system become responsive after trauma by balancing the nervous system's sensory-motor loop. Ordinarily, there is a split second where a healthy nervous system first "senses" a stimulus and then reacts to it ("motors out") in apt proportion. When this is not the case, a healthier response can be facilitated by bonding with other caring people and feeling part of a community. Healthy relationships help rebalance the nervous system. Training in bodily awareness—for example, somatic education—can facilitate this healthier response to trauma, conflict, and upset.

George P. Lakoff, linguistic theorist, viewed the attack on the World Trade Center in New York City as a "decapitation" because buildings are symbols of people. He contends that because of the "mirror neurons" that cause images to feel real, anyone exposed to the image of the Twin Towers falling[2] needed to heal, specifically in the neck and head region. We each felt a shock. Lakoff maintains it was the brain, high up in our bodies, that suffered most. Of course, the pain resonated everywhere.

Lakoff describes the connections from these "mirror neurons" to the emotional centers of our brain:

> Such neural circuits are believed to be the basis of empathy. This works literally—when we see a plane coming toward the building and imagine people in the building, we feel the plane coming toward us; when we see the building toppling toward others, we feel the building toppling toward us. It also works metaphorically. If we see the plane going through the building, and unconsciously we metaphorize the building as a head with the plane going through its temple, then we sense unconsciously but powerfully, being shot through the temple. Our systems of metaphorical thought, interacting with our mirror neurons systems, turn external literal horrors into felt metaphorical horrors. [...] To incorporate the new knowledge requires a physical change in the synapses of our brains, a physical reshaping of our neural system.[3]

When Lakoff claims the mind is "embodied," he is arguing that almost all of human cognition, up through the most abstract reasoning, depends on, and makes use of, such concrete and "low-level" faculties as the sensori-motor system and the emotions. "We are neural beings," he states. "Our brains take their input from the rest of our bodies. What our bodies are like and how they function in the world thus structures the very concepts we can use to think. We cannot think just anything—only what our embodied brains permit."[4] When a negative stimulus is strong or repetitive, we commonly respond by "freezing" with no expression at all or by numbing out. Another typical reaction is a sudden unconscious motoric response; this often backfires and damages our bodies or our psyches in another way.

The events on September 11 *were* "shocking." Of paramount importance for recovery from that shock was bonding with others in community and connecting with one's own resiliency through somatic processes. Practice with embodiment proved restorative. From the shock of an attack on our "peaceful" land, new communities were made—spontaneously and in overlapping and concentric circles, where people gathered both locally and worldwide to find out how to heal. Embodiment is an important skill for healing.

How Communities Educate:
The Democratic Paradigm

According to educator/social thinker John Dewey, a democratic community involves engagement in activity and engagement with others. There is no single, perfect community or even one way of being a community. Indeed, Dewey named all communities *communities-in-the-making.* We need skills that help us capitalize on the "making" process. Art educators are often comfortable with a "process." We can help to support communities-in-the-making through all of their stages—from the messy to the productive. By adding in somatic education, like BMC, we have tools for finding and including the "felt sense." As somatic educators, the subject and object of our shaping and our practice is the body-mind connection. We teach others to practice shifting governance from the brain to each and every part of the body—in other words, the body-as-a-whole. We make responsible decisions by listening to somatic cues from our entire body. BMC and other somatic practices can help deepen one's intentionality when making decisions—whether in everyday routines or in times of trauma. Somatic approaches to art-making can also serve to weave a web of resilience connections for a supportive community.

In times of conflict and violence, arts-based communities can address many types of human problems through metaphoric thinking. The arts, in general, can be used for "sneaky healing" in that they use symbolism and abstraction to approach difficult issues. Arts-based communities have opposing roles: both to perpetuate the conventions of the culture as it exists in the moment and to break down conventions of the culture in order to create new models. Art can be perceived as a method of change, of breaking through. Dewey saw art "as a way to shatter the crust of conventionalism and the routine consciousness."[5] Given that exposure to violence at varying levels (teasing, bullying, gangs, and media violence) pervades most schools, it is useful to know that art education activities can be used to directly confront bullying, avoid sexual harassment, practice conflict resolution, gain cross-cultural appreciation, and embody peace with self-presence.[6] We can use art-making as a form of balancing the nervous system and preparing for healthy decision-making. It is important to note that an authoritarian approach to art education and the competitive challenges of the art world are counter-productive. On the other hand, somatic approaches to art-making invest authority in the artist, whether child or adult. As artists, we decide what is right by tuning in to our own "felt experience," body awareness, and somatic attunement. As educators, we can consider what type of community we are making and invest in determining group values consistent with our educational philosophy.

A Peaceable Classroom

We are capable of using any conflict, mistake, or accident as a step toward healing and regenerating our communities and ourselves. From my work in New York City schools, it is extremely satisfying to convey the message that conflict itself is inevitable and that from conflict we can learn and fashion new solutions. Mistakes are also great sources of creativity, especially if we can stay relaxed enough when they happen and avoid conflict or trauma about failure. Those of us in long-term relationships can attest to the fact that the overcoming of conflict deepens intimacy. We are often hesitant as we approach the making of new friends, as we commonly prefer to spend time with people with whom methods for conflict are already established. Ultimately, we seek situations where our feelings are accepted and we feel our transgressions will be forgiven.

Somatic experiences with a wide range of movement styles can cross personal and cultural barriers to help us appreciate the other. Experiencing a somatization on the membranes of cells, for example, develops an awareness of permeable borders and healthy boundaries. These are rich metaphors for healing, conflict resolution, and being in community. Creating community has the potential to generate cliques, gangs, and hegemonic tiers of leaders. We should be alert to the formation of groups with rules defining who is an insider and outsider. Conflicts often develop from standing one's ground, by maintaining one's boundaries in a fixed way. Conflict resolution comes from yielding into shared space or redefining boundaries. As we experience the literal ability to move through membranes or to make changes in our membranes, we have embodied new ways of thinking and/or behaving.

From my own research, I have found that building a "peaceable community" is fostered by releasing trauma, reducing stress, and recognizing diverse metaphors for conflict transformation. It is important to practice embodied conflict resolution, confronting bullying of all types (personal, corporate, governmental, etc.), and to eliminate harassment based on gender, racial, ethnic, and class discrimination. We can cultivate cross-cultural appreciation and become peace activists.

The most effective peaceable classroom resides inside a peaceable school where the adults have found respectful ways to get their needs met, mature ways to deal with power struggles, and creative ways to appreciate one another. Adults model respect to one another and to each child—including those youth who do not act respectfully toward them. Excellent educational leaders recognize that children may come to school in pain, hungry, angry, neglected, bothered by someone, irritated, in a growth spurt and/or confused. As adults, we have more perspective on these issues than the students do; therefore, we need to model how to handle internal and/or external stressors gracefully. Adults who have experienced somatic education have the advantage of possessing more stress reduction skills, a wider palette of metaphors for change, and thus more conflict resolution methods.

The arts are formative in building empathy and can help us recuperate and connect to our inner selves. Art communicates our feelings and ideas, and so can help us build a connection to others. Aesthetic and symbolic depictions may convey innate understandings of "what is right" and certainly of what is possible. Appreciation of others' art can foster the ability to perceive, tolerate, and appreciate differences. This type of appreciation takes time to learn and is a developmental process, an unfolding. A large factor is letting going of "being right" by softening one's borders while still maintaining self-protective boundaries. Art educators who choose to infuse their teaching with socio-emotional intelligence can explore the realm of what is right for humanity instead of focusing on what is "right" in art. This process shifts classroom work toward deep cooperation. When students are asked to tune in to their "felt sense," using tools from somatic education, they also learn that finding one's personal best is more satisfying than squashing another person's sense of well-being. Having the somatic skills to physically feel what the "right decision" is on a body level can serve one well in moments of crisis.

Through the outward expression of collaborative effort, each individual is more able to grapple with conflict *and* cooperation. Using metaphors from the body, we learn that a community can be considered as a cell, defined in large part by its membrane. That membrane can become rigid or amorphous, or it can be well-defined, permeable, and resilient. The healthy membrane strives to keep what is needed for vitality in and to let toxins out. It also allows entry to the nourishing and defends against the toxic, keeping it out. Determining what to allow in or out is challenging.

As teachers we need to help our communities determine what is right, what is healthy, what is unfamiliar but indeed safe, what is too challenging, and even what is toxic. We can build these skills through discussion, but having the physical practice of each is what prepares us to handle ourselves in the split second after experiencing a traumatic stimulus. Embodied lessons that incorporate body awareness, movement practices, and cooperative art-making teach these "thinking-on-our-feet skills." When these contemplative somatic practices find their way into the daily rituals of our classrooms and lives, we are more resilient and more prepared to act wisely. As we find ways to experience our embodied selves *and minds* (to paraphrase Lakoff), we will be able to empathize and heal more often, creatively, and in connection with others.

Conclusion

How we go forward each day is in our hands. The processes of making anew, making art, and creating new symbols reshape our brain, our perceptions, and our experience. This helps our healing as individuals and as a world. As we grieve, we can also shine in our spontaneous eruptions of compassion. Each of the arts can be fully present in expressing our grief, our rage, and our call to action. The creation of sites for drama and dance filled with art/ifacts and music has been poignant in New York City since 9/11. I have seen the burgeoning of *peace* through dance programs ever since.[7]

A Fable

There was once a wise old man who could answer any question, no matter how difficult. One day, two people decided they were going to fool the old man. They planned to catch a bird and take it to the old man saying, "Is what we have in our hands alive or dead?" If he says "dead," we'll turn it loose, and it will fly away; if he says "alive," we'll crush it.

They caught a bird and went with it to the old man. They said, "Is what we have in our hands alive or dead?"

The wise old man considered them and smiled.

Then he said, "It's in your hands."

(Anonymous, taken from *A Call to Character*, Greer & Kohl)

Epilogue
Biographies, Historical Records, and Notes

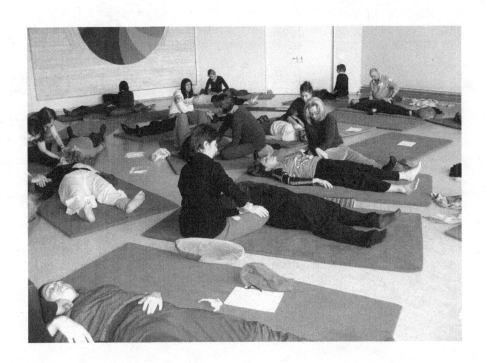

Bonnie Bainbridge Cohen: A Biography

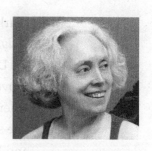

BONNIE BAINBRIDGE COHEN was born on New Year's Eve in 1941 in Miami, Florida. She comes from a family that lived in the world of the circus; her parents worked for Ringling Brothers and Barnum & Bailey Circus. Her childhood was full of travel, exotic animals, and people with unusual abilities and unconventional approaches to life. "I grew up believing the extraordinary was normal," she says. "The magic of the circus made nothing seem impossible, because in the circus everything is possible." Her mother was a dancer and they were "always dancing"; Bainbridge Cohen began dance classes at age three and "never really stopped." But she did not speak until she was three and until then, she felt the world coming to her in "vibration and current and awe," from which experience she grew her well-developed kinesthetic sense.

While still in high school, she began her research in anatomy by dissecting a cat in an advanced science research course and her work in movement therapy by exploring dance and music with children with cerebral palsy. She studied Occupational Therapy at The Ohio State University with Barbara Lockhart and Margaret Mathiott and learned the importance of seeing the whole person. Later, she trained with Betty Yerxa at Rancho Los Amigos Hospital in California in advanced approaches to rehabilitation, where she learned very detailed work with muscles as applied to children with severe polio and adults with spinal cord dysfunction. She studied Dance Therapy with Marion Chace, who taught her the process of teaching in the present, based upon the responses of the people with whom she was working. She learned neuromuscular reeducation with Andre Bernard and Barbara

Clark, who studied with Mabel Ellsworth Todd, author of *The Thinking Body*, a seminal work in body awareness. She learned Labanotation at the Dance Notation Bureau in New York and became a certified Laban Movement Analyst through the Laban Institute of Movement Studies, where she studied off and on for many years with Irmgard Bartenieff. She studied Action Profiling with Warren Lamb and Ellen Goldman and became a certified Kestenberg Movement Profiler with Judith Kestenberg.

In New York City she studied dance with Erick Hawkins, a leading choreographer and dancer of the twentieth century, who was a primary influence and "showed me effortless movement and the art of doing without doing." She taught dance at The Erick Hawkins School of Dance and at Hunter College. She studied voice with Sylus Engum and Herbert Doussaint, who had both studied with Douglas Stanley, the author of *Your Voice: Applied Science of Vocal Art.* She studied yoga with Yogi Ramira, who taught her "the techniques and power of yoga in the healing of organic imbalances and the effect it has on the mind."

Then, in 1968–69, she studied dance with Pauline de Groot and Jim Tyler and explored hands-on facilitation of movement at the University of Amsterdam Psychiatric Research Center in Holland. While she had always been doing hands-on work, it was during that year that Bainbridge Cohen realized the incredible power of touch. Because she didn't speak Dutch, she found that she had to transmit information primarily through touch without the aid of verbal language.

Bainbridge Cohen was certified as a Neurodevelopmental Therapist by Dr. Karl and Berta Bobath in England, leaders in the treatment of children and adults with brain dysfunction. From them, she learned the essential elements of the developmental process and how to repattern the nervous system based on that process. Mrs. Bobath told her, "If a person doesn't change directly under your hands, then you should do something else."

In January 1970, she and Leonard Cohen were married by Eido Roshi, who influenced them in Zen meditation. They then went to

Japan to pursue Len's serious interest in the martial art of Aikido. There, Bonnie helped to establish a school for occupational and physical therapy in Tokyo. She studied Katsugen Undo, a Japanese method of engaging in automatic movement developed by Haruchika Noguchi, the founder of Setai. These disciplines taught her the importance of looking within to discover the nature of her experience. She was also exposed to Asian medicine. Their son, Joshu, was born there in 1972.

Both before and after their time in Japan, she studied tai chi ch'uan with Professor Cheng Man-ch'ing, the "Master of Five Excellences" (in Chinese calligraphy, painting, poetry, medicine, and tai chi ch'uan). Bonnie and Len traveled back to New York City in 1973, where she founded The School for Body-Mind Centering. Their daughter, Basha, was born in New York in 1975. Then in 1976, the family moved to Amherst, Massachusetts, where their third child, Issa, was born in 1977. With The School for Body-Mind Centering established in Amherst, it continued to develop and grow for thirty-two years. Among her other teachers have been Drs. John Upledger and Richard McDonald in Craniosacral Therapy and Dr. Fritz Smith, who developed Zero Balancing.

In June 2009, they moved themselves and the School to El Sobrante, California. Currently, the School continues to evolve, and Bonnie teaches in Berkeley, where she and Len live with their three children, daughter-in-law Minami, and granddaughter Hana.

She has taught throughout the U.S., Canada, Europe, and Asia at colleges and universities, retreat centers such as Esalen, Kripalu, and Omega, and numerous conferences and festivals in dance, yoga, dramatic arts, body psychotherapy, children, music, and meditation. She maintains a private practice working with infants and toddlers with developmental challenges. She is the author of the book *Sensing, Feeling, and Action*, the DVDs *The Nervous System and Yoga* (2009) and *Four Special Children* (2005), and five VHS *Advanced Developmental Videos* (1992): three on *BNP and the Brain* and two on *BNP and the Organs*. Another DVD entitled *Dance and Body-Mind Centering* was produced in 2006 in Brussels,

Belgium, from her 2004 workshop, "Weight, Space, and Time." *The Origins of Movement: The Embodiment of Early Embryological Development* was produced in Cologne, Germany.

The School for Body-Mind Centering

In 1973, after Bonnie Bainbridge Cohen returned from Japan, she founded The School for Body-Mind Centering. Initially, she was working in her apartment on Waverly Place in New York City with a handful of students who explored with her an approach to movement from inner awareness of their own anatomy and developmental process. The six-person class limit was dictated by the size of her living room. They explored the relationships between the reflexes, righting reactions, and equilibrium responses and spinal, homologous, homolateral, and con-tralateral movements, which later became the basis of the Basic Neu-rological Patterns (BNPs.) These BNPs are unique to Body-Mind Centering and encapsulate the complete sequence of human movement development, from *in utero* to walking, showing the phylogenetic and ontogenetic influences and including the support of the various body systems. The curriculum also included the skeletal and muscular sys-tems, and breathing and vocalization. By the fall of 1976, the organ and endocrine systems were introduced.

Dancers Gale Turner and Beth Goren were among the early stu-dents.[1] They remember working one-on-one with Bainbridge Cohen and being "thrown around the living room" to elicit reflexive move-ment. Right away, they were required to explore the material through touch and repatterning by working with a partner for ten weeks; then they had to choose another partner for the next class series. They were also required to assist in classes and to teach what they had learned to newcomers. Turner and Goren recall that from the beginning, the emphasis was on maintaining the awareness of meeting and touching the whole person and not just the person's "problem." As interest increased, the classes were moved to student Kay Wylie's loft on 14th Street, which allowed for larger classes.[2]

Bainbridge Cohen was also teaching dance classes and offering workshops in particular subjects. One topic, for example, was the skull, which was explored once a week for a year. She focused on presenting somatizations in kinesthetic form, not just visualizations, so that people would keep their awareness in the body, and she learned to introduce material to people in a progression so that their learning would be supported by preparatory experience. She gradually developed a body-based language for movement awareness and expression. She taught people to look at the movement first and to see the potential in each person, rather than becoming fixated on difficulty, and to maintain a sense of the interrelatedness of all aspects of the person—physical, emotional, mental, and spiritual—as well as the person's relationships with others and their environment. The student or client was offered the opportunity to be an equal participant in the session, to exchange understanding with the teacher or therapist, and to co-create the experience. People were learning anatomy not just from books, but from living, breathing human beings, from their own bodies, and from their own personal experiences. The sharing of those experiences in the community of the class was creating a common pool of knowledge and understanding. Bainbridge Cohen offered traditional anatomy and physiology as well as touch and repatterning work, breathing exercises, and the use of vibrational sound in "toning." The material already codified was presented in the mornings; then Bainbridge Cohen's explorations of new material occurred in the afternoons. As the study material increased, the classes became larger and some of the advanced students began co-teaching classes with each other.

In the fall of 1976 Bainbridge Cohen moved with her family to Cape Cod and then to Amherst, Massachusetts. Shortly afterwards, Patricia Bardi moved to the Amherst area and, following the birth of Bonnie's third child, taught the majority of the BMC classes from 1977 to 1978. In addition to continuing the training material from New York, Bainbridge

Cohen began exploring other body systems and developmental work, including senses and perceptions, and finished all the systems (adding nervous system, fluids, ligaments, and fascia). She also began inviting infants and children with special needs to her classes, a practice which continued thereafter. Her own three children and Sandra Jamrog's four children were the first models of baby behavior in the classes, where observation was the main principle. The class was inspired by the children and the possibility for change they manifested through their direct experience. Since the infants and children were not filtering their behavior in any way, but responding in the moment, they actualized in movement the principles being taught in the class. Questions and comments from the students illuminated what was being embodied by the children, and through a community process of dialogue and sharing, mutual discovery and insight, the underlying principles were made clearer. The lessons learned from this process were incorporated into the training programs.

She continued to offer dance and movement workshops and classes in the Amherst area, with its five colleges, and in New York, and taught kinesiology in the Dance Therapy Master's Program at Antioch College in New Hampshire. She was collaborating with Randall McClellan, who was head of the Music Department at Hampshire College, on the dynamics of vocal expression. Beth Goren introduced the Contact Improvisation community to the BMC work in 1977, and soon after Nancy Stark Smith and Lisa Nelson, the editors of *Contact Quarterly*, moved to Massachusetts and began ongoing collaborations with Bainbridge Cohen, which continue to the present day. A collection of articles from this collaboration, previously published in *Contact Quarterly*, eventually became Bainbridge Cohen's book *Sensing, Feeling, and Action*, published by Contact Editions.

Several faculty members from the colleges in the Amherst area studied extensively with Bainbridge Cohen through the years: Andrea Olsen at Mt. Holyoke College; Daphne Lowell, Francia McClellan, Rebecca Nordstrom, and Peggy Schwartz at Hampshire College; and Susan Waltner at Smith College. And she traveled to teach for several summers at Naropa Institute in Boulder, Colorado, where she met Michael Ridge, who became her long-time student, collaborator, and friend and later created illustrations for her writings.

In 1978 she also began a more formal Baby Project by videoing her interactions with children with special needs, with Lisa Nelson acting as videographer, and added sessions with infants in 1979.

Leonard Cohen, Bonnie's husband, closed his chiropractic practice in 1985, and he began to travel and teach with her widely. They were seeking students for a new program and Len was encouraging men, in particular, to join the training. He had taken charge of administration for the school courses and programs, as well as offering touch and repatterning and professional issues. He also exposed students to Asian approaches to movement and mind through Aikido, meditation, and Katsugen Undo.

Bainbridge Cohen began a two-year morning-format training in September 1980 that concluded in May 1982. The students graduated as certified practitioners, and those who had begun studying with Bainbridge Cohen in New York and completed the Body Systems and Development trainings were designated certified teachers. Susan Peffley, Linda Tumbarello, and Sarah White had also moved from New York to the Amherst area and taught in the 1980–82 program. Tumbarello continued to teach later programs and was student coordinator for many years.

By 1982 the course material included the skeleton, muscles, organs, endocrine system, nerves, fluids, ligaments, senses and perception, and breathing and vocalization. The Basic Neurological Patterns were continuing to be developed, with the Yield and Push/Reach and Pull series coming into focus.[3]

Between 1982 and 1986 she continued offering courses and workshops that went deeper into the embodiment process. The new teachers were required to collaborate in writing manuals on the skeletal, organ, and muscular systems and on phylogenetic and ontogenetic development. Bainbridge Cohen chose what subject matter each teacher would write about. These manuals, along with Bainbridge Cohen's extensive study notes, were used in subsequent courses.

In 1986 she began a four-year summer training. About one hundred students from the U.S., Canada, Europe, Central America, and Asia gathered in St. Bridget's Church Hall in Amherst. Most of the students up until this time had been women, but now men comprised about ten percent of the group. The large size of the group fostered an intensity that led the work in new directions and allowed for different experiences of group dynamics, as the students took classes divided into varying sizes over the term. Although Bainbridge Cohen taught the main classes, the new teachers offered private sessions for integrative work during the 1986–89 training and led small group classes. The students had homework to do in between the terms, and they were required to work in partners and to receive sessions with advanced students and teachers. At this point Gale Turner moved to Amherst, assuming a major role in teaching and eventually advising students and coordinating summer classes.

All along, Bainbridge Cohen continued to explore new material; she would offer explorations and share the results, and the students would share their discoveries. The material already learned might change as new explorations revealed new understandings. In this way, the curriculum continued to expand, adding Cellular material. In 1986, cellular breathing and presence became a pivotal focus.

From 1987 to 1993 she taught experiential anatomy at a local school of dance, together with dancer Liana Ciaglo, where she developed her ideas for her two 2010 videos, *Experiential Anatomy in the Training of Young Dancers*, accompanied by two books, one on the pelvis and one on the feet.

Subsequent training programs continued the four-summer term format while simultaneously commencing a new September-to-May morning format (1988–1990.) A modular training program commenced in Berkeley, California, in 1995. In 1996, Bainbridge Cohen's health began to fail, as she dealt with post-polio syndrome left over from childhood. Her advanced students continued teaching the trainings under the direction of Myra Avedon, who further codified the curriculum. Avedon, a graduate of the 1989 practitioner program with extensive administrative, teaching, bodywork and embodiment experience, became Program Coordinator in 1995 and a few years later became Program Director, and then in 2005 became the Educational Director, coordinating programs internationally. In 2005–2006, Mark Taylor also participated fully. Myra Avedon was instrumental in bringing the international BMC community through the turbulent times during the ten years of Bainbridge Cohen's illness and recovery. Leonard Cohen continued to handle the administrative aspects of the programs. The program locations in the Pioneer Valley area included the Amherst Ballet Center, St. Bridget's Church Hall, and Hampshire College, all in Amherst; Thorne's Market and Smith College in Northampton; and Mt. Holyoke College in South Hadley.

By the middle 1990s, The School for Body-Mind Centering was running several practitioner training programs, including a 1992 teacher certification program that Bainbridge Cohen designed according to a specific and unique kind of pedagogy, represented here in the section "Applying Body-Mind Centering." The graduates of the practitioner program could go on to assist in subsequent programs and then take the teacher training program. In 1998, Myra Avedon directed the second teacher training program in collaboration with Bainbridge Cohen, Amelia Ender, Kate Tarlow Morgan, Gale Turner, and others, based on the self-reflexive nature of Body-Mind Centering in relation to fundamental principles of nature, nurture, and cognition. What became apparent during these first training cycles was the endless possibility for research, as if the educator in this body-mind work would unceasingly be the captain of a "fantastic journey." As the community grew in the United States, Europe, and other parts of the world, so too grew the range of the subject matter—from the study of body systems (bone, muscle, organ, etc.) and early movement development to specific experiential research into brain anatomy and function, the minute structures of the cell, and the mysteries of embryology. Primary to this work were certain lasting principles that could be applied in a variety of fields, including the arts, medicine, and education. Bainbridge Cohen began offering the workshops "Engaging the Whole Child" in 1994, Subcellular material in 1995, and Ontogenetic material in 2001. The Embryology material was introduced in 2004 with contributions from William Martin Allen, Thomas Greil, Amy Matthews, Vera Orlock, and Daniele Reihwald.

The U.S. programs had always attracted students from Europe; the large 1996 Amherst class was almost one-third European. Odile Roquet and Mark Tompkins brought Bainbridge Cohen to France to teach in 1990. Irene Sieben and others then arranged for her to teach in Germany. The programs expanded to Europe with a licensed program in Amsterdam running from 1995 to 1999, directed by Jacques Van Eijden. The School ran a program directed by Myra Avedon and Thomas Greil in Germany from 2003 to 2007; then Thomas Greil, Jens Johannsen, and Friederike Tröscher formed "moveus GbR" and began running licensed programs in Germany. In 2004 Gloria Desideri began bringing BMC into her work with the Public Health System of Viterbo, Italy, with children with severe disabilities and the training of educators in public day-care centers; in 2006 she began running licensed programs under the aegis of Leben. Thomas Greil and Vera Orlock expanded the licensed programs to France under the aegis of SOMA in 2006.

Meanwhile, back in the U.S., another licensed program began in 2007 in North Carolina sponsored by Kinesthetic Learning Centers and directed and taught by Maryska Bigos and Bob Lehnberg, with Janice Geller and Lisa Clark also teaching. In 2008 Katy Dymock began a licensed program under EmbodyMove in England, and Walburga Glatz began a licensed program with Anka Sedlakova through Sedlakova's Babyfit organization in Slovakia. Also in 2009, Adriana Almeida Pees started a licensed program in Brazil taught by her and Jens Johannsen.

During these years, as her health permitted, Bainbridge Cohen traveled to guest-teach in the programs and elsewhere. As her health improved, new programs were developed in addition to the practitioner and teacher trainings. In 2001 the School began a Somatic Movement Education training, which now comprises the first two years of the four-year practitioner program. Also in 2001, Bainbridge Cohen, together with Sandy Jamrog and Lenore Grubinger, initiated a training in Infant Development Movement Education for those wishing to focus on infants. Finally, in 2001, she began trainings in Embodied Anatomy and Yoga and Embodied Developmental Movement and Yoga, initially coordinated and taught with Lisa Clark. The yoga trainings are currently taught by Bainbridge Cohen and Amy Matthews in Berkeley, California, and by Amy Matthews and Roxlyn Moret in New York City.

Always, the emphasis in these trainings is on sharing the material through personal experience and learning by doing. The students are empowered through their own experiences in the material and learn by observing the embodiment of the material by the teacher, who models it in the teaching, and by sharing their experiences in the class. By offering this experiential, kinesthetic learning, and not just a mental "book" learning, the participants find their own embodiment, which is the empowerment they feel. Classes usually begin and end with a circle of students sitting quietly in the felt experience of community.

The School is presently based in El Sobrante, California. The trainings include an intensive four-year Practitioner Certification Program, a rigorous training requiring experiential and academic studies in anatomy, physiology, kinesiology, touch and repatterning, movement, psychophysical processing, the arts (dance, voice, and theater), and mind/spiritual practice. There is also a post-practitioner Teacher Certification program, a two-year Somatic Movement Education program, and three applications programs: an Infant Developmental Movement program, an Embodied Anatomy & Yoga program, and an Embodied Developmental Movement & Yoga program. About 600 people worldwide have graduated from these programs.

In recent years, Bainbridge Cohen has taught the yoga applications program while she creates a series of videos and books to document Body-Mind Centering. The licensed programs are now offered in the U.S. and other countries by qualified teachers of the work.

The Body-Mind Centering Association, Inc.

By 1985, many of Bonnie Bainbridge Cohen's students had created practices of their own and began to meet annually to compare their understandings of Body-Mind Centering as a practice. The School was planning to start a new cycle of the four-year program and expected at least 100 registrants, a very significant increase from prior years. Ellen Barlow and Sara Vogeler, both teachers in the program, foresaw the need for dialogue and support and developed the idea for the creation of an organization to support the expansion of the work and the professional development of its practitioners. Janice Geller, Beth Goren, Lenore Grubinger, Phyllis Krechevsky, and Linda Tumbarello spearheaded the incorporation of the not-for-profit organization in Northampton, Massachusetts, and comprised the first board of directors for The Body-Mind Centering Association, Inc. (BMCA), with Linda Tumbarello as President for the first six years.

At the School during this time, the greater number of students and the increasing amount of study material were driving a momentum toward more formal organization of the curriculum, more oversight of the actual teaching and learning, and more assessment of outcomes.

This more formalizing mind-shift was spreading out to the wider community as well. BMCA developed a Code of Ethics and Standards of Practice for practitioners and Teachers Guidelines, which the School later adopted for its students and teachers. As time went on, more attention was paid to the necessity for clarity around who was authorized to offer classes and sessions with Body-Mind Centering content; this was eventually addressed through professional membership requirements and a service mark licensing arrangement with the organization and its members. This clarity became more important as the School began opening licensed programs internationally.

The need for centralized dialogue and support has increased as the number of programs has grown. BMCA has held a conference in the U.S. every year since its founding. For the first fifteen years, these conferences always took place on the East Coast, but since then have mostly alternated between East and West coasts. Initially, graduates living in Europe preferred to work outside the USA-based BMCA in a loosely organized European-based BMCA, and conferences there were held sporadically over the years. There were numerous cross-border problems, however, and eventually it was agreed that the two organizations would combine and BMCA would sponsor conferences in Europe also, yearly if possible. The conferences provide an opportunity for direct exchange of new ideas and shared experience and maintain the sense of the community circle, an important concept in BMC learning.

BMCA's first publication, beginning in 1985, was its member newsletter, which initially contained mostly organizational news or member activity reports. After the large 1989 graduating class came into the organization, the newsletter expanded and began including essays and articles about the work itself, under the direction of successive editors Pat Ethridge, Gloria Desideri, and Wendy Sager-Evanson. By 1998, the journal *Currents* was created under the direction of Ditte Ruderman to focus more specifically on writing about Body-Mind Centering. The newsletter was maintained to disseminate information about the organization and the activities of its members. Both these publications were for members only, so their content circulated almost exclusively within the BMC community.

Don Hanlon Johnson, a primary thinker and author in the field of somatic studies, created The Somerville Symposium in 2001 to support the development of writing skills in practitioners from the various somatic fields. BMCA participated in this symposium, with Kimberly McKeever coordinating members' participation. The winner in the first symposium writer's contest was Piera Teatini, a BMCA member from

Italy who contributed the essay "A Shooting Smile," included in this volume. In the second year, the symposium was discontinued before a final winner was announced, but among the three finalists was Lee Saunders, a BMCA member from Canada, who contributed the essay "Simon, Jennifer, and Me: A Foot in a Sock in a Shoe," also in this volume.

The awareness of the importance of somatic writing that developed from the symposium encouraged BMCA to continue supporting the writing of its members. Member Susan Davidson, a professional editor, was the second editor of the journal and worked directly with the BMCA community to enrich their somatic writing skills. The subsequent and present managing editor, Kate Tarlow Morgan, has continued this tradition of direct editorial support and encouragement.

By 1998, the Body-Mind Centering community had grown beyond the Pioneer Valley around Amherst and small pockets of activity in other places. In an effort to reach those on the periphery, the Board determined to invite membership beyond the certified practitioners and teachers who were mostly local to New England. The goal was to integrate graduates in other geographical regions, especially the ones carrying the work to colleges and universities in research and writing practices in conjunction with other somatic practices, and those still studying at the School. Stretching both deeper and wider, BMCA also integrated the non-professional graduates who studied the work for their own personal development, with the intention of maintaining the continuity of the community circle. While the main purpose of the organization is to support the professional members in their teaching and practice, there is also a strong emphasis on inclusion of those who have studied the work but are not professionals.

In 2005, Ellen Barlow, a long-time BMC teacher and a founder of BMCA, created an initiative called the "Pool Project," convening a group of BMC teachers, practitioners, and students to pool their thoughts. She began drafting a summary statement of Body-Mind Centering methodologies, philosophies, theories, and principles. The scope of the project was intended to generate criteria for assessing best practices and not intended to be comprehensive. From this work and several BMCA conference sessions, Barlow and the group developed preliminary descriptions offered in "Articulating Our Experience," included in this volume. This project of description by the BMCA community is ongoing and reflects a maturing differentiation process with respect to a collective understanding of the work.

Personal experience and transformation are central to the notion of self-cultivation, a form of self-discipline and growth in ordinary, daily life which has its roots in ancient traditions from both East and West. Everyone who learns something from exploring in the BMC process may contribute that knowledge and experience to the wider circle, and everyone learns and grows from this sharing. Hence the inclusion here of essays conveying deeply personal experience as well as the more typical case studies and expositive descriptions more commonly found in professional compilations. The continuity of this "group mind" or mind-field derives from similar, shared exploratory experiences which awaken common understanding; group mind is consistently present in the school programs, the local groups, and the large conferences occurring around the world. Each student of BMC, at whatever level, feels himself or herself a part of it, whether by directly participating or by simply "holding" the mind within, which—this must be emphasized—is not a form of indoctrination or mind control but instead a recognition of shared experience and understanding. The importance of direct experience and individual self-cultivation in the work has required balancing over the years with BMCA's efforts to evolve beyond a very loose structure to a functional professional organization, as the "mind of the room" can be difficult to sense when people are not actually in the same room to conduct organizational business. The membership has consistently addressed the theme of balancing individual autonomy within the community circle, while respecting the business and regulatory needs of an organizational structure at the same time.

The range of people drawn to Body-Mind Centering is vast. The emphasis on movement as a method of learning has attracted dancers, actors, and athletes; the focus on early development has drawn child specialists, parents, and other caregivers; the attention to repatterning has addressed the disabled, trauma survivors, therapists, and teachers; and the focus on process has interested artists, therapists, and educators of all kinds. In the early days, students were more likely to be parents looking for help with their children's difficulties or dancers exploring movement processes. More recently, many professionals in related fields come for advanced training and often stay for deeper exploration.

Notes

Preface

[1] By 1978 Thomas Hanna had named this new field of endeavor Somatics and defined it as an approach to mind-body integration. The lineage of this work has roots that are centuries old.

[2] Body-Mind Centering is a registered service mark of Bonnie Bainbridge Cohen, used by The Body-Mind Centering Association with permission. Although the service mark symbol is not used with each mention herein to avoid visual clutter, it should be applied elsewhere. For questions, contact admin@bmcassociation.org.

Introduction to Body-Mind Centering

[1] The full text of this essay is available online at http://www.bodymind-centering.com/About/.

[2] Somatization: The word is used here to imply not a disorder but a process by which the body experience can be both visualized and enacted.

Articulating Our Experience

[1] Barlow began by consulting with a focus group consisting of Susan Aposhyan, Jan Cook, Cathy Crafton, Eileen Kinsella, and Mark Taylor. Subsequently, she formed the Methodology Focus Group, consisting of Cook, Gill Wright Miller, Wendy Sager-Evanson, and Karin Spitfire (who left the group in early 2006). All are teachers, practitioners, and students of Body-Mind Centering.

[2] Bonnie Bainbridge Cohen, "Introduction to Body-Mind Centering," in this volume.

Section One
The Active Role of the Baby in Birthing

[1] Bonnie Bainbridge Cohen, *Sensing, Feeling, and Action* (Northampton, MA: Contact Editions, 1993), p. 99.

[2] Bonnie Bainbridge Cohen, *Sensing, Feeling, and Action,* p. 103.

[3] Lennart Righard, MD, and Margaret Alade, RN, "Delivery Self-Attachment" (Self-published, 1995). Video based on a study in *The Lancet* 336 (1990): pp. 1105–07.

[4] Lennart Nilsson, *A Child Is Born* (New York: Delacorte Press/Seymour Lawrence, 1990).

[5] Bonnie Bainbridge Cohen, *Sensing, Feeling, and Action,* p. 106.

[6] Clare Welter, certified nurse-midwife. Dialogue regarding use of acupuncture in rotating a baby, 1998.

[7] Lewis Mehl, MD, PhD, "Hypnosis and Conversion of the Breech to the Vertex Presentation." *Archives of Family Medicine* 3 (October 1994): p. 880.

[8] Bonnie Bainbridge Cohen, *Sensing, Feeling, and Action,* p. 3.

[9] *Ibid.,* p. 124.

[10] *Ibid.,* p. 34.

[11] *Ibid.,* p. 35.

[12] *Ibid.*

[13] Sally Goddard Blythe, *Attention, Balance and Coordination: The A.B.C. of Learning Success* (Hoboken, NJ: John Wiley & Sons, Inc., 2009).

[14] Lennart Righard and Margaret Alade, "Delivery Self-Attachment."

[15] Bonnie Bainbridge Cohen, *Sensing, Feeling, and Action,* p. 124.

[16] Marilyn Habermas-Scher, teacher of voice, movement, and vocal healing.

[17] Mark McLean *et al.,* "A Placental Clock Controlling the Length of Human Pregnancy," *Nature Medicine* 1, no. 5 (May 1995): pp. 460–63.

[18] *Ibid.*

[19] A.G. Gillin, "Maintenance of High-Risk Pregnancies: Role of Prostaglandins and Other Mediators," *Australian and New Zealand Journal of Obstetrics and Gynaecology* 34, no. 3 (June 1994): pp. 351–56.

[20] Bonnie Bainbridge Cohen, *Sensing, Feeling, and Action,* p. 125.

[21] *Ibid.*

[22] According to Diane Elliot, BMC certified practitioner, and Gina Wray, certified practitioner of Alexander Technique and Kripalu yoga, ancient yogic and chanting traditions developed practices that employ toning to move into the intensity of poses. Kripalu yoga workshop, 1998.

[23] Bonnie Bainbridge Cohen, *Sensing, Feeling, and Action*, p. 57.

[24] *Ibid.*

[25] *Ibid.*

[26] Valerie el Halta of Birth Center, Dearborn, Michigan, quoted by Nancy Wainer Cohen in "Malpositioned Baby—Fix it!" *ICAN* Clarion, March 1997.

[27] *Ibid.*

[28] *Ibid.*

[29] Colleen Ahlers Moore, interview, 1988.

[30] Allen Ross and Mitakuye Oyasin, *We Are All Related* (Denver: Wiconi Waste, 1989).

[31] Joseph Campbell, *The Inner Reaches of Outer Space* (New York: Harper and Row, 1986).

[32] *Ibid.*

[33] Bonnie Bainbridge Cohen, *Sensing, Feeling, and Action*, p. 31.

[34] *Ibid.*, p. 107.

[35] Lennart Righard and Margaret Alade, "Delivery Self-Attachment."

[36] Bonnie Bainbridge Cohen, *Sensing, Feeling, and Action*, p. 127.

[37] *Ibid.*, p. 105.

[38] *Ibid.*, p. 122.

[39] Lenore Grubinger, comment in Infant Developmental Movement Educator class, Amherst, Massachusetts, The School for Body-Mind Centering, 2000.

Evoking the Fluid Body

[1] Emilie Conrad, *Life on Land: The Story of Continuum, the World-Renowned Self-Discovery and Movement Method* (Berkeley, CA: North Atlantic Books, 2007).

[2] See also Susan Aposhyan, "Molecules and Emotions," in *Currents* (Spring 2002).

[3] See Lynne McTaggart, *The Field: The Quest for the Secret Force of the Universe* (New York: Harper Collins, 2002).

Lumbrical Movement of the Feet and Hands

[1] David Gorman, *The Body Moveable*, 5th edition (Etobicoke, Ontario: Learning Methods Publications, 2002).

[2] Deane Juhan, *Job's Body: A Handbook for Bodywork*, 3rd edition (Barrytown, NY: Station Hill Press, 2002).

[3] Susan Aposhyan, *Natural Intelligence: Body-Mind Integration and Human Development* (Philadelphia: Lippincott Williams, and Wilkins, 1999); and Bonnie Bainbridge Cohen, *Sensing, Feeling, and Action* (Northampton, MA: Contact Editions, 1993).

[4] Annie Brook, *Contact Improvisation & Body-Mind Centering: A Manual for Teaching & Learning Movement* (Boulder, CO: Smart Books Publishing, 2000).

[5] Michael Miller, *The Elements of Pilates and the Michael Miller View* (Self-published, 2001).

Storming/Calming

[1] Marti Olsen Laney, *The Introvert Advantage* (New York: Workman, 2002), p. 22.

[2] Gerald J. Tortora and Sandra Reynolds Grabowski, *Principles of Anatomy and Physiology*, 9th edition (New York: John Wiley & Sons, 2000), p. 559.

[3] David E. Jones, *An Instinct for Dragons* (New York: Routledge, 2002), p. 110.

[4] Ken Grimes, "To Trust is Human," *New Scientist* 178, no. 2394 (2003): p. 34.

[5] Sophy Burnham, *A Book of Angels* (New York: Ballantine, 1990). Quotes in this paragraph are from pages 277, 49, and 111, respectively.

Seeing and Perceiving

[1] Lecture notes, Body-Mind Centering practitioner training program, Amherst, MA, Summer 1987.

[2] Carl Jung et al., *Man and His Symbols* (London: Aldous Books, 1964), pp. 273–74.

[3] Suzy Gablik, *Progress in Art* (New York: Rizzoli, 1977), p. 268.

[4] Matthew Fox and Rupert Sheldrake, *The Physics of Angels: Exploring the Realm Where Science and Spirit Meet* (San Francisco: HarperCollins, 1996), pp. 110–11.

Section Two
Meeting a Child

[1] Anthony Damasio, *The Feeling of What Happens: Body and Emotion in the Making of Consciousness* (New York: Putnam's Sons, 1999).

[2] Walter Freeman, *How Brains Make Up Their Minds* (London: Orion Books, 2000).

[3] Jean Ayres, *Sensory Integration and Learning Disorders* (Los Angeles: Western Psychological Services, 1979), pp. 52–53.

[4] Sandra Blakeslee, "Movement May Offer Early Clue to Autism" (*The New York Times*, 26 January 1999).

[5] Bonnie Bainbridge Cohen, *Sensing, Feeling, and Action* (Northampton, MA: Contact Editions, 1993), p. 4.

[6] Bonnie Bainbridge Cohen, "Introduction to Body-Mind Centering." Handout. Amherst, MA: The School for Body-Mind Centering, 1998: p. 4.

[7] *Ibid.*

[8] *Ibid.*

Playing Toward Healing

[1] Cohen is often quoted as saying: "The mind is like the wind, and the body is like the sand; if you want to know how the wind is blowing, look at the sand."

Dragon Riding through the Abyss

[1] The state of freeze has been recognized in the Body-Mind Centering work for many years. Trauma researchers and neuroscientists also recognize it. See, for example, Peter Levine, *Waking the Tiger: Healing Trauma* (Berkeley, CA: North Atlantic Books, 1997), and Stephen W. Porges, "Emotion: An Evolutionary By-Product of the Neural Regulation of the Autonomic Nervous System," in *The Integrated Neurobiology of Affiliation*, C.S. Carter *et al. Annual of the New York Academy of Science* 807 (1997).

[2] Shock is never really simple for the person experiencing it.

[3] The idea of a reversal in the nervous system is controversial, as impulses through neurons are considered to move in one direction

only. Recently, however, while studying a basic neuro-anatomy text, I saw a diagram of a collateral neuron from the sensory ganglia to the motor ganglia, and the authors mentioned "impulse-reversing." Note that there was no discussion of the possible stimulus for or impact of such a reversal.

Through its emphasis on the living experience of one's anatomy and physiology, Body-Mind Centering has identified this tendency for impulse reversal in the nervous system. As with much of what is experienced in the study of Body-Mind Centering, the empirical proof may be forthcoming, as the awareness of trauma is flowering in the mind of the world and as empirical researchers ask questions about the physiology of trauma.

Of Many Minds

[1] James Giordano, "Complementarity, Brain~Mind, and Pain," *Forsch Komplementarmed,* 15 (2008): pp. 71–73.

[2] Theodore M. Brown, "The Rise and Fall of American Psychosomatic Medicine," address to the New York Academy of Medicine, 29 November 2000. http://human-nature.com/free-associations/riseand-fall.html

[3] Susan Aposhyan, "Bringing Together Biology and Human Consciousness" in *Body-Mind Psychotherapy* (New York: W.W. Norton & Company, 2004).

[4] Bonnie Bainbridge Cohen, www.bodymindcentering.com/About/IntroToBMC.

[5] Dennis H. Novack, MD, "Realizing Engel's Vision: Psychosomatic Medicine and the Education of Physician-Healers," Psychosomatic Medicine 65 (2003): pp. 925–30.

[6] James Giordano, "Complementarity, Brain~Mind, and Pain."

[7] Rita Agdal, MA, "Diverse and Changing Perceptions of the Body: Communicating Illness, Health, and Risk in an Age of Medical Pluralism," *The Journal of Alternative and Complementary Medicine* 11 (2005): S67–S75.

A Shooting Smile

[1] Neuro-Linguistic Programming (NLP) defines itself as "the study of

the structure of subjective experience"—of humans, I'd like to add. Since subjective experience is what we take to be reality, meeting the processes we use to make up our own world brings forth an ability to transform them. Originally derived from modeling the communication patterns of excellent therapists such as Milton Erickson, Fritz Perls, and Virginia Satir, NLP now designates a whole set of models, tools, and theoretical frameworks seeking to enhance the quality of life of individuals and organizations—key lessons ranging from the honing of sensory acuity to the use of trance states, from alignment of one's values, identity, and beliefs to probing the depths of linguistic structures.

[2] Process Work is a cross-disciplinary approach to individual and collective change. It developed in the 1970s and 1980s when Dr. Arnold Mindell, a Jungian analyst in Zurich, Switzerland, began researching illness as a meaningful expression of the unconscious mind. Also known as Process Oriented Psychology and Dreambody work, Process Work offers new ways of working with areas of life that are experienced as problematic or painful. Physical symptoms, relationship problems, group conflicts, social tensions—all these experiences, when approached with curiosity and respect, can lead to new information that is vital for our personal or collective growth. With its roots in Jungian psychology, Taoism, and physics, Process Work is based on a belief that the solution to a problem is contained within the disturbance itself, and it provides a practical framework through which individuals, couples, families, and groups can connect with greater awareness and creativity. (This information comes from the PW Center of Portland, www.processwork.org.)

[3] Systemics is a broad term for a wide field that encompasses areas as diverse as management, health care, ecology, biology, family therapy, chaos theory, and more. It aims to understand and influence how systems form, develop, grow, create, evolve, and transcend themselves within an uninterrupted lattice of intercommunication and interdependence. It integrates feedback, self-regulatory processes, levels of organization, and the careful tracking of consequences from simple actions up to the system's choreography—and back.

[4] Underlying the forms of our expression through the body systems is the process of our movement development, both ontogenetic (human infant development) and phylogenetic (the evolutionary progression through the animal kingdom). Development is not a linear process but occurs in overlapping waves, with each stage containing elements of all the others. Because each previous stage underlies and supports each successive stage, any skipping, interrupting, or failing to complete a stage of development can lead to alignment/movement problems, imbalances within the body systems, and problems in perception, sequencing, organization, memory, and creativity. The developmental material includes primitive reflexes, righting reactions, equilibrium responses, and the Basic Neurological Patterns. These are the automatic movement responses that underlie our volitional movement. (This information comes from the SBMC website.)

[5] The reflexes, righting reactions, and equilibrium responses are the fundamental elements, or the alphabet, of our movement. They combine to build the Basic Neurological Patterns, which are based upon prevertebrate and vertebrate movement patterns. The first of the four prevertebrate patterns is cellular breathing (the expanding/contracting process in breathing and movement in each and every cell of the body), which correlates to the movement of the one-celled animals. Cellular breathing underlies all other patterns of movement and postural tone. Navel radiation (the relation and movement of all parts of the body via the navel), mouthing (movement of the body initiated by the mouth), and prespinal movement (soft, sequential movements of the spine initiated via the interface between the spinal cord and the digestive tract) are the other three prevertebrate patterns. The twelve vertebrate patterns are based upon spinal movement (head to tail movement), which correlates to the movement of fish; homologous movement (symmetrical movement of two upper and/or two lower limbs simultaneously), which correlates to the movement of amphibians; homolateral movement (asymmetrical movement of one upper limb and the lower limb on the same side), which correlates to the movement of reptiles; and contralateral movement (diagonal movement of one upper limb with the opposite lower limb), which

correlates to the movement of mammals. Development of the Basic Neurological Patterns establishes our foundational movement patterns and corresponding perceptual relationships—including spatial orientation and body image, and the basic elements of learning and communication. (This information comes from the SBMC website.)

Carrying the Message

[1] Paul Valery, "The Problem of the Three Bodies," from "Aesthetics," *The Collected Works in English,* Vol. 13, Bollingen Series 45 (Princeton: Princeton University Press, 1964).

[2] Jean Starobinski, "The Natural and Literary History of Bodily Sensation," *Fragments for the History of the Human Body, Part Two.* Michel Feher with Ramona Naddaff and Nadia Tazi, editors (New York: Zone, 1989), p. 355. The last definition is from a 1945 edition of Webster's dictionary.

[3] *Ibid.*

[4] *Ibid.,* p. 356.

[5] *Ibid.*

[6] *Ibid.*

[7] *Ibid.,* p. 364.

[8] Patricia A. Marek, "Laban Movement Analysis as a Tool for Psychological Assessment," unpublished Laban Movement Analysis Certification Project, Seattle, 1987.

[9] Eileen Heaney, "The Development of Infant Movement Behavior," Master's Thesis (New York, Bank Street College of Education, March 1991), p. 19.

[10] Bonnie Bainbridge Cohen, "Developmental Movement Repatterning," *Contact Quarterly* 14, no. 2 (1989).

[11] Bonnie Bainbridge Cohen, "The Evolutionary Origins of Movement," The School for Body-Mind Centering, pamphlet, 1989: pp. 12–14.

[12] D.W. Winnicott, "The Newborn and His Mother," *Babies and Mothers* (Beverly, MA: Addison-Wesley, 1987; originally published 1964), p. 19.

[13] *Ibid.,* p. 44.

[14] Bonnie Bainbridge Cohen, "The Evolutionary Origins of Movement," p. 12.

[15] *Ibid.*, p. 19.

[16] D.W. Winnicott, "The Newborn and His Mother," p. 44.

[17] Bonnie Bainbridge Cohen, "The Evolutionary Origins of Movement," p. 15.

[18] Claude Levi-Strauss, *Structural Anthropology* (New York: Basic Books, 1958, 1963), p. 200.

[19] D.W. Winnicott, "Basis for Self and Body," *International Journal of Child Psychotherapy* (January 1972).

Section Three

Postmodernism, Body-Mind Centering, and the Academy

[1] Don Hanlon Johnson, *Bone, Breath & Gesture: Practices of Embodiment* (Berkeley, CA: North Atlantic Books, 1995).

[2] Mirka Knaster, *Discovering the Body's Wisdom* (New York: Bantam Books, 1996), p. 242.

[3] I teach courses in cultural studies, movement analysis, and experiential anatomy, along with many first-year seminars on writing and identity and women's studies seminars on feminist theory and the arts.

[4] In feminist theory the term "dual-systems" refers to capitalism and patriarchy. Without overly belaboring the point, dual-systems theorists (such as Juliet Mitchell and Heidi Hartman—who interpret this work quite differently) believe that these two systems, although distinct, intersect in real life and oppress women in particularly egregious ways.

[5] *Postmodernism* is a larger, more general term than *poststructuralism*. The second is a subcategory of the first.

[6] See a more recent rebuttal of this in Ramsay Burt's *Judson Dance Theater: Performative Traces* (New York: Routledge, 2007), where in Chapter 1 he takes to task writings by Sally Banes attempting to define postmodernism (*e.g.*, *Writing Dancing in the Age of Postmodernism*, Middletown, CT: Wesleyan University Press [a subsidiary of University Presses of New England], 1994).

[7] See Chris Weedon in *Encyclopedia of Feminist Theories*, Lorraine Code, editor (London: Routledge, 2000), pp. 397–98.

[8] I am indebted to Dr. Eloise Buker, former director of Women's Studies at Denison University, and to a team of colleagues at Denison whose conversations and correspondence in 1997 brought me to the thumbnail sketch of postmodernism included in this essay.

[9] The card game Euchre is played by four players with a short deck of 24 cards (nines through Aces) instead of the more usual 52. "Trump" is determined through a bidding process after the hand has been dealt. The face value of the cards is based on which suit is named as trump. Since trump is not predetermined, assumptions of power are based on speculation about value and consequently present a risk.

[10] Simone de Beauvoir, *The Second Sex* (New York, Alfred A. Knopf, 1952; originally published in France, 1949), explains that we are all "others" in certain situations—like travelers in a foreign land. She continues to explain that the dominant male holds the subordinate female as "other" always.

[11] Mary Belenky *et al.*, *Women's Ways of Knowing: The Development of Self, Voice, and Mind* (New York: Basic Books, 1986).

[12] Richard Grossinger, *Planet Medicine: Modalities* (Berkeley, CA: North Atlantic Books, 1995), p. 339.

[13] See Chris Weedon in *Encyclopedia of Feminist Theories*, p. 171 (see note 7).

[14] The seven liberal arts comprise two groups of studies: the *trivium* and the *quadrivium*. Grammar, rhetoric, and dialectic (or logic) make up the trivium. The quadrivium consists of the studies of arithmetic, geometry, astronomy, and music. These liberal arts made up the core curriculum of the medieval universities. (http://en.wikipedia.org/wiki/Liberalarts) Colloquially, however, the term "liberal arts" has come to mean studies intended to provide general knowledge and intellectual skills in critical thinking and creativity, rather than occupational or professional skills.

[15] Margrit Shildrick in *Encyclopedia of Feminist Theories*, p. 63 (see note 7).

[16] Richard Grossinger, *Planet Medicine: Modalities*, p. 344.

[17] *Classic* refers to a body that is to be seen. Examples are the statue David and the photographs in fashion magazines. *Abject* refers to bodies that actually live: breathe, sleep, defecate, etc. These terms

come from Mikhail Bakhtin but have been used widely in body politics. See, for example, *Art and Answerability: Early Philosophical Essays* (Austin: University of Texas Press, 1990).

[18] Academic work on the difference of sight impairment often speaks about blindness as "black-blind," "legally blind," and "sight-impaired" but here I am making a statement about her functional sight/site in society. For this, the category of eyesight and its implication in legal definitions is not as important as the support her vision provided for choice-making life tasks.

[19] Of course, there is a phenomenon called *synesthesia* that is described in psychology books, but no one I knew could perform this condition, except perhaps my mother.

[20] Bonnie Bainbridge Cohen quoted in Stephanie Golden, "Body-Mind Centering," in *Yoga Journal* (September/October 1993): p. 89.

Learning the Fundamentals

[1] Arnold Gesell, *An Atlas of Infant Behavior* (New Haven: Yale University Press, 1934).

[2] Doman-Delacato: Glenn Doman (a physical therapist), together with Carl Delacato (an educational psychologist), developed an approach to treating children with brain injury, published in 1960 in the *Journal of the American Medical Association*. Their work drew heavily on the ideas of Temple Fay (a neurophysiologist), who was head of the Department of Neurosurgery at Temple University Medical School and president of the Philadelphia Neurological Society. Fay believed that the infant brain evolves (as with evolution of the species) through stages of development similar to a fish, a reptile, a mammal, and finally a human.

[3] Jean Ayres, *Sensory Integration and Learning Disorders* (Los Angeles: Western Psychological Services, 1979).

[4] Paul E. Dennison, *Brain Gym*, Teacher's Edition (Ventura, CA: Edu-Kinesthetics, Inc., 1998).

[5] Berte and Karel Bobath, *The Facilitation of Movement—The Bobath Approach* (Reprint: London: Bobath Centre, 1975).

[6] Elaine Abelson, *When Ladies Go A-Thieving: Middle-Class Shoplifting in*

the Victorian Department Store (New York: Oxford University Press, 1989).

7 This thought is replicated several places, notably in the author's own Practitioner Training Thesis written in 1993 (Kate T. Morgan, "Carrying the Message," Practitioner Training Thesis & BMCA, NP, 1993), as well as in a published essay three years later (Susan Shapiro, "The Embodied Analyst in the Victorian Consulting Room," *Gender and Psychoanalysis* 1, no. 3, 1996).

8 Sylvia Miller, *Rhythms* (published privately by M. Speer, 1996).

9 Similarly, Caroline Pratt, the founder and principal of the school, never trademarked her Wooden Unit Blocks that today are standard classroom material for preschools and kindergartens around the world. See Caroline Pratt, *I Learn From Children: An Adventure in Progressive Education* (New York: HarperCollins, 1990; originally published by Scholastic Press in 1940).

10 Stephen Jay Gould, *Ontogeny and Phylogeny* (Cambridge, MA: Belknap Press of Harvard University Press, 1977).

11 Irmgard Bartenieff with Dori Lewis, *Body Movement: Coping with the Environment*, was published in 1981 at the end of Bartenieff's life and includes a detailed description of the Bartenieff Fundamentals™ in an appendix.

12 Mabel Todd, *The Thinking Body* (Princeton, NJ: The Princeton Book Company, 1937).

13 Bonnie Bainbridge Cohen, *Sensing, Feeling, and Action* (Northampton, MA: Contact Editions, 1993).

14 Susan Aposhyan, *Natural Intelligence: Body-Mind Integration and Human Development* (Philadelphia: Lippincott, Williams, and Wilkins, 1999), p. 26.

15 Bonnie Bainbridge Cohen, "Embodied Yoga," Pamphlet. Amherst, MA: The School for Body-Mind Centering, 2007.

16 John Dewey, *The Essential Dewey: Volumes 1 and 2*, Larry Hickman and Thomas Alexander, editors (Bloomington, IN: Indiana University Press, 1998).

17 *Ibid.*

[18] This core principle is, without a doubt, a "progressive's" reaction to the doldrums of the factory (industrialization) and the dangers of Fascism. Ruth left specific directions *not* to include any military marches in the musical accompaniment choices for Rhythms.

[19] Joan Zuckerman Morgan, *Workshop for Teachers*, JZM Archives (property of the author), 2004.

[20] Ruth Doing, "Rhythmics" in *Progressive Education*, The City and Country School Archives, 1932.

[21] Sylvia Miller's handwritten notes from Ruth Doing's 1932 lecture.

[22] *Ibid.*

Mentoring from a Distance

[1] At the beginning of the semester, students were asked to list movement activities they had never done. I collated that list and calculated the activities that were least familiar to the majority of the students.

[2] The specific terms in italics I picked up several years ago from an email post by Piera Teatini on The Body-Mind Centering Association listserve. Teatini, an author in this text, named these as the stages of learning. This list of terms fairly typically parallels a university setting: problem statement (intention), purpose of the research (attention), methods to be used in the exploration (assimilation), interpretation of the data (retention), and future research that this work invites (extension).

[3] Elizabeth Behnke, "Matching," originally published in *Somatics* (Spring/ Summer 1988, pp. 24–32), and republished in Don Hanlon Johnson, editor, *Bone, Breath & Gesture: Practices of Embodiment* (Berkeley, CA: North Atlantic Books, 1995), pp. 315–37.

BMC and Yoga

[1.] See T.K.V. Desikachar, *The Heart of Yoga* (Rochester, VT: Inner Traditions International, 1995); A.G. Mohan, *Yoga for Body, Breath and Mind* (Portland, OR: Rudra Press, 1993); M. Pierce and M. Pierce, *Yoga for Your Life* (Portland, OR: Rudra Press, 1996).

[2.] "Yoga is the ability to direct the mind exclusively toward an object and sustain that direction without any distractions." Yoga Sutra of Patanjali, verse 1.2, translated by T.K.V. Desikachar, *The Heart of Yoga*.

3. Contact the author at www.brilliantbodywork.net for an audio somatization of this material.
4. For information on the primary respiratory mechanism, see H.
   Magoun, *Osteopathy in the Cranial Field* (Boise, ID: Northwest, 1966).

Yielding Toward Presence

1 Jay Seitz, "The Bodily Basis of Thought," *New Ideas in Psychology. An
   International Journal of Innovative Theory in Psychology*, vol. 18, no. 1
   (2000): pp. 23–40.
2 Bonnie Bainbridge Cohen, *Sensing, Feeling, and Action* (Northampton,
   MA: Contact Editions, 1993).

BMC and Dance

1 For more information about the Perceptual Action-Response Cycle,
   see Bonnie Bainbridge Cohen's essay in this volume.

Unfracturing

1 RoseAnne Spradlin quoted by Gia Kourlas, *The New York Times*, 2
   November 2003.
2 Athena Malloy, *The New York Times*, 2 November 2003.
3 Susan Reiter, *DanceViewNewYork*, 8 November 2003.
4 Chris Dohse, *the dance insider*, 12 November 2003.

Section Four
Body-Mind Centering, Mindfulness, and the Body Politic

1 Bonnie Bainbridge Cohen, *Sensing, Feeling, and Action* (Northampton,
   MA: Contact Editions, 1993), p. 1.
2 *Ibid.*
3 Joseph Goldstein, *One Dharma* (San Francico: Harper, 2003).
4 Anne Klein, *Meeting the Great Bliss Queen: Buddhists, Feminists, and the
   Art of the Self* (Boston: Beacon Press, 1995).
5 Jon Kabat-Zinn, *Coming to Our Senses: Healing Ourselves and the World
   through Mindfulness* (New York: Hyperion Press, 2005), p. 2.
6 *Ibid.*

Boundaries, Defense, and War

[1] Alfred Hässig, "Stress-Induced Suppression of the Cellular Immune Reactions: On the Neuroendocrine Control of the Immune System," *Medical Hypotheses* 46 (1996): pp. 551–55. See also Michael U. Baumgartner, "Too Much 'HIV'-Research, Not Enough AIDS-Research: An Introduction to the Work of Prof. Alfred Hässig," *Continuum* 3, no. 4 (1994): pp. 10–11.

[2] The "collective body" is the name given by Janet Adler to a form she developed within the discipline of Authentic Movement. I use it here in a different context and with slightly different meanings, with gratitude to Adler for the naming of this experience. See Janet Adler, *Offerings from the Conscious Body* (Rochester, VT: Inner Traditions, 2002).

[3] Wilhelm Reich, *Character Analysis* (New York: Farrar, Straus & Giroux, 1972).

[4] The School for Body-Mind Centering, Amherst, MA, 1986. Linda Hartley was a teacher in this program.

The Role of the Arts and Embodiment in Post-Trauma Community Building

[1] Other relevant integrative methods include Arnold Mindell's Process Oriented Psychology (also called "Process Work") and Ron Kurtz's body-centered psychotherapy, also called the Hakomi Method, or educational models such as those of Brazilian activist-educator Augusto Boal's "Theatre of the Oppressed" and the Laban/Bartenieff "movement analysis" work. My own research has used these embodiment methods together with the performing arts in schools. I call this work "Embodying Peace."

[2] Although seven buildings were ultimately destroyed, the lingering image that was played over and over again in the media was that of the World Trade Center's two tallest buildings, commonly known as "the Twin Towers," being struck and then collapsing.

[3] George Lakoff, *Don't Think of an Elephant! Know Your Values and Frame the Debate—An Essential Guide for Progressives* (White River Junction, VT: Chelsea Green Publishing Company, 2004), p. 54.

[4] George Lakoff, *Moral Politics: How Liberals and Conservatives Think* (Chicago: University of Chicago Press, 2002), pp. 143–76.

[5] John Dewey, *The Public and Its Problems* (New York: H. Holt and Company, 1927).

[6] Martha Eddy, *The Role of Physical Activity in Educational Violence-Prevention Programs for Youth.* Dissertation, Columbia University (Chelmsford, MA: UMI Press, 1998).

[7] See the website www.EmbodyPeace.org for further examples.

Epilogue

The School for Body-Mind Centering

[1] Sharna Allison, Patricia Bardi, Sandra Jamrog, Genevieve Kapuler, Dominique (Ruth) Leeds, Linda Tumbarello, Joan Whitacre, Sarah White, and Kay Wylie were also among the first advanced students.

[2] Some of the other early students were Morningstar Barbara Chenven, Joy Graham, Phoebe Neville, Susan Peffley, Stefanie Pukit, Kathy Rice, Eleanor Rosenthal, Gail Stern, Bill Weintraub, and Lydia Yohey.

[3] From 1977 to 1982, the students included Susan Aposhyan, Ellen Barlow, Maryska Bigos, Martha Eddy, Janice Geller, Bruce Hartley, Linda Hartley, Neala Haze, Patrice Heber, Sara Hostetler, Phyllis Krechevsky, Paul Langland, Francia McClellan (aka Tara Stepenberg), Susan Milani, Marghe Mills-Thysen, Jenna Rostek, Christine Tingskog, and Susan Waltner. In the 1982–86 period, Wendell Beavers, Erika Berland, Annie Brook, Jadwiga Rozanska Cataldo, Leslie Cerrier, Aria Edry, Lenore Grubinger, Eileen Kinsella, Antara Kyra Lober, Diane Madden, Sarah Shelton Mann, Rita Marquez, Diane Moore, Nancy Paré, Stephen Petronio, Beverley Stokes, Lou Stokes, Nancy Topf, Andy Warshaw, Randy Warshaw, and David Woodberry commenced their studies.

Bibliography

Abelson, Elaine. *When Ladies Go A-Thieving: Middle-Class Shoplifting in the Victorian Department Store.* New York: Oxford University Press, 1989.

Adler, Janet. *Offerings from the Conscious Body.* Rochester, VT: Inner Traditions, 2002.

Agdal, Rita. "Diverse and Changing Perceptions of the Body: Communicating Illness, Health and Risk in an Age of Medical Pluralism." *The Journal of Alternative and Complementary Medicine* 11, no. 1 (2005): S67–S75.

Aposhyan, Susan. "Bringing Together Biology and Human Consciousness." In *Body-Mind Psychotherapy.* New York: W.W. Norton and Co., 2004: pp. 20–65.

_____. "Molecules and Emotions." *Currents* (Spring 2002).

_____. *Natural Intelligence: Body-Mind Integration and Human Development.* Philadelphia: Lippincott, Williams, and Wilkins, 1999.

Ayres, Jean. *Sensory Integration and Learning Disorders.* Los Angeles: Western Psychological Services, 1979.

Bainbridge Cohen, Bonnie. "Introduction to Body-Mind Centering." Handout. Amherst, MA: The School for Body-Mind Centering, 1998.

_____. "Perceiving In Action." *Contact Quarterly* 9, no. 2 (1984).

_____. "The Alphabet of Movement, Part I." *Contact Quarterly* 14, no. 3 (1989).

_____. "The Evolutionary Origins of Movement." Pamphlet. Amherst, MA: The School for Body-Mind Centering, 1989.

_____. "Embodied Yoga." Pamphlet. Amherst, MA: The School for Body-Mind Centering, 2007.

_____. *Sensing, Feeling, and Action: The Experiential Anatomy of Body-Mind Centering.* Northampton, MA: Contact Editions, 1993.

Bartenieff, Irmgard, with Dori Lewis. *Body Movement: Coping with the Environment.* Philadelphia: Gordon & Breach, 1981.

Baumgartner, Michael U. "Too Much 'HIV' Research, Not enough AIDS

Research: An Introduction to the Work of Prof. Alfred Hässig." *Continuum* 3, no. 4 (1994): pp. 10–11.

Behnke, Elizabeth. "Matching." *Somatics* (Spring/Summer 1988): pp. 24–32.

Belenky, Mary, *et al. Women's Ways of Knowing: The Development of Self, Voice and Mind.* New York: Basic Books, 1986.

Blakeslee, Sandra. "Movement May Offer Early Clue to Autism." *The New York Times,* 26 January 1999.

Block, A. *I'm Only Bleeding: Education as the Practice of Violence Against Children.* New York: Peter Lang, 1997.

Blythe, Sally Goddard. *Attention, Balance and Coordination: The A.B.C. of Learning Success.* Hoboken, NJ: John Wiley & Sons, Inc., 2009.

Bobath, Berte and Karel. *The Facilitation of Movement—The Bobath Approach.* Reprint: London: Bobath Center, 1975.

Brook, Annie. *Contact Improvisation & Body-Mind Centering: A Manual for Teaching and Learning Movement.* Boulder, CO: Smart Books Publishing, 2000.

Brook, Annie. *From Conception to Crawling: Foundations for Developmental Movement.* Boulder, CO: Smart Books Publishing, 2001.

Brown, Theodore M. "The Rise and Fall of American Psychosomatic Medicine." Address to the New York Academy of Medicine, 29 November 2000. http://human-nature.com/free-associations/riseandfall.html.

Burnham, Sophy. *A Book of Angels.* New York: Ballantine, 1990.

Burton, J. *Transformations: Plots and Casts of Interior Dramas of Adolescents.* Drawing for the School's Conference Proceedings. Baltimore: Maryland Institute, College of Art, 1983.

Campbell, Joseph. *The Inner Reaches of Outer Space.* New York: Harper and Row, 1986.

Code, Lorraine (editor). *Encyclopedia of Feminist Theories.* London: Routledge, 2000.

Cohn, D. Personal communication. 13 September 2001.

Csikszentmihalyi, Mihaly. *Optimal Experience: Psychological Studies of Flow in Consciousness.* Cambridge, England: Cambridge University Press, 1992.

Damasio, Antonio. *The Feeling of What Happens: Body and Emotion in the Making of Consciousness.* New York: Putnam's Sons, 1999.

De Beauvoir, Simone. *The Second Sex.* New York: Alfred A. Knopf, 1952; originally published 1949.

Dennison, Paul. *Brain Gym,* Teacher's Edition. Ventura, CA: Edu-Kines-thetics, Inc., 1998.

Desikachar, T.K.V. *The Heart of Yoga.* Rochester, VT: Inner Traditions International, 1995.

Dewey, John. *Moral Principles in Education.* Boston: Houghton Mifflin Co., 1909.

_____. *The Public and Its Problems.* New York: H. Holt and Company, 1927.

_____. *Experience & Education.* New York: Collier Books, 1938.

_____. *The Essential Dewey: Volumes 1 and 2.* Larry Hickman and Thomas Alexander, editors. Bloomington, IN: Indiana University Press, 1998.

Dohse, Chris. "The Vandalized Lovemaps of RoseAnne Spradlin." *the dance insider* 12 (November 2003).

Doing, Ruth. "Rhythmics." *Progressive Education.* New York: The City and Country School Archives, 1932.

_____. "A Collection of Rhythms and Movement Education Articles, 1927–1940." Reprinted from unpublished *Progressive Education.* New York: Teachers College Publications.

Eddy, Martha Hart. *The Role of Physical Activity in Educational Violence-Prevention Programs for Youth.* Dissertation, Columbia University. (Chelmsford, MA: UMI Press, 1998).

_____ (editor). *Conflict Resolution Using Movement and Dance.* CustomBooks, 2001.

_____. "Dance and Somatic Inquiry in Studios and Community Dance Programs." *Journal of Dance Education* 2, no. 2 (2002): pp. 119–26.

_____. "Dynamic Embodiment." *Somatic Movement Therapy Training catalog,* 3rd edition, 2006. www.WellnessCKE.net

_____. "A Brief History of Somatic Education." *Journal of Dance and Somatic Practices* 1, no. 1 (June 2009): pp. 5–27.

_____. "The Role of Dance in Violence-Prevention Programs for Youth." *Dance: Current Selected Research* 7. Lynn Overby and Billie Lepczyk, editors. Brooklyn, NY: AMS Press, 2010.

el Halta, Valerie, of Birth Center, Dearborn, Michigan, quoted by Nancy Wainer Cohen in "Malpositioned Baby—Fix it!" *ICAN* Clarion, March 1997.

Engs, Ruth. *The Progressive Era Health Reform Movement: A Historical Dictionary.* Santa Barbara, CA: Praeger Publishing, 2003.

Fox, Matthew, and Rupert Sheldrake. *The Physics of Angels: Exploring the Realm Where Science and Spirit Meet.* San Francisco: HarperCollins, 1996.

Freeman, Walter J. *How Brains Make Up Their Minds.* London: Orion Books, 2000.

Fussell, Paul. *The Great War and Modern Memory.* New York: Oxford University Press, 1975.

Gablik, Suzy. *Progress in Art.* New York: Rizzoli, 1977.

Gardner, Howard. *Frames of Mind: The Theory of Multiple Intelligences.* 10th edition. New York: Basic Books, 1983.

Gesell, Arnold. *An Atlas of Infant Behavior.* New Haven: Yale University Press, 1934.

Gillin, A.G. "Maintenance of High-Risk Pregnancies: Role of Prostaglandins and Other Mediators." *Australian and New Zealand Journal of Obstetrics and Gynecology* 34, no. 3 (June 1994): pp. 351–56.

Giordano, James. "Complementarity, Brain-Mind, and Pain." *Forsch Komplementarmed* 15 (2008): pp. 71–73.

Goldstein, Joseph. *One Dharma.* San Francisco: Harper, 2003.

Gorman, David. *The Body Moveable.* 5th edition. Etobicoke, Ontario: Learning Methods Publications, 2002.

Gould, Stephen Jay. *Ontogeny and Phylogeny.* Cambridge, MA: Belknap Press of Harvard University Press, 1977.

Greene, M. *Releasing the Imagination: Essays on Education, the Arts, and Social Change.* San Francisco: Jossey-Bass, 1995.

Greer, C., and H. Kohl. *A Call to Character: A Family Treasury.* New York: HarperCollins, 1995.

Grimes, Ken. "To Trust is Human." *New Scientist* 178, no. 2394 (2003): p. 34.

Grossinger, Richard. *Planet Medicine: Modalities.* Berkeley, CA: North Atlantic Books, 1995.

Hässig, Alfred. "Stress-Induced Suppression of the Cellular Immune Reactions: On the Neuro-endocrine Control of the Immune System." *Medical Hypothesis* 46 (1996): pp. 551–55.

Heaney, Eileen. *The Development of Infant Movement Behavior.* Unpublished Master's Thesis, New York: Bank Street College of Education, March 1991.

Hellison, D. *Teaching Personal and Social Responsibility.* Champaign, IL: Human Kinetics, 1995.

Johnson, Don Hanlon. *Bone, Breath & Gesture: Practices of Embodiment*. Berkeley, CA: North Atlantic Books, 1995.

Jones, David E. *An Instinct for Dragons*. New York: Routledge, 2002.

Juhan, Deane. *Job's Body: A Handbook for Bodywork*. 3rd edition. Barrytown, NY: Station Hill Press, 2002.

Jung, Carl, *et al*. *Man and His Symbols*. London: Aldous Books, 1964.

Kendall, Elizabeth. *Where She Danced: The Birth of American Art Dance*. Berkeley: University of California Press, 1979.

Klein, Anne. *Meeting the Great Bliss Queen: Buddhists, Feminists, and the Art of the Self*. Boston: Beacon Press, 1995.

Knaster, Mirka. *Discovering the Body's Wisdom*. New York: Bantam Books, 1996.

Kourlas, Gia. "Dance: RoseAnne Spradlin Gives Sex a Realistic Crash and Giggle." *The New York Times*, 2 November 2003.

Kübler-Ross, Elizabeth. *The Wheel of Life: A Memoir of Living and Dying*. New York: Scribner, 1997.

Lakoff, George. Public Email. 11 September 2001.

_____. *Moral Politics: How Liberals and Conservatives Think*. Chicago: The University of Chicago Press, 2002.

_____. *Don't Think of an Elephant! Know Your Values and Frame the Debate: The Essential Guide for Progressives*. White River Junction, VT: Chelsea Green Press, 2004.

Laney, Marti Olsen. *The Introvert Advantage*. New York: Workman, 2002.

Lantieri, Linda, and Daniel Goleman. *Building Emotional Intelligence: Techniques to Cultivate Inner Strength in Children*. Louisville, CO: Sounds True, Inc., 2008.

Levi-Strauss, Claude. *Structural Anthropology*. New York: Basic Books, 1958, 1963.

Levine, Peter. *Waking the Tiger: Healing Trauma*. Berkeley, CA: North Atlantic Books, 1997.

Magoun, H. *Osteopathy in the Cranial Field*. Boise, ID: Northwest, 1966.

Marek, Patricia A. "Laban Movement Analysis as a Tool for Psychological Assessment," unpublished Certification Project, Seattle, 1987.

McLean, Mark *et al*. "A Placental Clock Controlling the Length of Human Pregnancy." *Nature* 1, no. 5 (May 1995): p. 460.

McTaggart, Lynne. *The Field: The Quest for the Secret Force of the Universe*. New York: Harper Collins, 2002.

Mehl, Lewis. "Hypnosis and Conversion of the Breech into the Vertex Presentation." *Archives of Family Medicine* 3 (October 1994).

Miller, Michael. *The Elements of Pilates and the Michael Miller View*. Self-published, 2001.

Miller, Sylvia. *Rhythms*. Self-published by Michael Speer, New York, 1996.

Mohan, A.G. *Yoga for Body, Breath and Mind*. Portland, OR: Rudra Press, 1993.

Morgan, Joan Zuckerman. *Rhythms: 1970–2005*. Unpublished private notes, The City and Country School Archives, New York.

Morgan, Kate Tarlow. "At Play In The Fields." *Body-Mind Centering Association Newsletter*. Northampton, MA (June 1991).

_____. "The Fundamentals and Basic Neurological Patterns," unpublished materials for Teacher Training Program at The Orchard School (2007). East Alstead, VT.

Nilssen, Lennart. *A Child is Born*. New York: Delacorte Press/Seymour Lawrence, 1990.

Novack, Dennis. "Realizing Engel's Vision: Psychosomatic Medicine and the Education of Physician-Healers." *Psychosomatic Medicine* 65 (2003): pp. 925–30.

Pierce, M. *Yoga for Your Life*. Portland, OR: Rudra Press, 1996.

Porges, Stephen W. "Emotion: An Evolutionary By-Product of the Neural Regulation of the Autonomic Nervous System." In *The Integrated Neurobiology of Affiliation*, C.S. Carter *et al. Annual of the New York Academy of Science* 807 (1997).

Pratt, Caroline. *I Learn From Children: An Adventure in Progressive Education*. New York: Simon and Schuster, 1940.

Reich, William. *Character Analysis*. New York: Farrar, Straus & Giroux, 1972.

Reiter, Susan. "under/world." *DanceView*. New York, 8 November 2003.

Righard, Lennart, MD, and Margaret Alade, RN. "Delivery Self-Attachment" (Self-published, 1995). Video based on a study in *The Lancet* 336 (1990): pp. 1105–07.

Ross, Allen, and Mitakuye Oyasin. *We Are All Related*. Denver: Wiconi Waste, 1989.

Seitz, Jay. "The Bodily Basis of Thought." *New Ideas of Psychology: An International Journal of Innovative Theory and Psychology* 18, no. 1 (2000): pp. 23–40.

Shapiro, Susan. "The Embodied Analyst in the Victorian Consulting Room." *Gender and Psychoanalysis* 1, no. 3 (1996).

Stanley, Douglas. *Your Voice: Applied Science of Vocal Art,* 3rd edition. New York: Pitman Publishing Corporation, 1945, 1950, 1957.

Starobinski, Jean. "The Natural and Literary History of Bodily Sensation." *Fragments for the History of the Human Body, Part Two.* Michel Feher with Ramona Naddaff and Nadia Tazi, editors. New York: Zone, 1989.

Todd, Mabel. *The Thinking Body.* Princeton, NJ: The Princeton Book Company, 1937.

Tortora, Gerald J., and Sandra Reynolds Grabowski. *Principles of Anatomy and Physiology.* 9th edition. New York: John Wiley & Sons, 2000.

Unrau, S. "Motif Writing in Gang Activity: How to Get the Bad Boys to Dance." *Congress for Research on Dance Conference Proceedings.* Washington, DC: Dancing in the Millennium Consortium, 2000.

Valery, Paul. "Aesthetics," *The Collected Works in English.* Vol. 13, Bollingen Series 45, Princeton University Press, 1964.

Winnicott, D.W. "The Newborn and His Mother." *Babies and Mothers.* Beverly, MA: Addison-Wesley, 1987.

Winnicott, D.W. "Basis for Self and Body" *International Journal of Child Psychotherapy* (January 1972).

Yenawine, P. The Arts Awareness Project. Teacher College Reserve Materials: Burton.

Bibliography

Image Credits

Cover and title page photo by Mishele Mennett taken at the Doane Dance
Performance Space, Denison University, Granville, Ohio

Index

J

jackknife movement sequence, 337

"Jacques" exercise, 46

jellyfish, 65–66

K

Kabat-Zinn, Jon, 375–76

karate, reflexes in, 281–84

Keeney, Bradford, 213

Kestenberg, Judith, 225

Kilpatrick, Howard, 277

kinesthetic knowledge, 24–25, 240

King, Alonzo, 355–56, 358

"knee-jerk reactions," 256, 384

Kroll, Susan, 28–29

L

Lakoff, George P., 392

Lamb, Warren, 225

Lamont, Bette, 135–37

learning

in the first year of life, 326

introverts and extroverts, differences
    in, 78

learning *vs.* psychological needs, 241–43

mentoring from a distance, 291–307

stages of, 432n 2

styles of, in group dynamics, 240–41

Levi-Strauss, Claude, 231

liberal arts education, 263–64, 296–98,
    429n 14

ligamentous system, 5

ligands, 42–43, 44

Lines ballet company, 355–56, 358

lumbrical movement of the feet and hands,
    67–74

Lyme disease, a case study, 159–76

lymphatic system, 379–80, 384–86

M

Mackenzie, Doug, 325–48

Maimonides, Moses, 312

martial arts training, 281–84

master-disciple (*rav-talmid*) relationship,
    309–23

matter as energy, 64

McGehee, Darcy, 121–43, 349–54

McGuire, Maggie, 369–76

meditation, goals of, 54

Mehl-Madrona, Lewis, 25

memory

flashback/memories, 192

introverts *vs.* extroverts, 78

as stored in the body, 271

traumatic, and the nervous system, 187–92

mentoring, 291–307, 309–23

metaphor, the reality of, 391–93

methodologies of BMC, 14

Methodology Focus Group, 13–14

midwives, 35

Miller, Gill Wright, 13–17, 247–67, 291–307,
    359–66, 428n 3

Miller, Sylvia, 272

mind

in BMC, 371–72

as motion *vs.* form, 64

responses to trauma, 188–89

shifting nature of, 43

Mindell, Arnold, 213

mindfulness, in Buddhism and BMC, 372–76

mirroring, case study with Camilla, 232–33

"mirror neurons," 392

About the Editors and Authors

Editors

Gill Wright Miller

Gill Wright Miller holds a BFA in dance performance from Denison University, an MA in Movement Studies from Wesleyan University, and a PhD in Dance Education and Women's Studies from New York University. She has been a professor of dance/dance studies at Denison University since 1981. During her tenure there, she trained extensively at the Laban/Bartenieff Institute for Movement Studies and The School for Body-Mind Centering.

Miller began investigating the work of BMC deeply after attending a two-week overview of all seven systems in 1991, followed by the first workshop titled "Engaging the Whole Child." She has been active in the BMC community for twenty years, serving on the Editorial Board for *Currents: The Journal of Body-Mind Centering*, co-coordinating the annual USA conferences for the past ten years, and hosting The Body-Mind Centering Association's Vision Weekend each year since 2001. In 2010, she envisioned, directed, and hosted a conference at Denison called *Somatic Pedagogies: A Cross-Talk* that specifically aimed to cross conversations of Body-Mind Centering with other somatic modalities, embodied cognition, and neurocognition.

Miller continues to teach at Denison University, specializing in embodied cultural studies in dance history, experiential anatomy/kinesiology, and movement analysis. She also choreographs and stages performances, creates conferences, pioneers embodied research methodologies, and publishes on pregnancy, dancing, and creativity in various journals including *Association for Research on Mothering* and *Contact*

Quarterly. In 2010, she was the invited author of two encyclopedic entries, one on "Motherhood and Creativity" and the other on "Women in Dance." Her current research on balancing critical and creative work in liberal arts curricula will be published as "Critically Re-Thinking Creativity," by TEAGLE in July 2011.

Pat Ethridge

Pat Ethridge earned a BA from Goucher College in Art History, an MA in dance from University of Illinois, and an MS degree in Asian Medicine from Pacific College of Oriental Medicine. She is also a licensed acupuncturist, bodyworker, and administrator who lives in New York City.

Pat first encountered BMC while she was a dancer and musician in New York City in the early 1980s through classes with various BMC teachers and an article written by Bonnie Bainbridge Cohen in *Contact Quarterly.* She was impressed by the body-based language used to describe movement and began studying at The School for Body-Mind Centering, graduating from the practitioner program in 1989. She has continued studying ever since.

Ethridge has been on the BMCA Board for sixteen years, seven of them as president. During that time she shepherded the organization's handling of both the profound (professional and service mark issues) and the mundane (email list serve and connections among practitioners living on various continents). She has also served on the Ethics Committee, as an editor of the BMCA Newsletter, and on the Editorial Board of the journal *Currents.* Along with Carolyn Rosenfield, Pat developed the Code of Ethics and Standards of Practice for BMC practitioners and teachers adopted by The School for Body-Mind Centering and The Body-Mind Centering Association.

Kate Tarlow Morgan

Kate Tarlow Morgan received her BA from City University of New York and her MA from New York University in Cultural History. Her dance training spans Graham and Hawkins, jazz, Congolese, and improvisation. Her bodywork background includes Ideokinesis, Alexander Technique, Topf Technique, and Zero Balancing. In 1986, Morgan enrolled at The School for Body-Mind Centering and completed both her practitioner and teacher trainings by 1991.

In the late 1970s, Morgan was part of the avant-garde movement that brought performance out of its traditional venue and into experimental spaces. She has worked as an urban archaeologist/historian and is founder of the Pinkster Festival based on a reconstruction of an eighteenth-century New York City event. As a movement artist and teacher, her interest in local place and its history has inspired her work, including a seven-year performance project and film about the NYC Subway. Morgan has lectured at The School for Body-Mind Centering, The Orchard School, The City and Country School, and has been a guest presenter at Denison University and Georgetown University. She is also a teacher and archivist of The Rhythms Technique.

Living in rural Vermont with her nine-year-old son, Morgan teaches Rhythms in the schools. She also serves BMCA as the managing editor of *Currents*, a somatics journal. Her book of short stories and essays on dance and urban history, *Circles and Boundaries*, was published by Factory School, New York, in 2009.

Authors

Ellen Barlow is a native of the Washington, DC, area where she lives and works as a movement education specialist. She holds a BA in Dance Education and yoga teacher certification in the Shivananda tradition. She also trained in the work of Irmgard Bartenieff, Lulu Sweigard, F.M. Alexander, and Moshe Feldenkrais before becoming a certified practitioner of Body-Mind Centering in 1982 and a certified teacher in 1985. Further influences have been Zero Balancing and Craniosacral Therapy. Barlow is a Certified GYROTONIC® Instructor and a Registered Somatic Movement Educator with the International Movement Education and Therapy Association (ISMETA). She was a cofounder of

The Body-Mind Centering Association (BMCA) and has served on the board and as president of ISMETA.

Annie Brook, PhD, LPC, is a certified BMC teacher and a BodyMind Psychotherapist, a certified Tantra teacher, a performance artist, and a licensed professional counselor. Annie is former Director of Body Psychotherapy at the master's level at Naropa University and now directs BodyMind Somanautics Training Program, which integrates BMC-based learning, early attachment, and pre- and perinatal psychology. Brook co-owns Colorado Therapies, where she maintains an ongoing private psychotherapy practice. She speaks and teaches nationally and internationally, is a published poet, wrote a column for *Tantra: the Magazine,* and has authored numerous audio and DVD products on movement education. Her books *From Conception to Crawling, Contact Improvisation and Body-Mind Centering, Sex and Spirit,* and *Attachment Imprints and Intimacy* are available at anniebrook.com.

Catherine Burns is a Registered Somatic Movement Therapist, Infant Developmental Movement Educator, Massage Therapist, Sage Femme Doula, and Lactation Educator. She incorporates principles of Body-Mind Centering in her therapy sessions and teaching. Catherine supports women throughout childbearing and children from infancy through school age. She offers staff development workshops in reflex integration for early childhood and for children with challenges, including autism. Catherine has been blessed with many extraordinary teachers including Diane Elliot, Suzanne River, Lenore Grubinger, Bonnie Bainbridge Cohen, and others in her lineage. Catherine has trained in craniosacral therapy with Carol Phillips and Benjamin Shields, reflex integration with Svetlana Masgutova, orofacial therapy with Anna Regner, and professional skills with Hakomi School of Psychotherapy. Catherine's practice can be viewed at www.mamabebe.org.

Naomi Duveen is a movement performer, a somatic movement therapist, and an educator. She completed her mime education in 1969 and performed with different theatre and mime companies in the Netherlands. She studied the dance release work with John Rolland and Nancy Topf. In 1994 she graduated as Body-Mind Centering practitioner at The School for Body-Mind Centering. She opened her practice (in which she worked with BMC) to different categories of clients. Currently she mainly works individually with clients. She has more than thirty years of experience as a movement teacher at the Amsterdam School of Higher Education in the Arts, and for sixteen years she taught an intensive two-year dance course in Den Haag. On occasion Ms. Duveen dances during openings of art exhibitions.

Naomi practices Healing Tao to continue her development and growth. Her website is www.naomiduveen.art-base.net.

Martha Eddy is an exercise physiologist and Registered Somatic Movement Therapist (RSMT) with a doctorate from Columbia University in Movement Science and Education. She works in private practice in New York City. Eddy served on the certification program faculty for both the School for BodyMind Centering® and the Laban/Bartenieff Institute of Movement Studies from 1984 to 1994. She founded the Somatic Movement Therapy Program (SMTT) in 1992 and renamed it Dynamic Embodiment-SMTT in 2008. She is also the founder and director of the Center for Kinesthetic Education (CKE) in New York, and a cofounder of and the director of Somatic Studies at Moving On Center in Oakland, California, and Moving For Life DanceExercise for Health, a nonprofit organization in New York City.

Diane Elliot, RSMT[SM,] is a spiritual teacher, ritual leader, dancer, choreographer, and somatic movement therapist. A Certified Practitioner/Teacher of Body-Mind Centering, she has studied and taught the work in group settings and private practice for more than thirty years. Following a twenty-five-year career in the movement arts, Diane entered rabbinic training at the Academy for Jewish Religion, California, where she earned a Master's degree in Rabbinical Studies and was ordained in 2006. She works in the San Francisco Bay Area and nationally, teaching, leading spiritual retreats, and working with individuals. She is a cofounder of *Merkavat Ha-Makhol* Institute for Embodied Spirituality and the author of numerous articles, essays, and poems. She can be reached at Rabbi.Diane18@gmail.com or visit her website www.WhollyPresent.org.

Michele Feldheim has been teaching movement and embodiment for more than twenty years. Michele integrates the BMC work into her Pilates Movement Classes, hands-on practice, and her music work. She has pioneered hands-on work called Autonomic Injury Release Technique (AIRT), which helps people heal from physical and emotional trauma, and teaches this work within and outside the Body-Mind Centering community. Michele is a professional jazz pianist, vocalist, and composer and taught Jazz Piano at Smith College and Amherst College from 1994 to 2007. Currently she teaches music at Putnam Vocational Technical High School in Springfield, Massachusetts, and performs in New England.

Her extensive training includes the following: Certified BMC Practitioner and Teacher, Certified Massage Therapist, Movement Therapist, Pilates Instructor, Yoga Instructor, Life Energy Fundamentals Training with Jeff Krock, and Polarity Therapy 1st Certification. She holds a BM from New England Conservatory and MM from University of Massachusetts at Amherst in Jazz Piano and Composition. She may be reached at yangsum@earthlink.net or at 413-584-7694 for information about bodywork, Pilates, AIRT, or for music education or performance.

Michelle Gay is the founder and executive director of the Society For Martial Arts Instruction, a not-for-profit dedicated to empowering people through martial arts and related movement studies. She is a Laban Certified Movement Analyst, Registered Somatic Movement Educator/Therapist, and 4th-degree black belt. In addition to teaching karate to children and adults, she created and regularly teaches "Good Guy/Bad Guy Self-Defense" workshops at Broadway Dance Center, Anatomy and Kinesiology at the Manhattan Center for Alexander Technique, and martial arts to Dalton High School seniors. She is a five-time World Oyama Knockdown Karate Champion and a student of Body-Mind Centering. Her first book, *Brain Breaks for the Classroom*, was released by Scholastic Teaching Resources in 2009.

Thomas Greil has been working in the somatics field for more than ten years and is involved in yoga and meditation practice. He is a Certified Teacher and Practitioner of Body-Mind Centering and studied many years with Bonnie Bainbridge Cohen to develop his work with babies and children with special needs. He was originally trained as a journalist, and it remains his passion to write about movement and bodywork. He organized the first Body-Mind Centering program in Germany and founded moveus, a somatic training school in Germany, with Jens Johannsen and Friederike Tröscher. As the co-director (with Vera Orlock) of the BMC Certification Program in France, he teaches in and coordinates BMC programs in France, Italy, and Germany. In his private practice he works with babies, children, and adults with structural and neurological challenges. Contact Thomas at www.somatic-movement.de.

Lenore Grubinger, RSMT, is the Director of Amajoy Developmental Movement and Bodywork Center in Massachusetts. She is a Certified Teacher of Body-Mind Centering with more than thirty years of experience, and a practitioner of craniosacral therapy. A Registered Somatic Movement Therapist, Ms. Grubinger received her BA from the University of Massachusetts. She serves infants, families, and professionals through individual sessions and consulting. A contributor to the curriculum of the Infant Developmental Movement Education program of The School for BMC, she is the author of *Seven Recommendations for You and Your Baby* and *Neurological Movement Patterns and the Central Nervous System*, both available on her website. She is a member of the

International Somatic Movement Therapy and Education Association, and founder of the Early Care Providers of Pioneer Valley. Contact Lenore at www.amajoy.net.

Linda Hartley is a certified practitioner and teacher of Body-Mind Centering, UKCP-registered Transpersonal Psychotherapist, senior registered Dance Movement Psychotherapist, and ISMETA Registered Somatic Movement Therapist. She has an MA in Somatic Psychology, and has studied Authentic Movement with Janet Adler, and Process Oriented Psychology. Linda taught and worked as a therapist for many years in the UK and internationally, and currently practices in Norfolk, England. As founding director of the Institute for Integrative Bodywork and Movement Therapy, she has run training programs based on Body-Mind Centering, Authentic Movement, and Somatic Psychology since 1990. She is the author of *Wisdom of the Body Moving: An Introduction to Body-Mind Centering, Servants of the Sacred Dream,* and *Somatic Psychology: Body, Mind and Meaning,* and editor of *Contemporary Body Psychotherapy.* Hartley can be reached at www.ibmt.co.uk or www.lindahartley.co.uk.

Douglas MacKenzie, founder of BrilliantBody™, is a Certified Practitioner of Body-Mind Centering, a craniosacral therapist, a Registered Somatic Movement Therapist, and instructor of Gyrotonic® and Gyrokinesis®. He has worked in private practice since 1990, and at Canyon Ranch in Lenox, Massachusetts (1995–2007), where he also trained staff therapists. He graduated from Wesleyan University and the Connecticut Center for Massage Therapy. Doug draws from his study of Viniyoga, Chi K'ung, Acutonics, World Music, Falconry, and Movement Improvisation. His gentle work benefits infants and elders; those who suffer chronic/acute injury or various complex syndromes; and professional athletes, dancers, and musicians. Also a musician, Doug plays contemporary guitar and traditional *mrdangam,* the principal drum in South Indian classical music. For more about Doug see: www.brilliantbodywork.net.

Darcy McGehee holds an MFA in dance and theatre and is associate professor of dance at the University of Calgary. She incorporates training in theatre, voice, anatomy, kinesiology, and somatics in her approach to dancing, choreographing, and teaching. She is a Registered Somatic Movement Therapist and Infant Developmental Movement Educator and researches human development, the use of somatic techniques in dance training, and the application of somatic therapy to developmental delays.

Maggie McGuire, PhD, began studying with Bonnie Bainbridge Cohen in 1984. A student of Buddhism and Native American spiritual practices, and formerly an early childhood/special education teacher who switched into experiential, body-centered psychotherapy and family systems work, she is immersed in the field of body-based approaches to education and psychotherapy. Maggie is a licensed clinical psychologist with a private practice in Hardwick, Vermont, and a certified practitioner of Body-Mind Centering.

Michael Ridge is a native of Australia with strong interests in surfing, Aikido, and philosophy who came to the U.S. in the mid-1980s, where he studied at Naropa College in Boulder, Colorado, and then at The School for Body-Mind Centering. Ridge co-taught with Leonard Cohen the Aikido training that was an element in the SBMC curriculum during the 1990s. During this time, Ridge worked closely with Ms. Cohen and was the illustrator of several of her teaching manuals.

Lee Saunders, BMC-certified teacher, works nationally and internationally as a dance voice artist, Somatic Movement Educator/Therapist, and naturopathic doctor. Based in Canada, she promotes wellness through voice, movement, touch, and nutrition. Her clients range from newborns to seniors, at all levels of movement ability. Lee has received the Prix Éloizes—Artist of the Year in Dance; was nominated for the Somerville Award for writing on somatic methods; and was published in *Self & Society,* the Journal for the British Society of Humanistic Psychology. With her husband Ruell Sloan, BSC, BEd, MSc, and certified practitioner of BMC (SBMC '89), she founded the non-profit Tycheco Voice and Movement Productions, and established a somatic movement studio on their farm and another within Théâtre l'Escaouette, where Lee is dance artist-in-residence.

Karin Spitfire, Director of Moving Matters, is a Registered Somatic Movement Therapist & Educator, a certified teacher and practitioner of Body-Mind Centering, a faculty member of The School for Body-Mind Centering, the Institute for Somatic Movement Studies in the Netherlands, and Green River Dance for Global Somatics in Minneapolis, and holds an MA in Women's Studies. Spitfire began in 1982 utilizing her experience in the arts, somatics, feminist analysis, and action to guide many in the release of trauma from the physical, emotional, and spiritual body. Spitfire has been equally engaged in producing art in many forms of media. Her performance piece "Incest: It's All Relative" toured nationally from 1982 to 1986. She was Poet Laureate of Belfast, Maine, and her poetry book *Standing with Trees* was published in 2005.

Mark Chandlee Taylor directs the Center for BodyMindMovement, a somatic movement education program with sites in Pittsburgh, Pennsylvania; Lorane, Oregon; and Mexico City (www.bodymindmovement.com). A Registered Somatic Movement Therapist, he teaches movement and embodiment practices in the U.S., Europe, Asia, and Central and South America, maintains a private practice in Pittsburgh, and serves on the board of directors of the International Somatic Movement Education and Therapy Association (ISMETA). He was artistic director and choreographer for Dance Alloy in Pittsburgh and for Mark Taylor & Friends in New York, and served as a member of the Princeton University dance faculty. He was U.S. Program Director for The School for Body-Mind Centering and taught in its programs in Massachusetts, Germany, Slovakia, and France.

Piera Nina Teatini is deeply in love with the force that through the green fuse drives the flower (and thanks Dylan Thomas for the vivid phrasing). In her small way, she's served it by plowing, seeding, watering the field of creativity, communication, and personal development for the past thirty years. She has worked as a copy and scriptwriter, as a trainer in Communication Skills and Creativity, and as a Somatically Oriented Coach for individuals, groups, and organizations, in Italy and abroad. Since the birth of her daughter in 2005, she has drastically reduced traveling and devoted herself to staying put, writing science, of all things, plus a little poetry-with-humor, and singing. Her main influences, besides Body-Mind Centering, include Arnold and Amy Mindell's Process Oriented Psychology and Process Work, based in Portland, Oregon (www.aamindell.net).

About North Atlantic Books

North Atlantic Books (NAB) is an independent, nonprofit publisher committed to a bold exploration of the relationships between mind, body, spirit, and nature. Founded in 1974, NAB aims to nurture a holistic view of the arts, sciences, humanities, and healing. To make a donation or to learn more about our books, authors, events, and newsletter, please visit www.northatlanticbooks.com.

North Atlantic Books is the publishing arm of the Society for the Study of Native Arts and Sciences, a 501(c)(3) nonprofit educational organization that promotes cross-cultural perspectives linking scientific, social, and artistic fields. To learn how you can support us, please visit our website.